S0-AZQ-259

Photodynamic Therapy

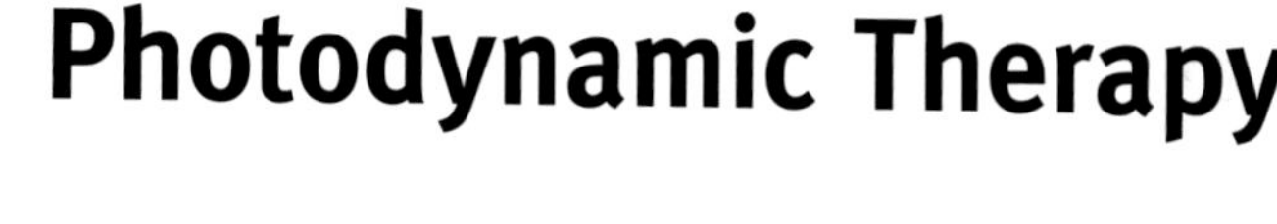

Procedures in Cosmetic Dermatology

Series Editor: Jeffrey S. Dover MD FRCPC
Associate Editor: Murad Alam MD

Botulinum Toxin, second edition 
Alastair Carruthers MA BM BCh FRCPC FRCP(Lon) and Jean Carruthers MD FRCSC FRC (OPHTH) FASOPRS
ISBN 978-1-4160-4213-6

Soft Tissue Augmentation, second edition
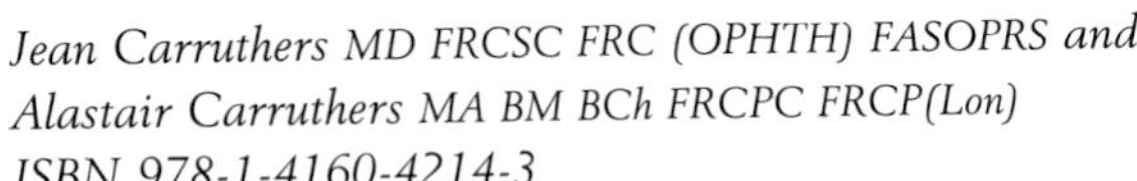
Jean Carruthers MD FRCSC FRC (OPHTH) FASOPRS and Alastair Carruthers MA BM BCh FRCPC FRCP(Lon)
ISBN 978-1-4160-4214-3

Cosmeceuticals
Zoe Diana Draelos MD
ISBN 978-1-4160-0244-4

Lasers and Lights: Volume I 
Vascular • Pigmentation • Scars • Medical Applications
David J. Goldberg MD JD
ISBN 978-1-4160-2386-9

Lasers and Lights: Volume II, second edition
Rejuvenation • Resurfacing • Treatment of Ethnic Skin • Treatment of Cellulite
David J. Goldberg MD JD
ISBN 978-1-4160-4212-9

Photodynamic Therapy, second edition
Mitchel P. Goldman MD
ISBN 978-1-4160-4211-2

Liposuction 
C. William Hanke MD MPH FACP and Gerhard Sattler MD
ISBN 978-1-4160-2208-4

Scar Revision
Kenneth A. Arndt MD
ISBN 978-1-4160-3131-4

Chemical Peels 
Mark Rubin MD
ISBN 978-1-4160-3071-3

Hair Transplantation 
Robert S. Haber MD and Dowling B. Stough MD
ISBN 978-1-4160-3104-8

Treatment of Leg Veins 
Murad Alam MD and Tri H. Nguyen MD
ISBN 978-1-4160-3159-8

Blepharoplasty 
Ronald L. Moy MD and Edgar F. Fincher
ISBN: 978-1-4160-2996-0

Advanced Face Lifting 
Ronald L. Moy MD and Edgar F. Fincher
ISBN 978-1-4160-2997-7

Towards the prevention and treatment of the most common form of cancer affecting the most people worldwide – skin cancer

Towards the treatment of the most common skin condition affecting teenagers worldwide – acne

Towards the advancement of patient care in dermatology

Mitchel P. Goldman

Procedures in Cosmetic Dermatology

Series Editor: Jeffrey S. Dover MD FRCPC

Associate Editor: Murad Alam MD

Photodynamic Therapy

Second edition

Edited by

Mitchel P. Goldman MD

Associate Clinical Professor of Dermatology/Medicine, University of California, San Diego; Medical Director, La Jolla Spa MD, La Jolla, CA, USA

Series Editor

Jeffrey S. Dover MD FRCPC

Associate Professor of Clinical Dermatology, Yale University School of Medicine, Adjunct Professor of Medicine (Dermatology), Dartmouth Medical School, Director, SkinCare Physicians, Chestnut Hill, MA, USA

Associate Editor

Murad Alam MD

Chief, Section of Cutaneous and Aesthetic Surgery, Department of Dermatology, Northwestern University, Chicago, IL, USA

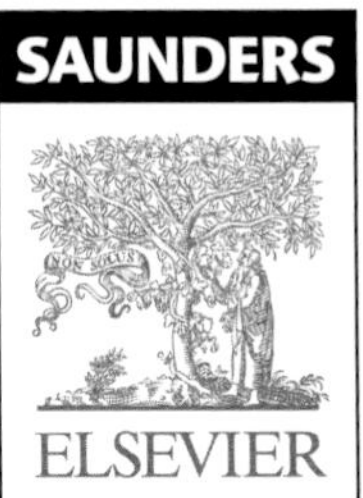

SAUNDERS
ELSEVIER

An imprint of Elsevier Inc

First edition 2005
Second edition 2008
ISBN: 978-1-4160-4211-2

British Library Cataloguing in Publication Data
A catalogue record for this book is available from the British Library

Library of Congress Cataloging in Publication Data
A catalog record for this book is available from the Library of Congress

Note
Neither the Publisher nor the Editors and Authors assume any responsibility for any loss or injury and/or damage to persons or property arising out of or related to any use of the material contained in this book. It is the responsibility of the treating practitioner, relying on independent expertise and knowledge of the patient, to determine the best treatment and method of application for the patient.

The Publisher

Commissioning Editors: Claire Bonnett, Karen Bowler
Development Editor: Anne Bassett
Project Manager: Anne Dickie
Design Direction: Charlotte Murray
Illustration Manager: Merlyn Harvey
Illustrator: Richard Prime

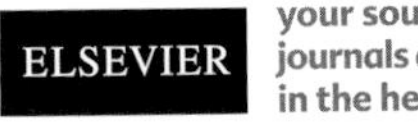

Printed in China

Last digit is the print number: 9 8 7 6 5 4 3 2 1

Contents

Series Preface ix
Series Preface First Edition x
Preface xi
List of Contributors xiii

1 Mechanism of Action of Topical Aminolevulinic Acid 1
Brian D. Zelickson

2 Treatment of Acne with Systemic Photodynamic Therapy 11
Yoshiyasu Itoh

3 Treatment of Acne with Topical Photodynamic Therapy 31
Macrene Alexiades-Armenakas

4 Treatment of Hidradenitis Suppurativa 37
Michael H. Gold

5 Treatment of Sebaceous Hyperplasia 45
Dore J. Gilbert

6 Treatment of Skin Cancer Precursors 53
Sari M. Fien, James Ralston, Joyce B. Farah, Nathalie C. Zeitouni, Allan R. Oseroff

7 Treatment of Skin Cancer 69
Sigrid Karrer, Rolf-Markus Szeimies

8 Treatment of Basal Cell Nevus Syndrome 81
Dany J. Touma

9 Treatment of Human Papilloma Virus 87
Ida-Marie Stender

10 Treatment of Cutaneous T-Cell Lymphoma, Psoriasis, and Port Wine Stain Birthmarks 97
Tanya Kormeili, Kristen M. Kelly

11 Prevention of Skin Cancer 107
Catherine Maari, Robert Bissonnette

12 Photodynamic Rejuvenation with Methyl-Aminolevulinic Acid 117
Ricardo Ruiz-Rodriguez, Laura Lopez-Rodriguez

Contents

13	Photodynamic Therapy for Photorejuvenation Pavan K. Nootheti, Michael H. Gold, Mitchel P. Goldman	125
14	Treatment of Vascular Lesions Zhou Guoyu	137
15	Clinical Application of Fluorescence Diagnosis Wolfgang Bäumler, Tino Wetzig	149
Index		161

Second edition

Series Preface

Procedures in Cosmetic Dermatology

Four years ago we began a project to produce 'Procedures in Cosmetic Dermatology', a series of high quality, and practical, up-to-date, illustrated manuals on procedures in cosmetic dermatology. Our plan was to provide dermatologists and dermatologic surgeons with detailed books accompanied by instructional DVD's containing all the information they needed to master most, if not all of the leading edge cosmetic dermatology techniques. Thanks to the efforts of our superb book editors, chapter authors, and the tireless and extraordinary publishing staff at Elsevier, the series has been more successful than any of us could have hoped. Over the past 3 years, thirteen volumes have been introduced, which have been purchased by thousands of physicians all over the world. Originally published in English, many of the texts have been translated into different languages including Italian, French, Spanish, Chinese, Polish, Korean, Portuguese, and Russian.

Our commitment to you is to convey information that is practical, easy to use, and up to date. Since new devices and minimally invasive techniques are continually being refined in this rapidly changing area, the time has now come to inaugurate second editions of these books. During the next few years updated texts will be released. The most time-sensitive books will be revised first, and others will follow.

This series is an ever evolving project. So in addition to second editions of current books, we will be introducing entirely new books to cover novel procedures that may not have existed when the series began. Enjoy and keep learning.

Jeffrey S. Dover MD FRCPC and Murad Alam MD

First edition

Series Preface

Procedures in Cosmetic Dermatology

While dermatologists have been procedurally inclined since the beginning of the specialty, particularly rapid change has occurred in the past quarter century. The advent of frozen section technique and the golden age of Mohs skin cancer surgery has led to the formal incorporation of surgery within the dermatology curriculum. More recently technological breakthroughs in minimally invasive procedural dermatology have offered an aging population new options for improving the appearance of damaged skin.

Procedures for rejuvenating the skin and adjacent regions are actively sought by our patients. Significantly, dermatologists have pioneered devices, technologies and medications, which have continued to evolve at a startling pace. Numerous major advances, including virtually all cutaneous lasers and light-source based procedures, botulinum exotoxin, soft-tissue augmentation, dilute anesthesia liposuction, leg vein treatments, chemical peels, and hair transplants, have been invented, or developed and enhanced by dermatologists. Dermatologists understand procedures, and we have special insight into the structure, function, and working of skin. Cosmetic dermatologists have made rejuvenation accessible to risk-averse patients by emphasizing safety and reducing operative trauma. No specialty is better positioned than dermatology to lead the field of cutaneous surgery while meeting patient needs.

As dermatology grows as a specialty, an ever-increasing proportion of dermatologists will become proficient in the delivery of different procedures. Not all dermatologists will perform all procedures, and some will perform very few, but even the less procedurally directed amongst us must be well-versed in the details to be able to guide and educate our patients. Whether you are a skilled dermatologic surgeon interested in further expanding your surgical repertoire, a complete surgical novice wishing to learn a few simple procedures, or somewhere in between, this book and this series is for you.

The volume you are holding is one of a series entitled 'Procedures in Cosmetic Dermatology'. The purpose of each book is to serve as a practical primer on a major topic area in procedural dermatology.

If you want to make sure you find the right book for your needs, you may wish to know what this book is and what it is not. It is not a comprehensive text grounded in theoretical underpinnings. It is not exhaustively referenced. It is not designed to be a completely unbiased review of the world's literature on the subject. At the same time, it is not an overview of cosmetic procedures that describes these in generalities without providing enough specific information to actually permit someone to perform the procedures. And importantly, it is not so heavy that it can serve as a doorstop or a shelf filler.

What this book and this series offer is a step-by-step, practical guide to performing cutaneous surgical procedures. Each volume in the series has been edited by a known authority in that subfield. Each editor has recruited other equally practical-minded, technically skilled, hands-on clinicians to write the constituent chapters. Most chapters have two authors to ensure that different approaches and a broad range of opinions are incorporated. On the other hand, the two authors and the editors also collectively provide a consistency of tone. A uniform template has been used within each chapter so that the reader will be easily able to navigate all the books in the series. Within every chapter, the authors succinctly tell it like they do it. The emphasis is on therapeutic technique; treatment methods are discussed with an eye to appropriate indications, adverse events, and unusual cases. Finally, this book is short and can be read in its entirety on a long plane ride. We believe that brevity paradoxically results in greater information transfer because cover-to-cover mastery is practicable.

We hope you enjoy this book and the rest of the books in the series and that you benefit from the many hours of clinical wisdom that have been distilled to produce it. Please keep it nearby, where you can reach for it when you need it.

Jeffrey S. Dover MD FRCPC and Murad Alam MD

Second edition

Preface

Photodynamic therapy (PDT) dates its onset to 1400 BC when a variety of botanical products were used to improve phototherapy. PDT was first used as a treatment for skin cancer 100 years ago in 1905 by Drs Von Tappeiner and Jodblauer. Over this past century physicians have been experimenting with a variety of compounds that can localize in various internal and external tumors or benign structures such as hair follicles and sebaceous glands and be activated by light to provide localized destruction. Wide varieties of such compounds have been tested and are effective in treating a variety of tumors. However, prolonged photosensitivity and the lack of specificity hampered the widespread acceptance of PDT as a viable treatment modality.

To overcome the adverse effects of systemically administered photosensitizing agents, topical agents were studied. In 1999, 5-aminolevulinic acid (ALA; Levulan, DUSA Pharmaceuticals) was the first topical agent to receive approval by the USA Food and Drug Administration (FDA). In 2006, the methylated form of ALA, Metvix (which will be launched as Metvixia [Galderma]) was approved by the FDA. Levulan was approved for the treatment of actinic keratosis and Metvixia was approved for the treatment of actinic keratosis and basal cell carcinoma. Although approved for limited indications as stated above, as with most pharmacologic agents, researchers worldwide realized that ALA could be used to treat a wide variety of dermatologic conditions. Even though it has only been 3 years since the publication of the first edition of this text, the rapid advancement of treatment modalities warrants a second edition. This second edition expands the outstanding contributions of the first edition's authors and adds additional chapters on the treatment of sebaceous hyperplasia, hidradenitis suppurativa, treatment of vascular lesions, clinical application of fluorescence diagnosis, and a separate chapter on photorejuvenation with methyl-ALA.

This text brings together some of the leading medical research scientists from the United States, Japan, Canada, Germany, Spain, China, and Denmark, who present their published research and hypothesize on future applications of PDT. Our purpose is to present the reader with an up-to-date account on the use of topical PDT in the treatment of a wide variety of cutaneous disorders.

The future of ALA-PDT looks bright. This text provides evidence that ALA-PDT has left the laboratory setting and should become part of our everyday practices. In addition to therapeutic efficacy in treating cutaneous disease, cosmetic improvements are seen in a variety of cutaneous concerns, including photorejuvenation and acne vulgaris. The introduction of short-contact, full-face/broad-area ALA-PDT treatment makes this therapy very attractive for the dermatologic community—it is safe, efficacious, and relatively pain-free, without significant adverse effects, and commercially available for widespread use. Clinicians should be ready for this new therapeutic approach which may rethink how dermatologists treat photodamage, sebaceous hyperplasia, acne vulgaris, and a variety of other conditions bridging the world of medical dermatology and cosmetic dermatologic surgery.

Mitchel P. Goldman MD

To the women in my life

My grandmothers, Bertha and Lillian

My mother, Nina

My daughters, Sophie and Isabel

And especially to my wife, Tania

For their never-ending encouragement, patience, support, love, and friendship

To my father, Mark – a great teacher and role model

To my mentor, Kenneth A. Arndt for his generosity, kindness, sense of humor, joie de vivre, and above all else curiosity and enthusiasm

At Elsevier, Sue Hodgson who conceptualized the series and brought it to reality and Claire Bonnett for polite, persistent, and dogged determination.

Jeffrey S. Dover

Elsevier's dedicated editorial staff has made possible the continuing success of this ambitious project. The new team led by Claire Bonnett, Anne Bassett and the production staff have refined the concept for the second edition while maintaining the series' reputation for quality and cutting-edge relevance. In this, they have been ably supported by the graphics shop, which has created the signature high quality illustrations and layouts that are the backbone of each book. We are also deeply grateful to the volume editors, who have generously found time in their schedules, cheerfully accepted our guidelines, and recruited the most knowledgeable chapter authors. And we especially thank the chapter contributors, without whose work there would be no books at all. Finally, I would also like to convey my debt to my teachers, Kenneth Arndt, Jeffrey Dover, Michael Kaminer, Leonard Goldberg, and David Bickers, and my parents, Rahat and Rehana Alam.

Murad Alam

List of Contributors

Macrene Alexiades-Armenakas MD PhD
Assistant Clinical Director, Yale University School of Medicine, New York, NY, USA

Wolfgang Bäumler PhD
Department of Dermatology, University of Regensburg, Regensburg, Germany

Robert Bissonnette MD FRCPC
President, Innovaderm Research, Montreal, QC, Canada

Joyce B. Farah MD
Dermatology Resident, Department of Dermatology, Roswell Park Cancer Institute, Buffalo, NY, USA

Sari M. Fien MD
Photodynamic Therapy Research Fellow, Roswell Park Cancer Institute, Buffalo, NY, USA

Dore J. Gilbert MD
Associate Clinical Professor of Dermatology, University of California, Irvine, CA, USA

Michael H. Gold MD
Medical Director, Gold Skin Care Center, Tennessee Clinical Research Center, Clinical Assistant Professor, Department of Medicine, Department of Dermatology, Vanderbilt University School of Medicine, School of Nursing Nashville, TN, USA

Mitchel P. Goldman MD
Clinical Professor of Dermatology/Medicine, University of California, San Diego; Medical Director, La Jolla Spa, La Jolla, CA, USA

Zhou Guoyu MD
Associate Professor of OMS, Deputy Director of Medical Laser centre, Ninth People's Hospital, Shanghai Jiaotong University Medical College and Deputy Director of Lasers Medicine and Engineering Committee, Shanghai Laser Society, Shanghai, China

Yoshiyasu Itoh MD PhD
Director, Daikanyama Clinic of Dermatology and Plastic Surgery, Tokyo, Japan

Sigrid Karrer MD PhD
Assistant Professor, Department of Dermatology, University of Regensburg, Regensberg, Germany

Kristen M. Kelly MD
Associate Clinical Professor of Dermatology, Beckman Laser Institute and Medical Clinic, University of California, Irvine, CA, USA

Laura Lopez-Rodriguez MD
Dermatology Department, Clinica Ruber, Madrid, Spain

Tanya Kormeili MD APC
Westwood Medical Plaza
10921 Wilshire Blvd, Suite 410
Los Angeles, CA, USA

Catherine Maari MD FRCPC
Clinical Instructor, Department of Dermatology, University of Montreal Hospital Center, Montreal; Innovaderm Research, Montreal, QC, Canada

Pavan K. Nootheti MD
Cosmetic Dermatologist, La Jolla SpaMD, La Jolla, CA, USA

Allan R. Oseroff MD PhD
Professor and Chair of Dermatology, Roswell Park Cancer Institute, Buffalo, NY, USA

James Ralston MD
Resident and Assistant Clinical Instructor, Department of Dermatology, Roswell Park Cancer Institute, Buffalo, NY, USA

Ricardo Ruiz-Rodriguez MD PhD
Chief of Dermatology, Clinica Ruber, Madrid, Spain

Ida-Marie Stender MD PhD
Private Practice, Charlottenlund Dermatology Clinic, Copenhagen, Denmark

Rolf-Markus Szeimies MD PhD
Associate Professor, Department of Dermatology, University of Regensburg, Regensburg, Germany

Dany J. Touma MD
Adjunct Associate Proefssor of Dermatology, Boston University School of Medicine and Private Practice, Boston, MA, USA

Tino Wetzig MD
Department of Dermatology, Universty of Leipzig, Leipzig, Germany

Nathalie C. Zeitouni MDCM FRCPC
Chief of Dermatologic Surgery; Associate Professor of Clinical Dermatology; Director of Dermatologic Surgery Training, Roswell Park Cancer Institute, State University of New York, Buffalo, NY, USA

Brian D. Zelickson MD
Assistant Professor, Department of Dermatology, University of Minnesota, Minneapolis, MN, USA

1 Mechanism of Action of Topical Aminolevulinic Acid

Brian D. Zelickson

INTRODUCTION

Heliotherapy, the use of sunlight to treat various medical disorders, dates back to the ancient Egyptians, Greeks, and Indians. The use of exogenous photosensitizers to improve the efficacy of phototherapy was described in the *Atharva Veda*, a sacred Indian book dating back to 1400 BC. These historical descriptions point to the use of sunlight in combination with a photosensitizing plant containing psoralens to treat a variety of skin conditions, such as vitiligo and psoriasis. Just over 100 years ago the Nobel Prize in Medicine was awarded to Niels Finsen for his research in the use of light to treat lupus vulgaris. It was not until the early 1900s that a German medical student, Oscar Raab, demonstrated the lethal effects of the combination of acridine orange and light on a protozoan. This oxygen-dependent, light-sensitive reaction was termed "photodynamic" by Dr Raab's teacher, Von Tappeiner. Three years later, Jesionek and Tappeiner used the dye eosin and light to successfully treat skin cancer. In the early 1960s, Lipson and Schwartz of the Mayo Clinic brought photodynamic therapy (PDT) into the modern era. They injected hematoporphyrins—a fluorescent mixture of porphyrins—into a patient undergoing surgery and noted fluorescence in neoplastic tissue, demonstrating the photosensitizer's localization in tumors. Its widespread use in dermatology was propagated by the seminal work of Kennedy and colleagues (1990) and the development of PDT with topical 5-aminolevulinic acid (ALA).

GENERAL OVERVIEW: MECHANISM OF ACTION

In PDT, a chemical reaction activated by light energy is used to selectively destroy tissue. The reaction requires three basic elements: (1) a photosensitizing compound, (2) light, and (3) oxygen. For a clinical effect, the photosensitive chemical (photosensitizer) and a light source that emits wavelengths absorbed by the chemical must be localized in the target tissue. The reaction produces singlet oxygen ($^1O_2$) and other free radicals that are cytotoxic (Box 1.1). Singlet oxygen's radius of cytotoxic action is greater than 0.02 μm and its lifetime in biologic systems is less than 0.04 μs. Niedre and colleagues (2005) provided the first direct evidence that PDT-induced skin damage is related to singlet oxygen production. After exposing ALA-photosensitized hairless mouse skin to 635-nm laser radiation, they found that skin damage was associated with cumulative oxygen production.

PDT has many applications in medicine because the photosensitizer accumulates preferentially in abnormal tissue, thus localizing the cytotoxic effects of the reaction products. Temporary cutaneous photosensitivity is the most frequent adverse effect of PDT.

In order to best employ PDT in the clinical setting it is important to have a good understanding of the unique chemical reaction involved. The individual components of the PDT reaction, including the photosensitizers, the activating light sources, along with the biochemical reactions that take place, will be discussed in more detail to give a better understanding of the mechanism of action.

PHOTOSENSITIZERS

Photosensitizers are compounds that have a stable electronic configuration, which at ground state energy is in a singlet state. However, with exposure to light, the absorbed photons convert the compound into a higher energy state. Many different types of photosensitizers have been used for PDT. These include porphyrins, porphyrin precursors, phthalocyanines, porphycenes, chlorines, and pheophorbides (Table 1.1). Despite this long list, only a few are used for treating cutaneous conditions.

Many factors relate to the efficacy of a photosensitizer. An ideal photosensitizer is (1) minimally toxic, (2) taken up more quickly by abnormal (target) tissue than by normal tissue, (3) cleared rapidly from normal tissue, (4) activated at wavelengths that penetrate the target tissue, and (5) capable of producing large amounts of cytotoxic product. Photosensitizers in use or showing promise for cutaneous indications are shown in Table 1.2.

• Localization

Photosensitizers useful in PDT are taken up by both normal and rapidly dividing (malignant) cells, but are cleared less rapidly from neoplastic cells. This difference in clearance rate may be due to the greater number and permeability of blood vessels and slower lymphatic drainage in rapidly dividing neoplastic cells. Photosensitizers are believed to localize in blood vessels, lysosomes, mitochondria, plasma membranes, and nuclei of tumor cells. PDT kills tumor cells by (1) direct destruction by singlet oxygen, (2) damage to blood vessels, and (3) activation of an immune response.

The rate at which the photosensitizer is localized in the target tissue and then cleared from the target tissue and the surrounding structures helps to determine the timing and dosing of the light exposure. These pharmacokinetics are significantly dependent upon the type of photosensitizer and its mode of delivery.

Box 1.1 Production of cytotoxic singlet oxygen and other free radicals

$$\text{Photosensitive chemical} + \text{light} \longrightarrow {}^1O_2 + \text{free radicals}$$

For cutaneous applications, the photosensitizer is usually produced endogenously by first applying photosensitizing agent to the skin. For example, ALA can act as a photosensitizing agent. Though not photosensitive, ALA applied to the skin penetrates into underlying tissue where it is converted to protoporphyrin IX (PpIX), a photosensitive compound (see below).

• Porphyrins

Porphyrin-based photosensitizers, especially porfimer sodium (Photofrin, QLT Phototherapeutics Inc, Vancouver, BC, Canada), have been used to treat cancers of the bladder, lung, esophagus, stomach, skin, and cervix by PDT. Porphyrins absorb maximally at the Soret band

Table 1.1 Photosensitizers and their precursors used in experimental and clinical PDT applications

Porphyrins	Porphyrin precursors	Phthalocyanines	Porphycenes
Hematoporphyrin derivative	δ-Aminolevulinic acid (ALA)	Chloroaluminum tetra-sulfonated phthalocyanine	9-Acetoxy-2,7,12,17-tetra-N-propylporphycene
Dihematoporphyrin ether/ester	δ-Aminolevulinic acid (ALA)-methyl-, propyl-, hexyl-esters	Zinc(II)phthalocyanine	2-Hydroxyethyl-7,12,17-tris(methoxyethyl) porphycene
Porfimer sodium		Silicone naphthalocyanine	23-carboxy-24-methoxycarbonylbenzo(2, 3)-7,12, 17-tri(methoxyethyl)-porphycene
Tetrasodium-meso-tetraphenylporphyrin-sulphonate		Aluminum sulfonated phthalocyanine	
Metallotetra-azaporphyrin			
Chlorines	**Pheophorbides**	**Other**	
Monoaspartyl chlorine e_6, diaspartyl chlorine e_6	Pheophorbide a	Fluoresceins (fluorescein sodium, tetrabromofluorescein-eosin)	
Chlorine e_6 sodium	Bacteriopheophorbide	Anthracenes (anthraquinone, acridine orange, yellow)	
Bacteriochlorin a		Hypericin	
Benzoporphyrin derivative monoacid ring A		Furocoumarin (5-methooxypsoralen, 8-methoxypsoralen) Chlorophyll derivatives Purpurins (metallopurpurin, tin etiopurpurin SnET2) Phenothiazines Methylene blue, violet green Azure C, thionine, Nile blue A Lutetium texaphyrin Hypocrellin Rose Bengal Rhodamine 123	

Adapted from Luksiene Z 2003 Photodynamic therapy: mechanism of action and ways to improve the efficiency of treatment. Medicina (Kaunas) 39:1137–1150

Table 1.2 Photosensitizers and their potential indications for cutaneous malignancies

Sensitizer	Trade name	Potential indications	Activation wavelength (nm)
BPD-MA	Verteporfin	BCC	689
ALA	Levulan	BCC	410–650
MAL	Metvix	BCC	635
SnET2	Purlytin	BCC, cutaneous metastatic breast cancer	664
HPPH	Photochlor	BCC	665
Phthalocyanine-4	Pc 4	Cutaneous/subcutaneous lesions from diverse solid tumor groups	670

BPD-MA = benzoporphyrin derivative monoacid ring A; ALA = 5-aminolevulinic acid; MAL = methyl-aminolevulinate; SnET2 = tin etiopurpurin dichloride; HPPH = 2-[1-hexyloxyethyl]-2-devinyl pyropheophorbide-a
Adapted from Dolmans DE, Fukumura D, Jain RK 2003 Photodynamic therapy for cancer. Nature Review of Cancer 3:380–387

(360–400 nm) and have four smaller peaks between 500 and 635 nm. Cutaneous applications of porphyrin sensitizers are limited because clearance of porphyrins is slow, leading to cutaneous photosensitivity for 4–6 weeks.

Porfimer sodium, a purified mixture of porphyrins, was the first photosensitizer for PDT to obtain US governmental clearance for human use. When administered intravenously, porfimer sodium is selectively retained in tumors as compared to normal tissue. This property makes it possible to treat tumors that can be illuminated, such as those in the skin and the gastrointestinal, genitourinary, and pulmonary tracts. Porfimer sodium's main drawback is cutaneous photosensitivity; patients must avoid sun exposure for weeks after treatment. A major advantage of topically applied ALA is that cutaneous photosensitivity is limited to the treated area and lasts only a few days.

• Nonporphyrins

Other photosensitizers under investigation include benzoporphyrin derivative (used to treat basal cell carcinoma [BCC]), SnET2 (BCC, cutaneous metastatic breast cancer, Kaposi's sarcoma, prostate cancer), chorin derivatives (BCC), and phthalocyanine-4 (cutaneous and subcutaneous lesions of many solid tumors).

• Topical aminolevulinic acid and methyl aminolevulinate

A natural precursor to photosensitive PpIX, ALA is widely used in PDT for cutaneous disorders. The formation of ALA from glycine and succinyl CoA in tissue (in the presence of ALA synthase) is the first and rate-limiting step in heme biosynthesis (Box 1.2). Two molecules of ALA condense enzymatically to form porphobilinogen (PBG), then four PBG molecules are converted to uroporhyrinogen I (UROP I). This leads to the formation of PpIX to which iron is added in the presence of ferrochelatase to form heme. When ALA is applied to tumors of epidermal origin such as BCC and SCC, strong fluorescence due to PpIX is observed.

Box 1.2 Steps in heme biosynthesis

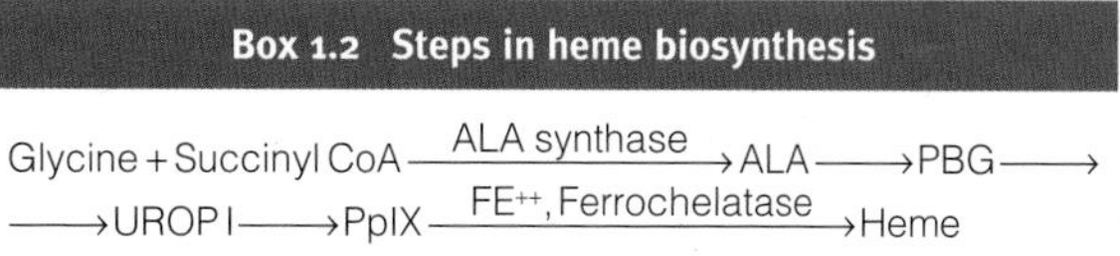

BIOSYNTHESIS OF HEME

In the absence of exogenous ALA, the concentration of free heme controls the amount of ALA produced in tissue by feedback inhibition of ALA synthase. When a large amount of ALA is applied to the skin and absorbed by rapidly dividing (abnormal) cells, PpIX concentration increases more rapidly than it can be converted to heme by the available ferrochelatase, leading to a temporary build-up of PpIX. The preferential accumulation of PpIX in certain types of cells (by mechanisms not fully understood) is the basis for the clinical use of ALA in PDT.

PENETRATION INTO SKIN

The effectiveness of a photosensitizing agent depends partly on how deeply and how selectively the agent penetrates the skin. The penetration efficiency of ALA is influenced by skin thickness, and ALA penetrates skin of benign abnormalities (e.g. actinic keratoses [AKs], sun damage, abrasions, inflammation, psoriasis) more readily than normal skin. The generally thicker skin of Native Americans and Asian people is less permeable to ALA than the thin skin of Europeans.

The rate that PpIX accumulates and is distributed in cutaneous tumors depends on the type of lesion. Superficial BCC and squamous cell carcinoma (SCC) produce abnormal keratin which is more easily penetrated by ALA than nearby normal skin, suggesting that ALA can be liberally applied on and around the lesion unless the patient has unusually thin or sun-damaged skin. It has been estimated the ALA requires 3–15 h to penetrate 2.5–3.0 mm into various types of tissue; however, it works into AKs within as little as 60 min. Physicians can verify that ALA has entered tissue and become PpIX by observing fluorescence under ultraviolet light (Wood's lamp). With prolonged exposure to light (>13 h), ALA-treated lesions become irritated, edematous, and erythematous.

Because ALA is hydrophilic and does not readily penetrate the stratum corneum, a large amount must be applied to skin to assure sufficient absorption for PDT. This drawback stimulated the development of lipophilic esters of ALA (e.g. methyl-aminolevulinate [MAL]) to promote more rapid absorption.

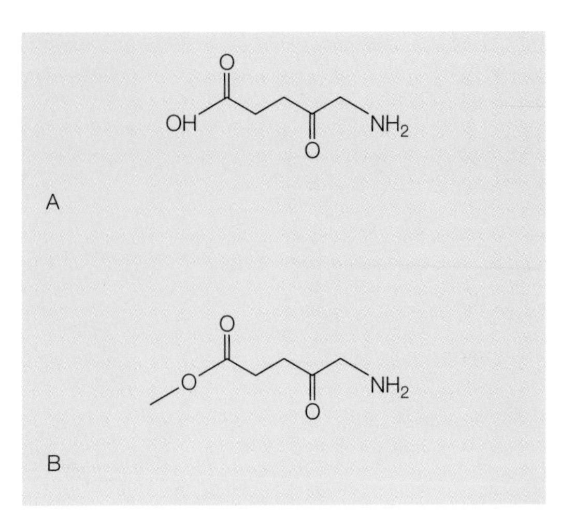

Fig. 1.1 Structures of (**A**) 5-aminolevulinic acid HCL (ALA; Levulan® Kerastick®, DUSA Pharmaceuticals, Wilmington, MA) and (**B**) methyl-aminolevulinate (MAL; Metvix®, PhotoCure ASA)

TREATMENT EXPERIENCE

When ALA has penetrated deeply enough and has been converted into PpIX, the patient is ready for light treatment. Less than 1 min after exposure to light, most patients report a burning, tingling, or itching that peaks in a few minutes and subsides to the level of a "mild sunburn" in the treated area. The sensation disappears within 24 h but the treated area may be tender for a few days.

ADVERSE EFFECTS

When treatment is completed, the treated area may be slightly edematous and erythematous. In heavily freckled patients, a histamine-like reaction may occur, with erythema extending up to 10 cm outside the treated lesion. Some patients may develop superficial erosions with weeping and crusting. Patients should be instructed to avoid sun exposure for 24–48 h due to temporary cutaneous phototoxicity associated with treatment.

LEVULAN AND METVIX

Research in topical photosensitizing agents resulted in the 1999 US Food and Drug Administration (FDA) clearance of Levulan® Kerastick® (5-aminolevulinic acid HCl, DUSA Pharmaceuticals, Wilmington, MA) for the treatment of multiple AKs on the scalp and head, and the 2001 European approval of Metvix® (methyl-aminolevulinate, PhotoCure ASA) PDT for the treatment of AK and BCC. Figure 1.1 shows the structures of both products.

LIGHT–TISSUE INTERACTIONS

In PDT, a source that emits light at wavelengths within the absorption spectrum of the photosensitizer must be available.

Three basic events occur when light is exposed to the skin: (1) the light is reflected from the surface of the skin, (2) the light is scattered by the skin after penetrating it, and (3) the light is absorbed by structures within the skin. Reflected light can be used for diagnostic purposes; however, it does not have a direct clinical effect. Scattered light also has no clinical effect. Light absorbed by specific structures in the skin is the only light that can lead to a clinical effect. When light is absorbed it is converted into different types of energy, such as heat or acoustical waves, or as in PDT, the excitation of other atoms.

The absorption of light and its effects on tissue are related to several factors: (1) wavelength of the light, (2) energy or intensity of the light, and (3) chromophores in the tissue. A detailed analysis of these factors is outside the scope of this chapter; however, there are some simple concepts that should be grasped in order to better understand PDT. For any therapeutic effect to occur the light must reach the targeted tissue, be absorbed by it, and have enough energy to cause the desired response.

In general, the longer the wavelength, the deeper the light penetrates tissue. Light at 630 nm penetrates up to 5 mm while 700–800-nm light may reach up to 2 cm. However, it is important to note that once the light is absorbed, by the photosensitizer or any other chromophore, it will not penetrate any deeper. For example, green light with a wavelength of 532 nm can penetrate up to 1 mm into nonpigmented tissue, while the much longer 10 600-nm infrared light can only penetrate 20–30 μm into tissue due to its water absorption. It is important to choose an activation light that not only has deep penetration so it can reach the target but also that has no other competing absorbers in the surrounding tissue.

Most light used in cutaneous PDT is in the visible or near infrared spectrum. The reason for this is that all available sensitizers have absorption spectra within these wavelengths. Absorption peaks for porphyrins are at 410 (maximum), 505, 540, 580, and 630 nm. The amount of photoactivation depends on the amount of absorbable light that reaches the photosensitizer in the target tissue. The advantage of longer wavelengths is limited by how strongly the photosensitizer absorbs light at these long wavelengths. For example, 630-nm light penetrates more deeply into tissue than 410-nm light, but absorption by a porphyrin photosensitizer is much stronger at 410 nm than at 635 nm. This decreased absorption can be partially overcome by extending the time of light exposure or increasing the amount of light energy. Thus, the appropriate wavelength and dosage of light delivered depends on the depth of the target tumor as well as how well it is absorbed by the photosensitizer.

• Nonlasers

Lasers and nonlasers have been used with success in PDT for dermatologic conditions. Visible light sources such as halogen, xenon, and fluorescent lamps—even slide projectors—are less expensive and more effective than lasers in treating large lesions or lesions in which depth of penetration is unimportant (e.g. AKs). Nonlaser light sources also do not require the use of safety glasses. In addition, irradiation with multiple wavelengths, as with broadband visible light, can improve efficacy. For example, 630–675-nm light is frequently used in lasers to activate PpIX, but a source that also provides 675-nm light also activates photoprotoporphyrin, a photoproduct of PpIX. The result is greater therapeutic benefit. Dosimetry with visible light, however, may be less accurate than with a laser and stray infrared light from the broadband source may heat the skin, causing pain.

Three blue light sources—the BLU-U® PDT Illuminator (DUSA Pharmaceuticals, Wilmington, MA) for the treatment of AK lesions, the ClearLight™ System (Lumenis) for the treatment of moderate inflammatory acne, and the Omnilux (Photo Therapeutics Ltd)—have been cleared by the FDA. Intense pulsed light (IPL) at 560–1200 nm has been used for simultaneous skin rejuvenation and removal of AK lesions.

• Lasers

With lasers, users can more easily target specific areas, minimize exposure times, and select wavelengths. Pulsed gold vapor, continuous-wave argon pumped dye, copper vapor, KTP. and pulsed-dye lasers (PDLs) have been used in dermatologic PDT.

• Alternative light dosing

There have been several reports of using high-energy, very short pulsed exposures of light (PDLs, pulsed KTP lasers, and IPL devices) to activate PpIX after topically applying ALA. Figure 1.2 and Table 1.3 show the relative PpIX activation doses of various lasers and light sources. These studies have shown significant clearance of AK, actinic chelitis, and acne, as well as significant improvement in the fine lines, dyspigmentation, and erythema of photodamaged skin (Fig. 1.3). The advantage of using these devices is that the treatment is relatively fast and these devices, unlike ALA-PDT alone, can clear vessels and pigmentation.

Other investigators have shown that very low-dose chemiluminescent light patches (each patch emits 431–515-nm wavelength light for a total of 55.6 mJ/cm^2 over 20 min) over a long exposure time (45–60 min) can produce significant clearing in AK and inflammatory acne. Local treatment effect using topical ALA with a low-energy light source shows an early inflammatory response with long-term clearing of AK (Fig. 1.4). The main potential benefit of this procedure is that these light sources are very inexpensive, disposable, and may be perfect for home use.

Both of these types of activations, although they work in the clinical setting, have not been shown to produce a PDT reaction in in vitro studies. In vitro phototoxicity assays have been performed using tumor cell cultures incubated with ALA and exposed to a PDL using 595 nm, 10-mm spot size, 6-ms pulse duration (5 J/cm^2) pulsing 10 times (50 J/cm^2), and the low energy light patch as described above. These in vitro experiments resulted in no significant cell killing (DUSA Pharmaceuticals, personal communication).

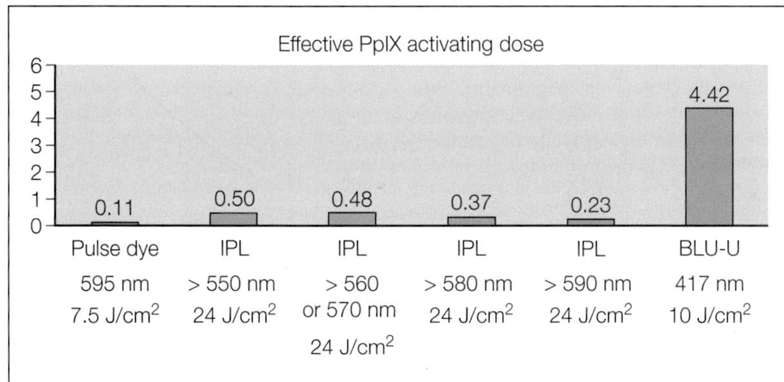

Fig. 1.2 Effective PpIX-activating doses

Table 1.3 Effective PpIX-activating doses for various IPL filter settings

	Dose (J/cm²)	PAE coefficient	Effective dose (J/cm²)	Dose to equal pulsed dye (J/cm²)
Pulsed dye	7.5	0.0150	0.11	7.5
IPL—550 nm	24	0.0207	0.50	5.4
IPL—560 or 570 nm	24	0.0198	0.48	5.7
IPL—580 nm	24	0.0152	0.37	7.4
IPL—590 nm	24	0.0095	0.23	11.9
BLU-U	10	0.4425	4.42	0.3

IPL = intense pulsed light; PAE = PpIX activating energy
Courtesy of DUSA Pharmaceuticals, Inc

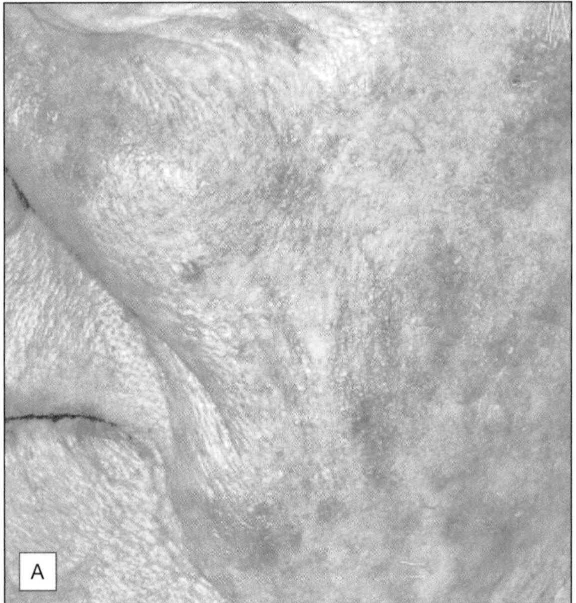
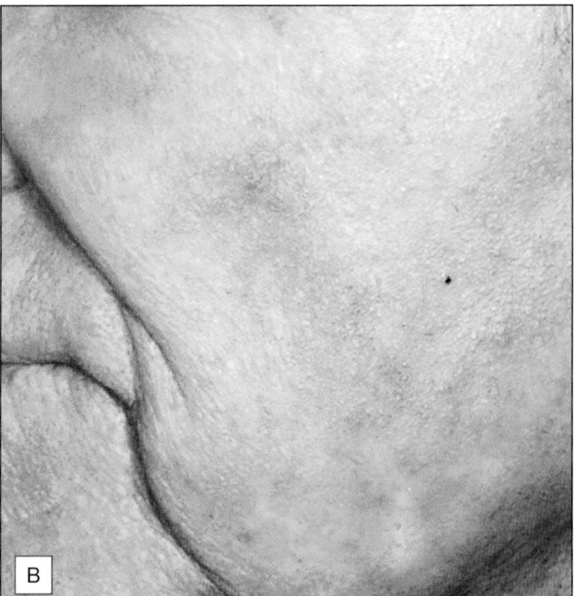

Fig. 1.3 Severe photodamage pre-treatment (left) and 3 months after treatment with topical ALA (60-min incubation) and PDL exposure with 595 nm, 6-ms pulse duration, 10-mm spot size)

This gives rise to the question of how this light activation works. It appears to be different from the way most PDT works. There may be enough activation of PpIX in order to stimulate a host immune response against the surrounding structures, or other mechanisms may be occurring that we are not aware of. One simple explanation is that since most of the areas studied are on the face, which cannot be adequately protected from light exposure, these short-pulsed and low-level long-pulsed exposures do not activate much of the PpIX and the reaction mostly occurs over the next several days by incidental exposure to light. However, Victor Ross has shown very good PpIX activation on sun-protected skin after IPL exposure (Fig. 1.5).

PHOTODYNAMIC THERAPY REACTION

To achieve a successful clinical response there needs to be the simultaneous presence of accumulation of photosensitizer, appropriate light exposure, and oxygen within the target tissue. Once this set of events takes place a chemical reaction occurs which gives rise to the clinical effects. There are several key elements to this reaction: excitation of the photosensitizer, reaction of the excited photosensitizer within the target tissue, response of the target tissue, and response of the surrounding tissue (host response).

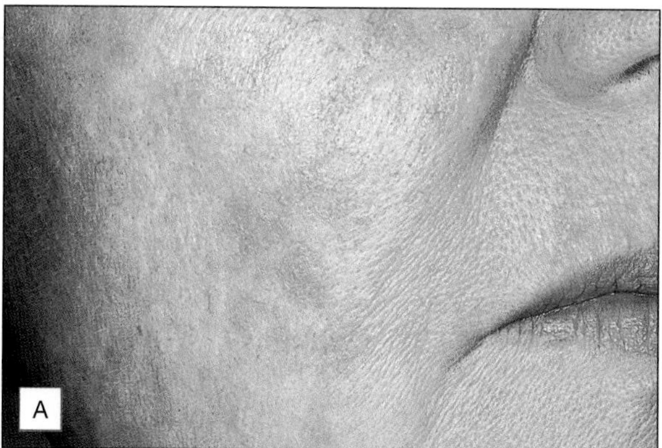

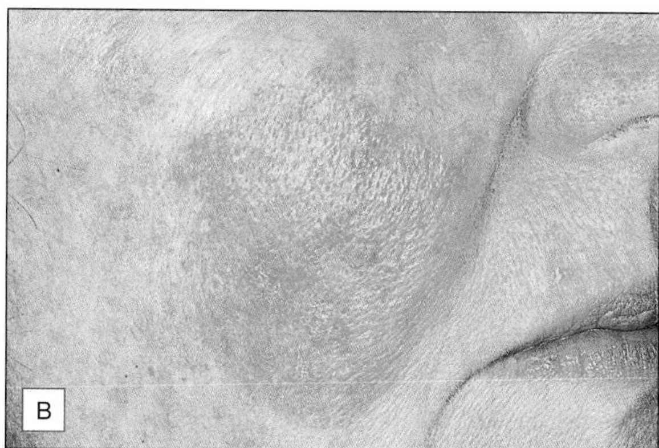

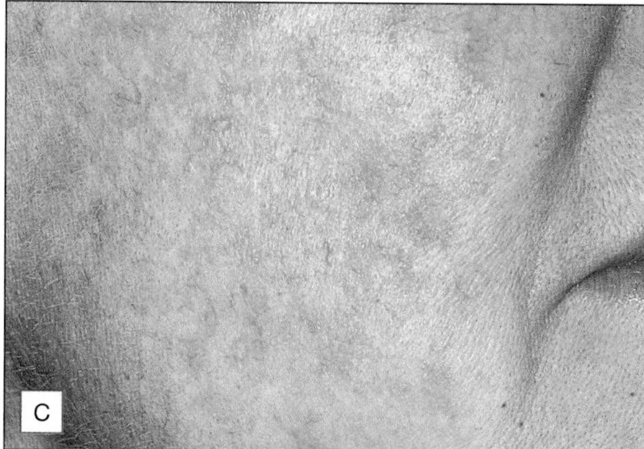

Fig. 1.4 (**A**) Pre-treatment showing diffuse actinic keratosis. (**B**) 1-week follow-up after 45 min ALA incubation and 45-min exposure using a topical light patch showing erythema and urtication. (**C**) 3-month follow-up showing resolution of the keratosis

• Excitation

Upon absorption of photons the ground-state photosensitizer is excited to a singlet-state molecule. There is little to no photodynamic damage caused by this singlet-state molecule because its lifetime, in the nanoseconds, is much too short to react with the surrounding structures. It can, however, dissipate its energy by emitting it as fluorescence or nonradiative decay. This latter event results in the generation of thermal energy and may be an important mechanism of cellular injury. Alternatively, it can convert into the longer-lasting triplet state. Compared to the singlet state, the triplet state molecule has a lifetime in the micro- to milli-seconds (Fig. 1.6). These longer-acting excited molecules react with the surrounding structures to create the cytotoxic effects of the photodynamic reaction.

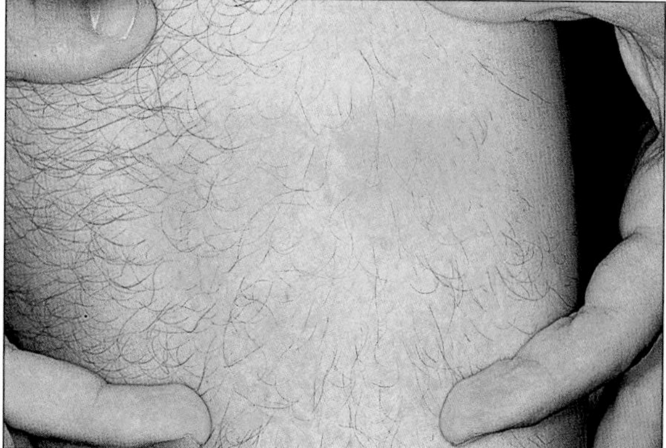

Fig. 1.5 Image of the upper thigh after a 24-h ALA incubation and treatment with the violet hp (Lux V) (Palomar medi lux) using 9 J/cm^2. Note erythema and urtication confined to treated area (Courtesy of Dr E Victor Ross)

The triplet-state molecule dissipates its energy by either radiative emission causing phosphorescence or by going through a quenching reaction. This latter reaction leads to the production of most of the cytotoxic products causing the biologic response and occurs as either a type I or type II mechanism. The type I mechanism yields radical ions by an electron transfer from the excited triplet-state photosensitizer to a nearby molecule. The resulting radical species can then readily react with oxygen to generate reactive oxygen species (ROS) that result in cytotoxic effects by oxidative damage to the surrounding cellular structures. The type II mechanism occurs when the triplet-state photosensitizer reacts with ground-state molecular oxygen. This energy transfer gives rise to highly reactive singlet-state oxygen that can react with biologic structures to cause oxidative cellular injury and death.

• Oxidative reactions

It has been well established that anoxic conditions can completely abolish any PDT effect. In dermatology oxygen is supplied mostly by the flow of blood to the targeted cells, but also through passive absorption from the surface of the skin. Molecular oxygen is critical for the cytotoxic effect in both type I and type II mechanisms. Local oxygen is consumed as the PDT reaction occurs. It is thus important to control the rate of the reaction so that it does not outpace the available oxygen. High-fluence, continuous-wave light exposure has been shown to cause significant reduction in PDT effects by the depletion of oxygen. This effect can be reduced or negated by using a lower rate of light exposure or pulsed light.

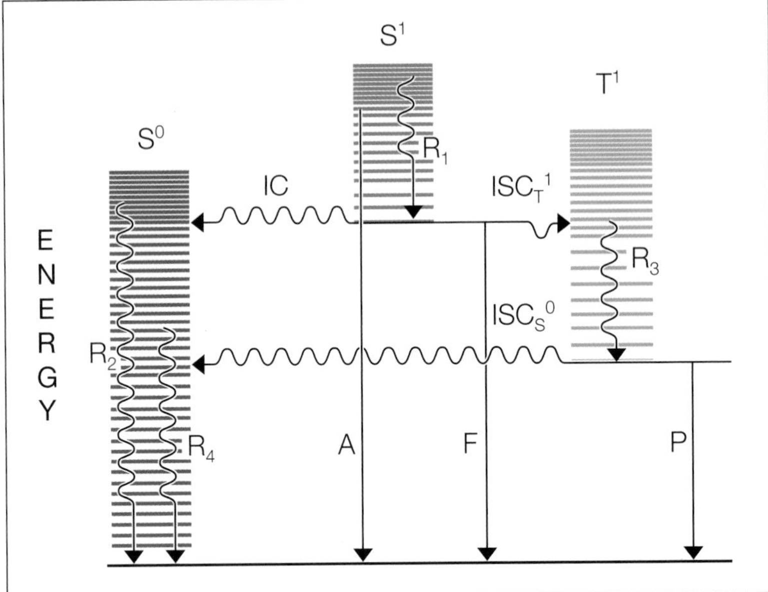

Fig. 1.6 Jablonski diagram illustrating some of the physical processes that can occur after a molecule absorbs a photon, excited state levels, and transitions. S^0 is the ground electronic state of the molecule. S^1 and T^1 are the lowest excited states—singlet and triplet states, respectively. Straight arrows represent processes involving photons, wavy arrows represent radiationless transitions. A = absorption; F = fluorescence; P = phosphorescence; IC = internal conversion; ISC = intersystem crossing; R = vibrational and rotational relaxation (Reproduced from Phillips D 1997 Progress in Reaction Kinetics 22:175. Adapted with permission from Sharman WM, Allen CM, van Lier JE 2000 Role of activated oxygen species in photodynamic therapy. Methods in Enzymology 319:376–400)

Weishaupt and colleagues were the first to report singlet oxygen as the primary cytotoxic agent causing tumor cell death. Subsequently, other ROS, such as superoxide anion, hydrogen peroxide, and hydroxyl radicals, have been shown to be produced by type I and/or type II mechanisms. These ROS then react with a number of biologic targets. The main tissue constituents include water, amino acids, pyrimidine and purine bases, and phospholipids. All but water are targets for cell death and can be significantly altered by reacting with reactive oxygen. This reaction is considered to be the main cytotoxic component of PDT.

• Cellular reactions

The cellular response to ROS formed from the PDT reaction is basically thought of either as an apoptotic or a necrotic event. Many events occur as a result of the reaction, and the ultimate response is determined by the localization and amount of the newly formed ROS. Many different cellular structures are affected, including amino acids (cystine, histidine, tryptophane, tyrosine, methionine), nucleosides (guanine), and unsaturated lipids. Many factors, such as mode of administration, incubation times, size of the sensitizer, affinity toward lipids, and tissue structure, play a role in the localization of the photosensitizer which, in turn, determines which cell structures are oxidatively damaged.

In general, photosensitizers penetrate deeper into the cell structures the longer the incubation time. Short incubation times, minutes to hours, lead to more reaction at the cellular membranes, while with progressively longer periods the reactions occur inside cellular structures such as liposomes, mitochondria, and the nucleus. When the reaction oxidizes lipid membranes, the integrity of the membrane is lost as well as its transport system, causing rupture of the membrane itself. The membrane-associated peptides, including cell-surface receptors, ionic channels, and surface enzymes can also be deactivated by oxidative cross-linking.

Longer incubation times and more lipophilic photosensitizers are prime ways to target mitochondria. This organelle is critical for cellular function. It is the cell's powerhouse for producing energy through ATP synthesis and its damage has been linked to condensation of nuclear chromatin and apoptosis. Photofrin is well localized within the mitochondria, while the conversion of ALA to PpIX takes place in the mitochondria. Although breaks in nuclear DNA have been seen with PDT, these are not frequent and thus there mutative damage is not a concern with PDT.

• Cytotoxicity

Photodynamic cytotoxicity results in necrosis or apoptosis of the cell. In general, when the oxidative destruction is localized to the mitochondria, apoptosis occurs, and when it is in the cell wall, necrosis predominates. Apoptotic cell death is a unique form of cellular injury first described in the early 1970s. It is a naturally occurring process involving a genetically programmed series of events leading to the death of a cell. Another hallmark of apoptosis is the paucity of inflammatory response. PDT has been shown to rapidly induce apoptotic cell death. It is interesting to note that some malignant cells are unable to undergo apoptosis, making them unresponsive to chemotherapy. This resistance is not transferred to PDT. An apoptotic response to PDT is not always observed. This might be a

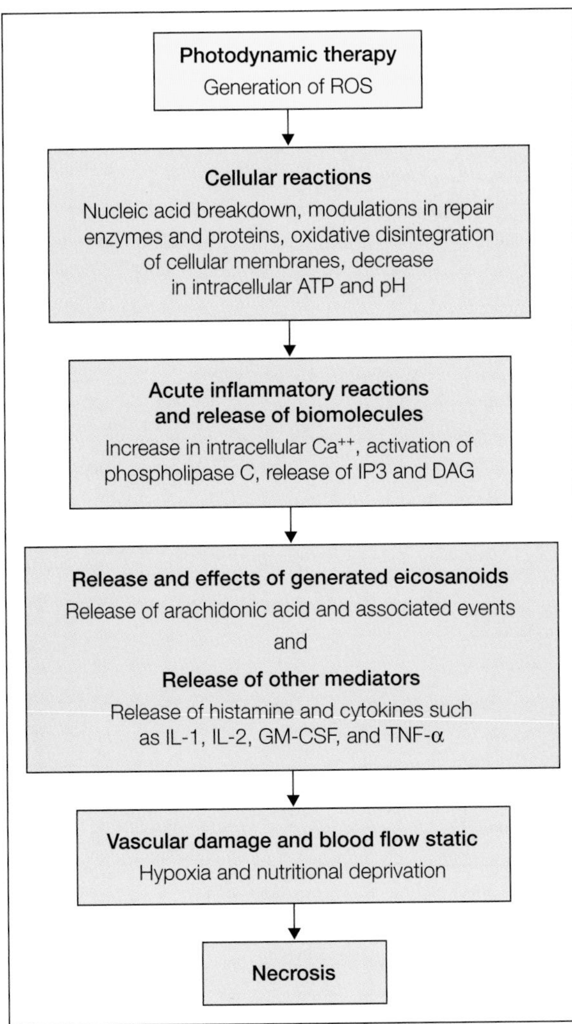

Fig. 1.7 Proposed mechanism for necrosis by PDT. DAG = diacylglycerol; GM-CSF = granulocyte-macrophage colony stimulating factor; IL = interleukin; IP3 = inositol triphosphate; ROS = reactive oxygen species; TNF = tumor necrosis factor (Reproduced with permission from Ahmad N, Mukhtar H 2000 Mechanism of photodynamic therapy-induced cell death. Methods in Enzymology 319:342–358)

result of insensitive detection devices or alternative cytotoxic pathways. As previously discussed, if the localization of the sensitizer is near the cell membrane, cellular necrosis is most likely to occur.

Cellular necrosis occurs with PDT as a result of many different mechanisms—from a direct cellular response leading to an intense inflammatory reaction, to a direct attack on the tumor's blood supply causing hypoxia and necrotic cell death. The proposed scheme is shown in Figure 1.7. After the injury the body then takes over either to remove the cellular debris after apoptosis or to create an inflammatory response to remove the injured tissue and repair the resulting environment. The cascade of cytotoxic and inflammatory mediators, as well as the wound healing mechanisms that repair the damage, are well outlined. The extent of this response is dependent upon the type and extent of tissue damage and is primarily a result of the PDT reaction mechanisms noted above, as well as the extent of susceptible or neoplastic tissue. This is an inherent difficulty of this therapy. The clinical response can be quite variable and is not always predictable. Given the same photosensitizer, dosage, incubation time, and light exposure (time and energy), very different results can be achieved depending on the tissue being treated. For example, in treating patients for multiple AKs with photodamaged skin, the PDT response depends solely on the extent of background photodamage: in a patient with multiple but discrete AKs and little or no background actinic damage, the PDT phototoxic reaction will be very small compared to a patient with little or no discrete AKs but widespread photodamage with large areas of susceptible cells.

CONCLUSION

The mechanisms described will be helpful in selecting the appropriate sensitizer, incubation time, and activator for a given clinical situation.

• Acknowledgment

We would like to acknowledge Fred Wilson for his editorial support.

FURTHER READING

Ahmad N, Mukhtar H 2000 Mechanism of photodynamic therapy-induced cell death. Methods in Enzymology 319:342–358

Alexiades-Armenakas M 2006 Laser-mediated photodynamic therapy. Clinics in Dermatology 24:16–25

Baum CL, Arpey CJ 2005 Normal cutaneous wound healing: clinical correlation with cellular and molecular events. Dermatologic Surgery 31:674–686

Dolmans DE, Fukumura D, Jain RK 2003 Photodynamic therapy for cancer. Nature Reviews Cancer 3:380–387

Dover JS, Bhatia AC, Stewart B, et al 2005 Topical 5-aminolevulinic acid combined with intense pulsed light in the treatment of photoaging. Archives of Dermatology 141:1247–1252

Kalka K, Merk H, Mukhtar H 2000 Photodynamic therapy in dermatology. Journal of the American Academy of Dermatology 42:389–413

Kawauchi S, Morimoto Y, Sato S et al 2004 Differences between cytotoxicity in photodynamic therapy using a pulsed laser and a continuous wave laser: study of oxygen consumption and photobleaching. Lasers in Medical Science 18:179–183

Kennedy JC, Pottier RH, Pross DC 1990 Photodynamic therapy with endogenous protoporphyrin IX: basic principles and present clinical experience. Journal of Photochemistry and Photobiology B 6:143–148

Kerr JF, Wyllie AH, Currie AR 1972 Apoptosis: a basic biological phenomenon with wide ranging implications in tissue kinetics. British Journal of Cancer 26: 239–257

Luksiene Z 2003 Photodynamic therapy: mechanism of action and ways to improve the efficiency of treatment. Medicina (Kaunas) 39:1137–1150

Nestor MS, Gold MH, Kauvar AN et al 2006 The use of photodynamic therapy in dermatology: results of a consensus conference. Journal of Drugs in Dermatology 5:140–154

Niedre MJ, Yu CS, Patterson MS et al 2003 Singlet oxygen luminescence as an in vivo photodynamic therapy dose metric: validation in normal mouse skin with topical amino-levulinic acid. British Journal of Cancer 92:298–304

Sharman WM, Allen CM, van Lier JE 2000 Role of activated oxygen species in photodynamic therapy. Methods in Enzymology 319:376–400

Weishaupt KR, Gomer CJ, Dougherty TJ 1976 Identification of singlet oxygen as the cytotoxic agent in photoinactivation of a murine tumor. Cancer Research 36:2326–2329

2 Treatment of Acne with Systemic Photodynamic Therapy

Yoshiyasu Itoh

INTRODUCTION

Acne vulgaris is a common skin disease in adolescents and young adults. Although a small number of acne lesions may be tolerable and easily treated, repeated recalcitrant acne is hard to cure and has a tendency to lead to scarring, causing further distress. Complete freedom from the chronic pimpled condition is very difficult to achieve, although many methods have been introduced. In order to attempt to solve this problem, 5-aminolevulinic acid (ALA)-photodynamic therapy (PDT) treatment can be used as a primary regimen. Post-treatment management is necessary to preserve the improvements achieved by ALA-PDT. This chapter provides guidance on how to treat acne with ALA-PDT and how to successfully diminish apparently incurable acne.

Hyperpigmentation after topical ALA-PDT has been observed with very high frequency in Asian patients because of melanogenesis and epidermal exfoliation, which occurs via photodynamic action due to the accumulation of protoporphyrin IX (PpIX) in the epidermis (Figs 2.1, 2.2). More recently, oral administration of ALA has been used for treating acne, and this technique is described in this chapter (Figs 2.3, 2.4).

A major cause of acne inflammation is believed to be an increase in perilesional pathogenic bacteria, especially *Propionibacterium acnes*. Patients undergoing long-term dosage with antibiotics are frequently infected with a number of bacteria, but not always *P. acnes* (Tables 2.1, 2.2), which may be seen more frequently in more seriously infected patients. However, ALA-PDT treatment is more successful at eradicating *P. acnes* than other bacteria because the available photosensitizers in acne patients infected with *P. acnes* are endogenous coproporphyrin and PpIX associated with external dosage of ALA, while in patients with other bacteria the only operative photosensitizer is PpIX. Before ALA-PDT treatment, it is important to know whether the main bacterium in lesions is *P. acnes*, as eradication of bacteria apart from *P. acnes* may require more PDT procedures. To answer this question, ultraviolet examination is useful (Box 2.1).

Box 2.1 Ultraviolet examination

Ultraviolet pictures can easily show the amount of porphyrin as fluorescence and are very useful for judging the bacterial conditions of the patient's skin. If there is no dosing with photosensitizers, the presence of fluorescence means the appearance of endogenous porphyrin (mostly coproporphyrin) produced by *P. acnes*. Healthy controls and most patients undergoing treatment with antibiotics at a low dosage demonstrate fluorescence well (Figs 2.5, 2.6, see page 16). On the other hand, patients with a serious acne condition frequently present less fluorescence, which means that acne lesions are caused by bacteria other than *P. acnes* (Figs 2.7, 2.8, see page 16). The oral administration of external ALA produces an accumulation of PpIX in the pilosebaceous units and induces more production of coproporphyrin to *P. acnes*. As a result, enhancement of fluorescence is seen (Fig. 2.9, see page 17). On topical application of ALA, fluorescence caused by the accumulation of PpIX in the upper half of the epidermis is seen.

Table 2.1 Acne grading by Burton scale

Grade	Description
Grade 0	Total absence of lesions
Grade I	Subclinical acne—few comedons visible only in close examination
Grade II	Comedonal acne—comedons with slight inflammation
Grade III	Mild acne—inflamed papules with erythema
Grade IV	Moderate acne—many inflamed papules and pustules
Grade V	Severe nodular acne—inflamed papules and pustules with several deep nodular lesions
Grade VI	Severe cystic acne—many nodular cystic lesions with scarring

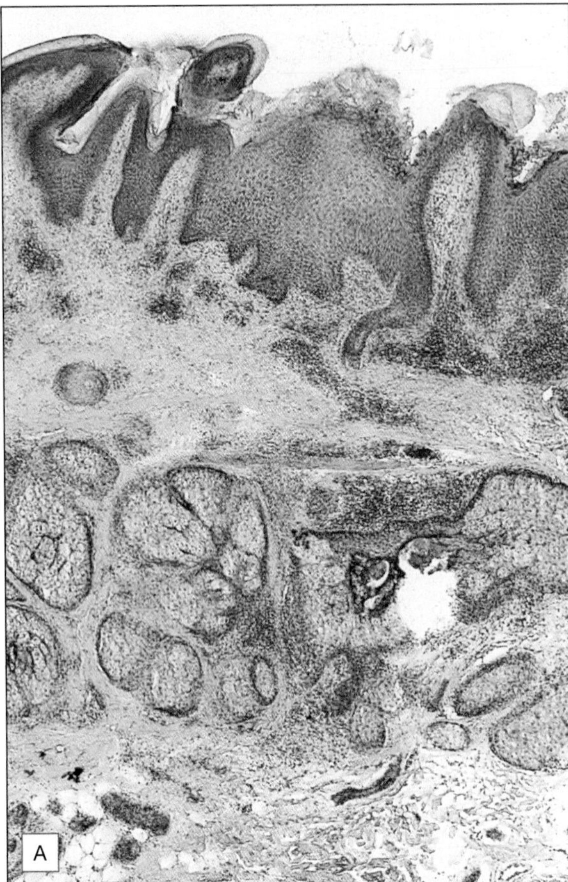

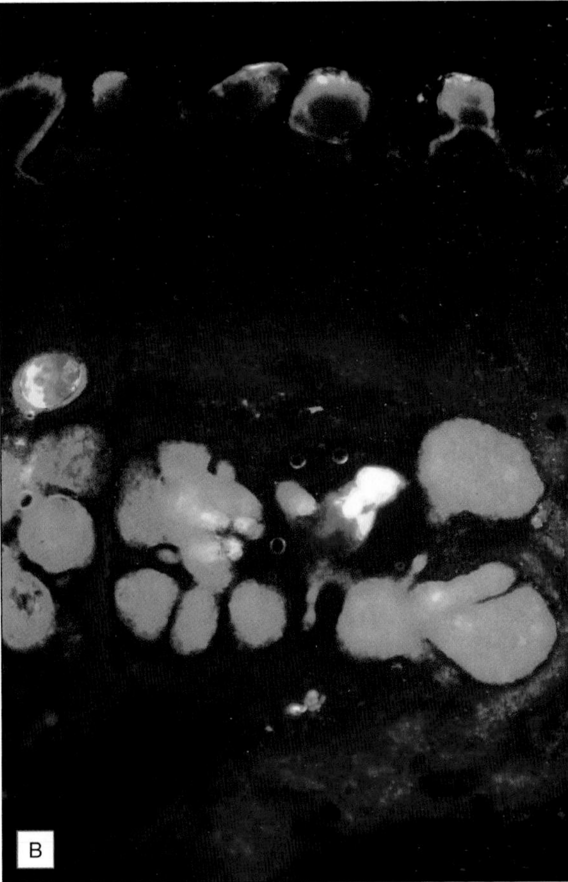

Fig. 2.1 Twelve hours after topical application of 20% ALA ointment, the upper half of the epidermis (**A**) and the whole sebaceous gland (**B**) in sebaceous nevus show fluorescence due to accumulation of PpIX. The eccrine gland does not show fluorescence

Table 2.2 Species of bacteria in 39 serious acne patients (Grades IV–VI on the Burton scale)

Species of bacteria	Number
P. acnes	3
P. acnes + *S. epidermis*	12
P. acnes + MSSA	3
P. acnes + MRSA	3
P. acnes + *S. epidermis* + MSSA	1
P. acnes + *S. epidermis* + MRSA	2
S. epidermis	6
MSSA	1
MRSA	3
MSSA + *S. epidermis*	2
MRSA + *S. epidermis*	2
P. acnes + *S. epidermis* + *S. capitis*	1
P. acnes + *S. epidermis* + *S. hominis*	1

PATIENT SELECTION

A major effect of ALA-PDT treatment of acne is bactericidal. The secondary effect is damage to the sebaceous glands. ALA-PDT treatment can be used for all types of acne and acne in all areas. Moreover, folliculitis, rosacea, and seborrhea are also likely to respond to PDT (Fig. 2.10, see page 17). Although most acne patients have accompanying seborrhea, patients with dry skin or atopic dermatitis may have a more complicated treatment regimen. Patients with dry skin need adequate moisturizing skin care as sebaceous glands are destroyed. Generally, sebum secretion is restored 1 month after one session of ALA-PDT treatment. Monthly repeated ALA-PDT treatments can improve seborrhea.

EXPECTED BENEFITS

The results of 96 acne patients treated with orally administered ALA-based PDT are shown. All patients, 30 men and 66 women, were grades IV–VI on the Burton scale (see Table 2.1) and underwent PDT after a 4-week

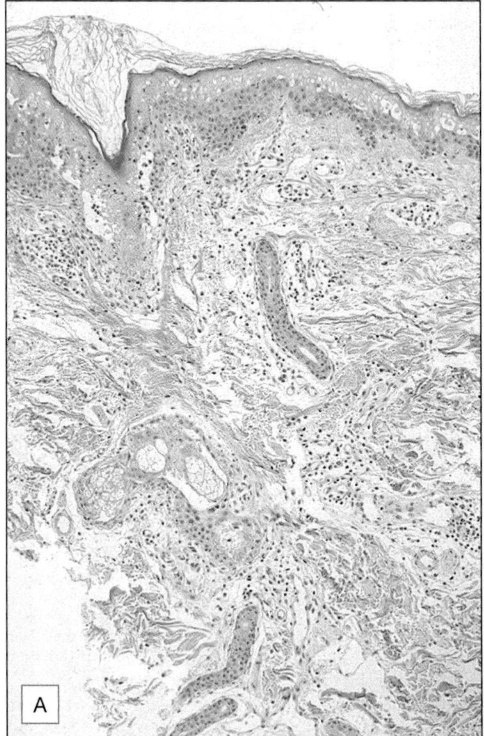

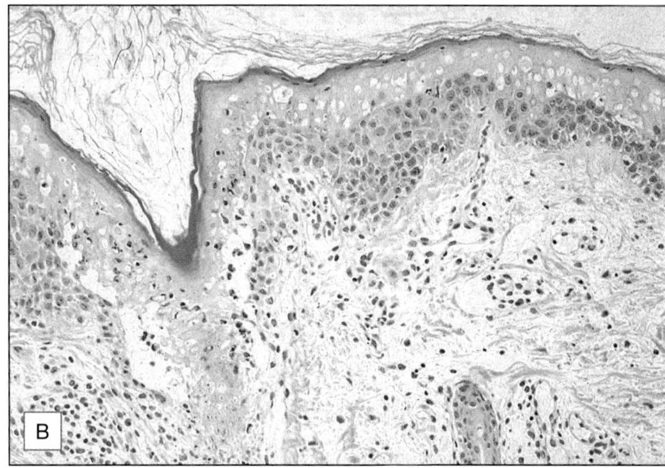

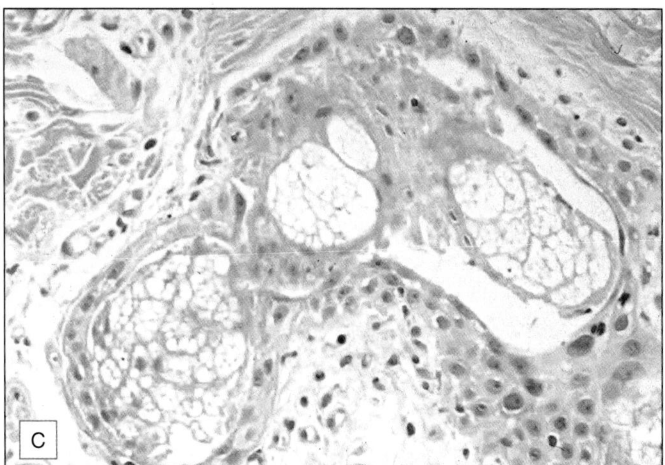

Fig. 2.2 Two days after PDT treatment to the sebaceous nevus in Figure 2.1, the upper half of the epidermis (**A**) and the inner sheath of the hair follicle (**B**) show apoptosis, and damage to the sebaceous gland (**C**) is seen. The basal pigmentation in the epidermis is observed

washout period. The average age of the patients was 28 years. As 38 patients were treated on both the face and body, the total numbers of patients treated for facial acne and body acne were 83 and 51, respectively. Four hours after the oral administration of ALA at 10 mg/kg of body weight (BW), acne lesions were exposed to polychromatic visible light by a metal halide lamp. All patients underwent between two and four sessions of PDT (one PDT series) and received no other treatments. Each PDT course lasted between 2 and 4 weeks. Based on the photographs before and 3 months after the final PDT treatment, the numbers of papulopustular lesions, but not comedonal lesions, were counted, and the physician's rating assessment of "worsened", "unchanged", "improved", or "markedly improved" was obtained. All patients were interviewed about adverse effects.

The average reductions in papulopustular lesions before and after ALA-PDT treatments were 12% for facial acne and 18% for body acne, respectively (Figs 2.11–2.13, see page 18). The rating assessments for the facial and body acne are summarized in Table 2.3. In the rating assessment for facial acne, 0 patients (0%) had worsened, 7 (8.4%) were unchanged, 26 (31.3%) had improved, and 50 (60.3%) were markedly improved. In the rating assessment for the body acne, the relevant scores were 0 (0%), 4 (7.8%), 16 (31.4%), and 31 (60.8%) patients, respectively.

Table 2.3 Clinical assessments

Assessment	Face (number)	Body (number)
Worsened	0	0
Unchanged	7	4
Improved	26	16
Markedly improved	50	31

In this study, almost all patients tolerated the light irradiation, while five patients complained of discomfort, burning, and stinging during the irradiation. Of 96 patients,

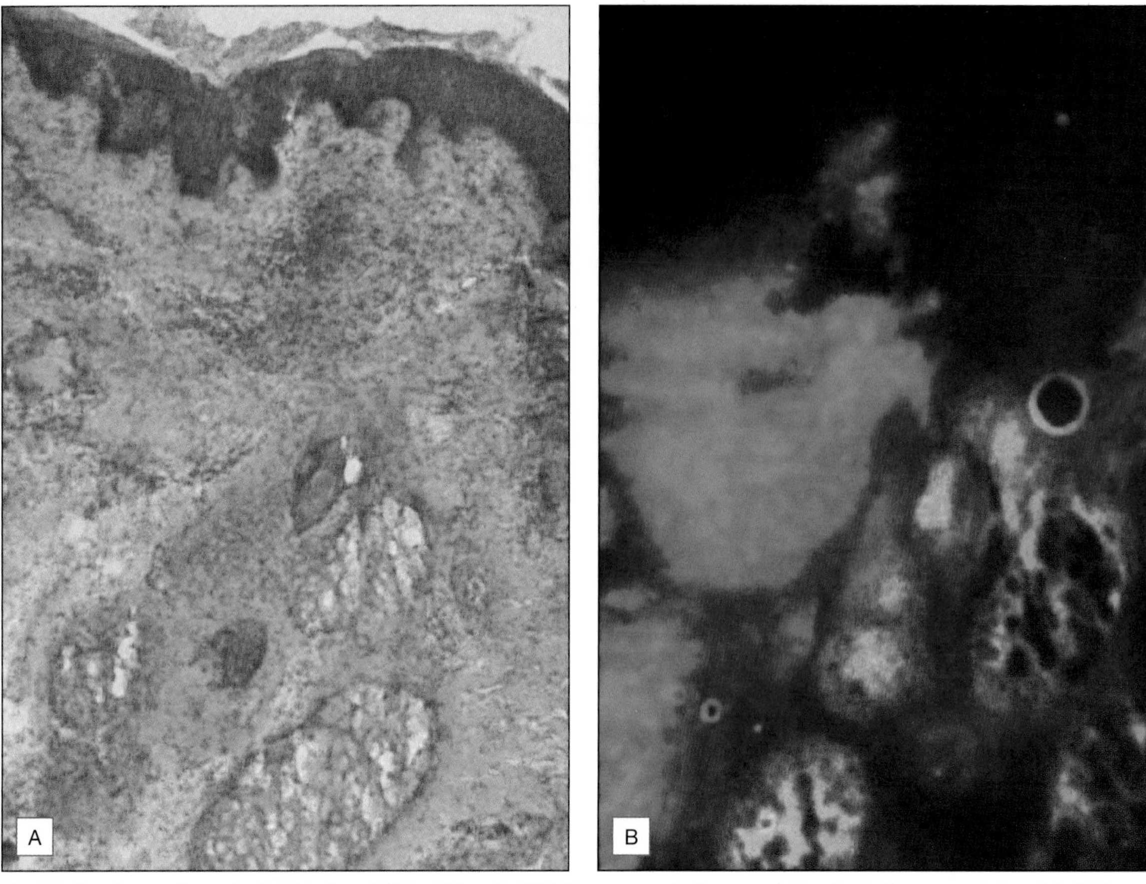

Fig. 2.3 Four hours after oral administration of ALA of 10 mg/kg BW, fluorescence in the normal skin, due to the accumulation of PpIX, is seen in the pilosebaceous unit but not the epidermis

eight complained of transient nausea for several hours. Almost all patients developed erythema immediately after PDT treatment. Erythema of the face continued for 1–5 days, although most patients recovered within 2 days. Erythema of the body was very mild in most cases and disappeared within 1 day. Five percent of the affected faces showed swelling lasting for 1–5 days. A high degree of erythema and swelling were more often seen in patients with fair skin. Two days after a PDT session, new acne, new pustules, and/or hypersecretion of sebum were observed, and were expected as a treatment reaction consisting of a massive discharge of bacteria and destruction of the sebaceous glands (Figs 2.14–2.16, see page 20). Typical reactive acne entails several spots that heal within 1 week, and this occurs frequently in the peri-oral area. Healing is fast because bacteria in reactive acne are already dead. High-degree reactive acne is caused by excessive irradiation from the light source but the extent of reactive acne is usually in proportion to the degree of acne severity. Excessive reactive acne should be avoided because it can give rise to disfiguring acne scars. Almost all facial acne patients treated with PDT noticed reactive sebum for several days afterwards, following which they became aware of a rapid decrease in sebum. Generally, the degree of reactive sebum depends on the degree of seborrhea. Erythema, swelling, reactive acne, and reactive sebum appear most profusely after the first PDT session. On repeat PDT treatment, these reactions decrease.

We reported a series of ALA-PDT treatments on over 5000 acne patients from 1998 to 2004. Since 1999, orally administered ALA-PDT has been the preferred route in this group, with the oral dosage used being 10 mg/kg BW. No patient has suffered from liver dysfunction (Figs 2.17–2.20, see page 21). Five patients have developed herpes simplex on the lip within 2 days after a PDT session, but all of these patients had a past history of herpes simplex. Among these five, two received topical ALA and three orally administered ALA. Very frequently, hyperpigmentation and epidermal exfoliation were observed in Asian patients treated with topically applied ALA-PDT. Pigmentation change persisted over 1 week to 2 months; epidermal exfoliation lasted from the fourth to the tenth day. To avoid pigmentation and epidermal exfoliation, orally administered ALA-PDT may be preferable when treating patients with skin phototypes IV and V.

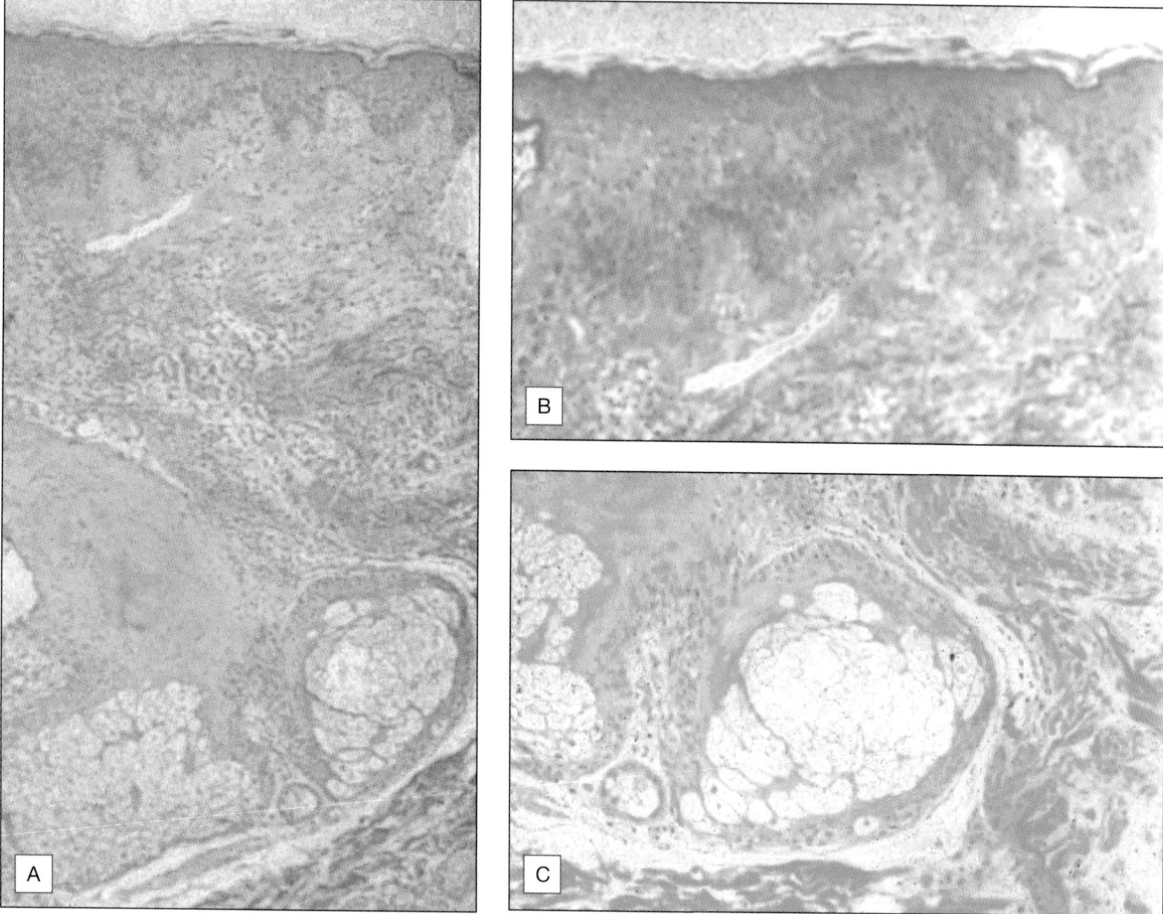

Fig. 2.4 Two days after PDT treatment to the normal skin in Figure 2.3, damage to the sebaceous gland is seen (**C**) but the epidermis is intact (**A**,**B**)

Pigmentation after topically applied ALA-PDT is caused by melanogenesis, which is a photodynamic reaction to the accumulation of PpIX in the epidermis. Pigmentation after orally administered ALA-PDT may be postinflammatory, because it is recognized in patients showing high levels of erythema and swelling. While a decrease in sebum secretion often leads to dry skin, 1 month after a PDT session, the level of sebum secretion recovers. We have never encountered any patients with persistent, problematic photosensitivity after PDT. Adverse effects and complications are summarized in Box 2.2.

Optimal PDT treatment can lead to the eradication of etiological bacteria to acne and the suppression of new papulopustular lesions for over 6 months. Comedonal lesions are restrained because sebum is controlled. In patients with seborrhea, persistently repeated PDT procedures improve skin texture and decrease the secretion of sebum and pore size.

Box 2.2 Adverse effects and complications

After oral administration of ALA:

- Nausea and vomiting

During irradiation:

- Discomfort, burning, and stinging

After PDT:

- Erythema, swelling, "reactive acne", "reactive sebum", hyperpigmentation, dry skin, epidermal exfoliation (only topical application of ALA), and herpes simplex

OVERVIEW OF TREATMENT STRATEGY

• Treatment approach

In acne patients receiving PDT, high levels of irradiation from light sources may completely eradicate bacteria in only one treatment. However, complications such as ery-

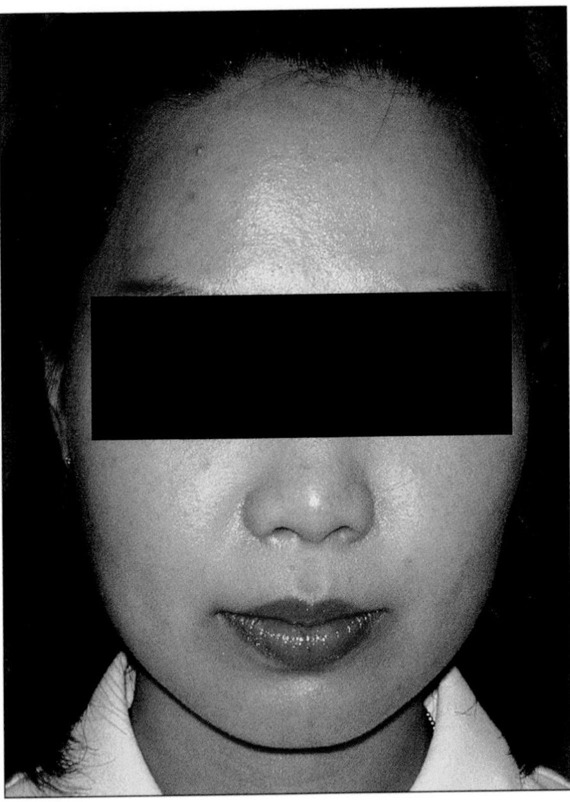

Fig. 2.5 Patient shows a very mild acne condition which was evaluated as grade I on the Burton scale. There is no treatment history

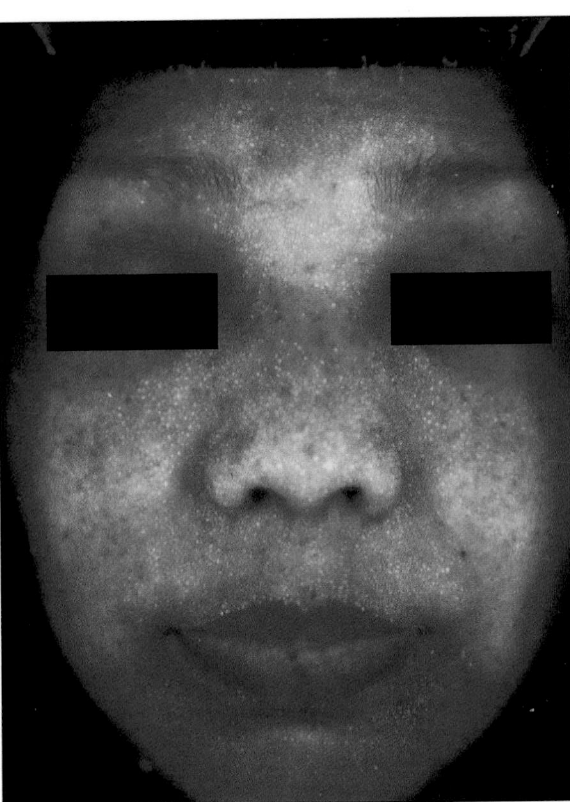

Fig. 2.6 In the ultraviolet picture, the patient in Figure 2.5 reveals an abundant fluorescence as a dot shape, which is due to endogenous coproporphyrin by *P. acnes*

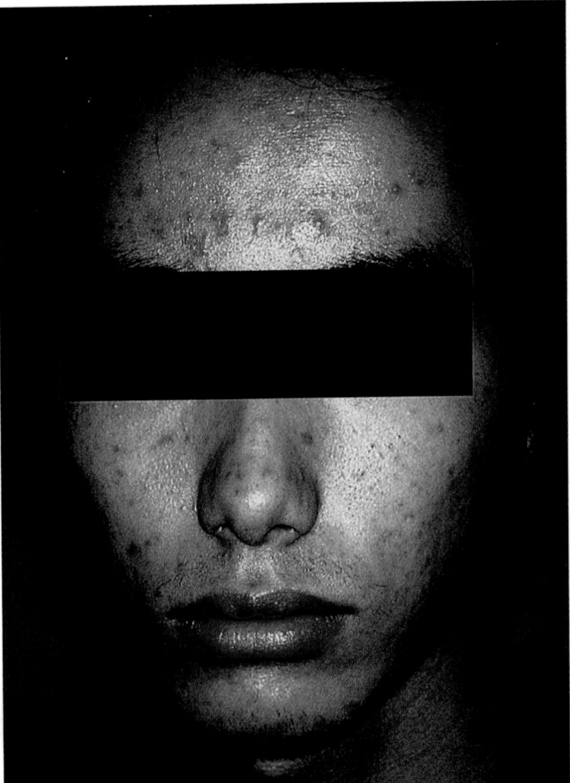

Fig. 2.7 Patient with acne of grade IV on the Burton scale, revealing many papulopustular lesions. The patient had continuously undergone several typed doses of antibiotics for 1 year

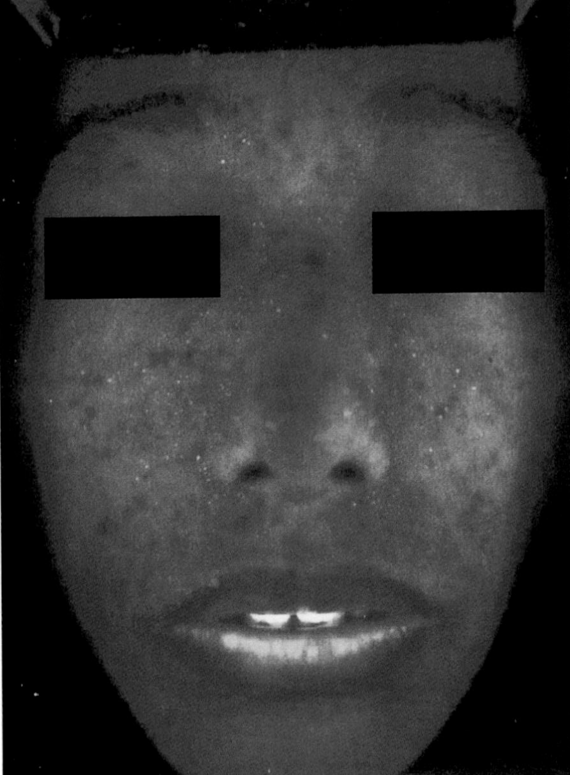

Fig. 2.8 In the ultraviolet picture, the patient in Figure 2.7 reveals a slight degree of dot-shaped fluorescence caused by *P. acnes*-based endogenous porphyrin

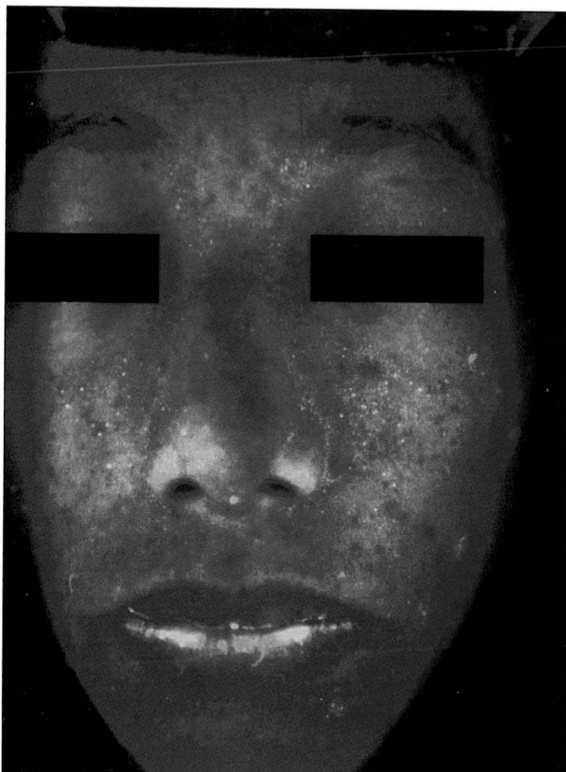

Fig. 2.9 Four hours after oral administration of ALA of 10 mg/kg BW, the ultraviolet picture of the patient in Figure 2.7 demonstrates the enhancement of dot-shaped fluorescence from the accumulation of external ALA dosage-based PpIX

thema, swelling, reactive acne, and pigmentation may be prominent if the irradiation is too strong. To continue treatments with no downtime, lower level irradiation is recommended for initial treatments. At subsequent PDT treatments, a step-by-step increase of the light energy is possible. For instance, if a patient is expected to receive four PDT treatments in one PDT series, the light energy dosage for the second PDT session may be set at 1.2 times that in the first PDT, that of the third PDT may be 1.4 times, and that of the fourth 1.6 times. In a given PDT series, the number of treatments may be based on the seriousness of the acne and the types of etiologic bacteria. To reduce acne slightly, two treatments may be appropriate. However, it is sometimes necessary to deliver treatments three times or more. As sensitivity to ALA-PDT treatment is different for *P. acnes* compared with other bacteria, ultraviolet examination before starting a PDT series is important. For acne of grade IV or more on the Burton scale, four treatment sessions are routinely planned. In the final PDT treatment, if reactive acne is still apparent, an additional PDT procedure may be desired. A promising treatment result can be expected when no more reactive acne appears.

The interval between each PDT treatment is usually from 10 days to 4 weeks. If a very long interval is used,

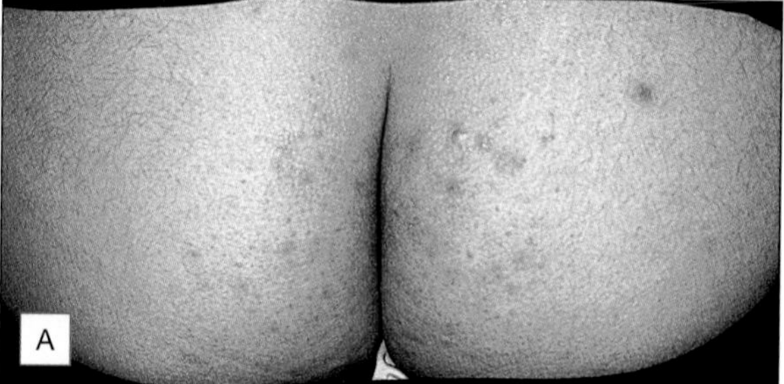

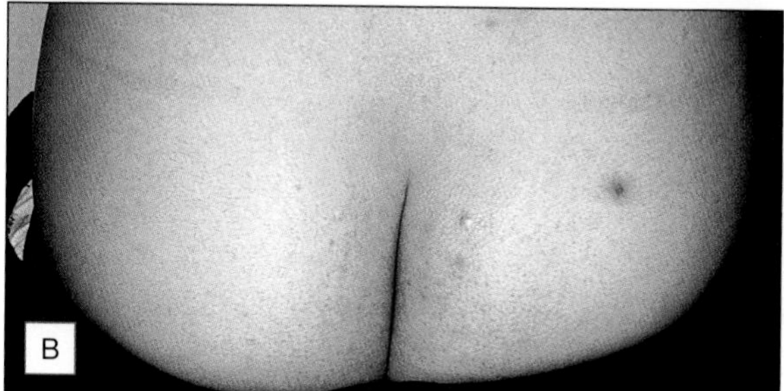

Fig. 2.10 (**A**) Folliculitis on the buttock. (**B**) Two weeks after two PDT sessions with a 2-week interval, the lesion shows an excellent result

the efficiency decreases because the bacteria propagate. If a treatment schedule is consistent and if the skin is in reasonable condition, an interval of 10 days is best.

For complete recovery from recurrent recalcitrant acne, treatment with ALA-PDT only may not be sufficient, although an improvement will be seen for a time. In patients with chronic acne, red acne scars remain for a long time even if papulopustular lesions disappear. Moreover, a hair follicle with redness can easily produce a papulopustular lesion again (Fig. 2.21, see page 23). If one PDT series can stop new lesions for 6 months, the remaining red scars should return to normal color within this period. If the red acne scars remain after 6 months following one PDT series, those treated hair follicles have a likelihood of inducing acne recurrence. To remove redness, iontophoresis with vitamin C and intense pulsed light (IPL) treatment are effective (Figs 2.22–2.26, see page 23). Acne scars without redness may be associated with dimpling but do not produce recurrent acne lesions.

PDT treatments spaced 1 month apart can reduce sebaceous glands. However, more than 10 treatments may be necessary.

Figure 2.27 depicts the treatment approach.

• Patient interviews

It is important to confirm a past history of treatment:

- Have antibiotics been used?
- What was the dosage and how long was the treatment course?
- Is there a past history of herpes simplex?
- How long has the patient been suffering from acne?

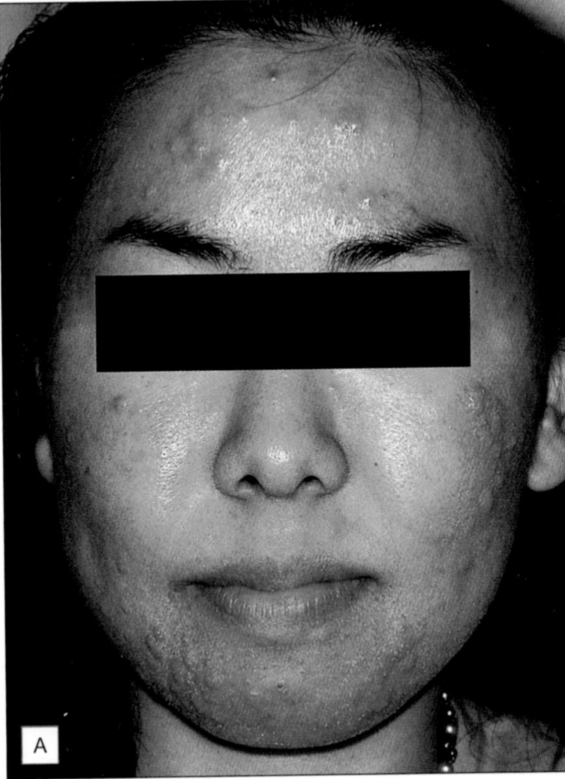

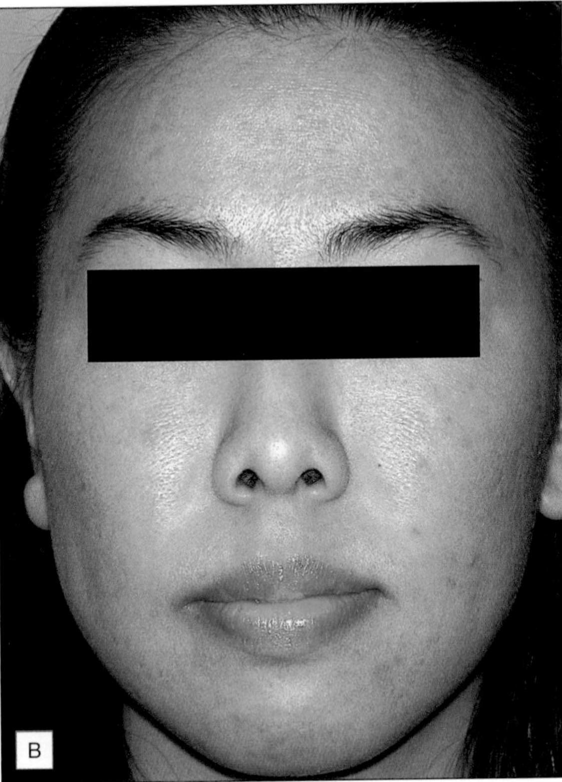

Fig. 2.11 (**A**) Acne patient of grade V on the Burton scale, with many papulopustular lesions and several large cystic lesions. (**B**) Three months after one PDT series (four PDT sessions), the patient demonstrates an apparent improvement

A check of the skin phototype is also needed:

- Is there a history of photosensitivity?
- Is there a history of drug-induced photodermatitis?
- Is the skin seborrheic, normal, or dry?

TREATMENT TECHNIQUES

• Patients

Acne, rosacea, seborrhea, folliculitis, and infection of the pilosebaceous units are indications for ALA-PDT treatment. Previously, application of tretinoin cream is useful to recover skin condition after PDT treatment. Medicines that could give rise to drug-induced photodermatitis should be washed out for several weeks prior to initiation of PDT. In patients with a past history of herpes simplex, a prophylactic antiviral drug should also be administered.

• Equipment

The fluorescence excitation spectrum of PpIX has its peaks at 410 (the Soret band), 510, 545, 580, and 630 nm. Down to 2 mm from the skin surface, 410-nm light provides the largest degree of photoactivation, whereas at depths exceeding 2 mm, 630-nm light is more effective. In flat normal skin, the depth of the sebaceous gland may be less than 2 mm. However, when treating an elevated acne papule or cystic acne, depths exceeding 2 mm are common and treatment should use the 630-nm wavelength. Moreover, in our experience, compared with red light, blue light may produce stronger inflammation, erythema, swelling, and reactive acne after a PDT session.

The light source for PDT can be supplied by several types of lasers and light sources. We have used a 630-nm pulsed excimer dye laser (PDT-EDL 1, HAMAMATSU, Hamamatsushi, Japan) for acne treatment. However, lasers with larger spot sizes or even an incoherent light source may be more efficient at treating larger areas. Theoretically, incoherent light sources are able to produce uniform skin-surface illumination because the shape of the face is an uneven sphere, although affected areas of the chest and the back are flat. As energy density will be increased four times if the distance between a light source and the surface of the affected area doubles, uniformity of energy density in treating large areas is very important to achieve the expected outcome. Uneven irradiation causes excessive reactive acne, erythema, swelling, hyperpigmentation, and uncertain results. It is also important that the light source be movable because it is difficult to

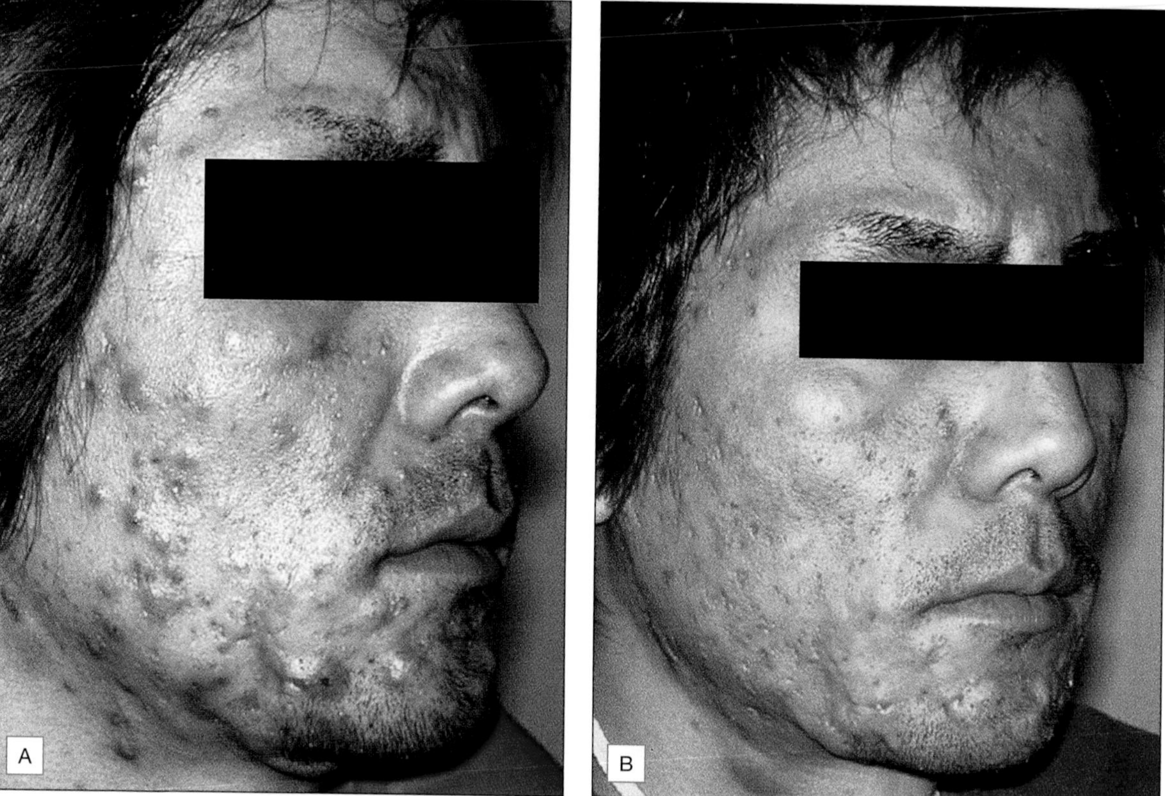

Fig. 2.12 (**A**) Acne patient of grade VI on the Burton scale, with many large cystic lesions. (**B**) Three months after one PDT series—four PDT sessions with 2-week intervals—the patient demonstrates an apparent improvement but deep dimples remain

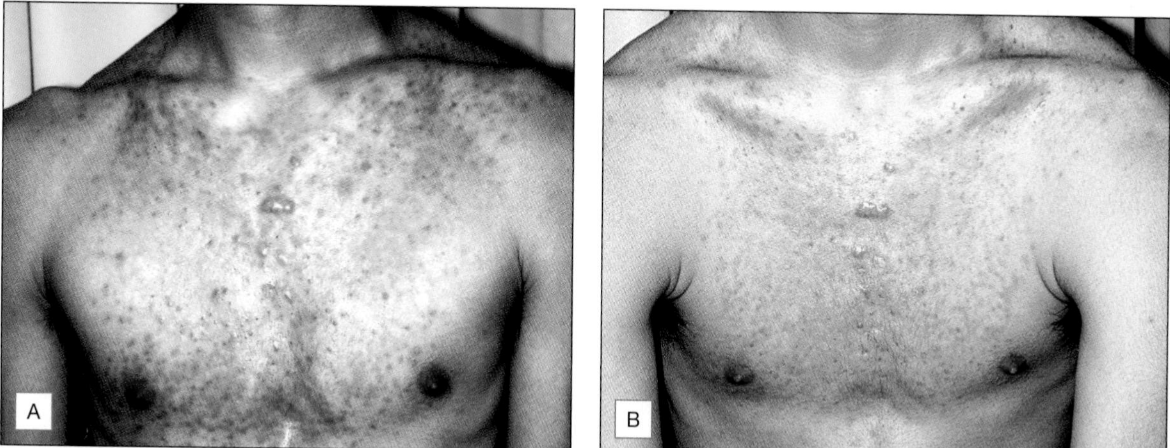

Fig. 2.13 (**A**) A severe acne condition on the chest. (**B**) Three months after one PDT series—two PDT sessions with 2-week intervals—the patient demonstrates an apparent improvement

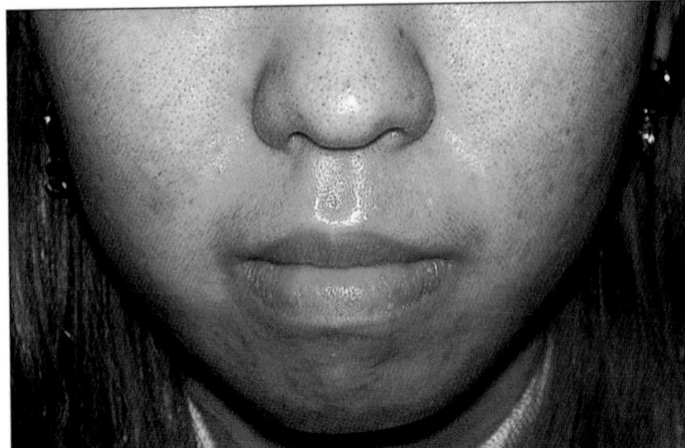

Fig. 2.14 Acne patient of grade IV on the Burton scale just before the first PDT

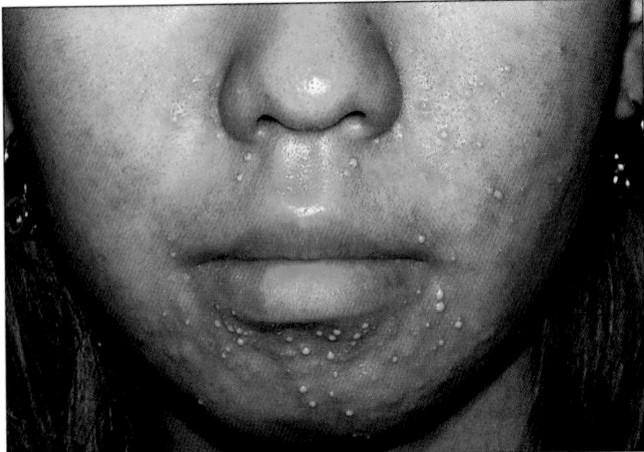

Fig. 2.15 Three days after the first PDT treatment for the patient in Figure 2.14, severe "reactive acne" is seen. Reactive acne consists of many papules and pustules. It is caused by the irradiation being too strong. Strong irradiation is able to kill many bacteria but can produce severe reactive acne, which may lead to prolonged red acne scars. This case of reactive acne lasted for 1 week

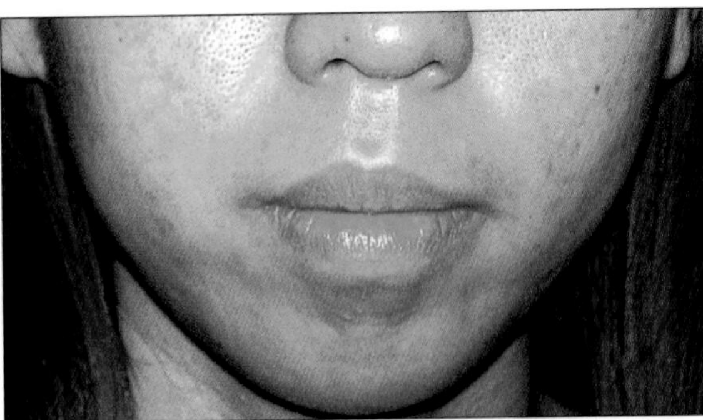

Fig. 2.16 Three months after one PDT series (three PDT treatments), the patient in Figure 2.15 demonstrates an apparent improvement. It was necessary to leave a 5-week interval between the first and second PDT because of a delay in skin recovery due to excessive reactive acne

irradiate the region from the lower jaw to the neck if the patient is in the supine position.

We use two light sources. One is a polychromatic visible light source with four-lamp boxes with metal halide lamps (Usio Inc, Tokyo, Japan; Fig. 2.28, see page 24). Although the highest peak is at 610 nm, the spectrum also efficiently covers the 545-, 580-, and 630-nm wavelengths absorbed by PpIX, as well as 670 nm (Fig. 2.29, see page 25). Excitation at the 670-nm peak is helpful since it too leads to the development of activated photoproducts. This device has circular spots with diameters of 5 and 10 cm. When the distance between the lamp and the affected surface is 13 cm, the average fluence rate and the energy-density uniformity of the light are 69.2 mW/cm^2 with a tolerance of ± 11.5% using the 10-cm spot (Fig. 2.30, see page 25). The precise maneuverability of this light source permits accurate planning of treatment and makes it suitable for the treatment of facial acne.

The second light source used frequently is a light-emitting diode (LED) device (Omnilux pdt, Photo Therapeutics, UK), which can emit both blue and red light. An LED may be the optimal light device because it is inexpensive and provides a wide irradiated area with selectively narrow wavelengths (Fig. 2.31, see page 25). The spectrum output of the red light in our LED light source (Omnilux pdt) emits along a narrow band centering on 630 nm. Because the power is high, we usually leave a 20-cm distance between the lamp and the target surface. Although this equipment can irradiate an extremely wide area, regrettably the energy-density uniformity can be suboptimal with an irradiation distance of 20 cm (Fig. 2.32, see page 25). Therefore, we prefer this equipment for treating body acne because the energy dosage needed in that case is twice that for treating facial acne, and thus precision in delivered energy density is less important.

TREATMENT ALGORITHM

Several weeks of pre-treatment with tretinoin cream or daily iontophoresis using vitamin C derivatives is frequently used so that recovery after PDT treatment is more brisk.

Four hours after oral administration of ALA at 10 mg/kg BW, acne lesions are exposed to the light source. The ALA powder is mixed with water or orange juice for dosing. At the first PDT session, the patient should be watched in the clinic from the start of oral administration of ALA to complete irradiation because nausea is frequently observed. Nausea is almost always seen within 2 h after ALA is taken. Vomiting is rarely noted. When nausea occurs, an antiemetic should be administered and the PDT sessions stopped for a time. However, precautionary treatment with an antiemetic should be avoided if possible because this may impair the stability of ALA. Starting with the second PDT session, patients may take ALA at home before coming to the clinic. Patients develop photosensitivity 2 h after oral administration. Therefore, from

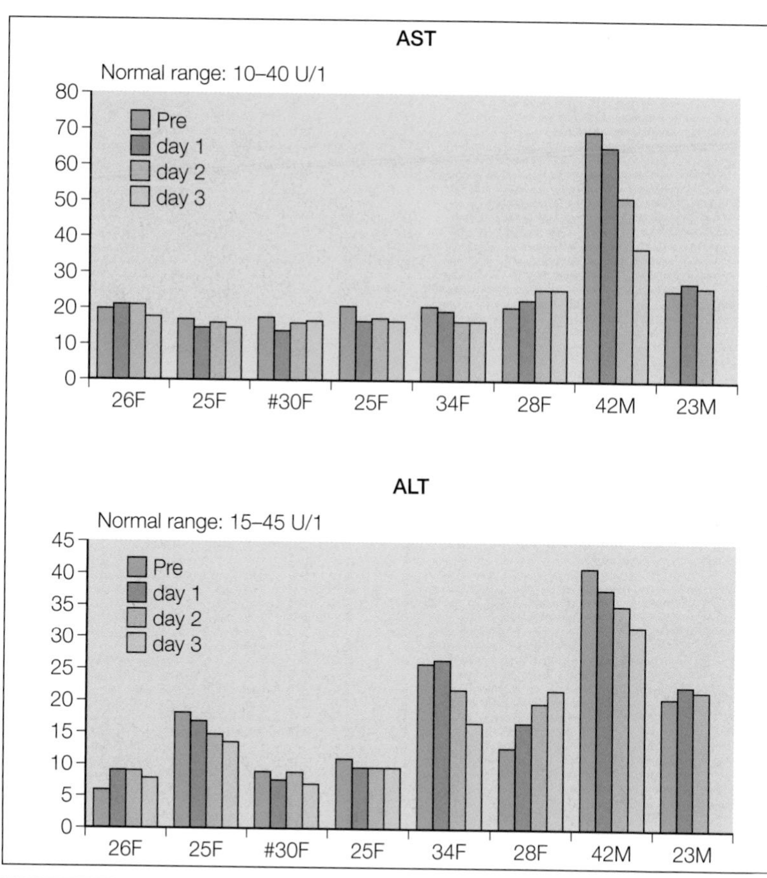

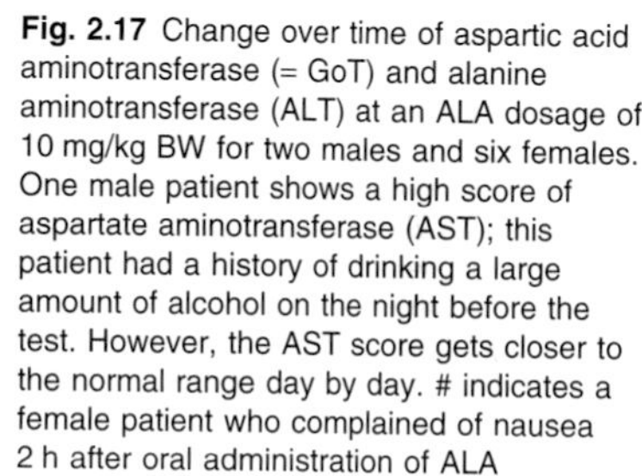

Fig. 2.17 Change over time of aspartic acid aminotransferase (= GoT) and alanine aminotransferase (ALT) at an ALA dosage of 10 mg/kg BW for two males and six females. One male patient shows a high score of aspartate aminotransferase (AST); this patient had a history of drinking a large amount of alcohol on the night before the test. However, the AST score gets closer to the normal range day by day. # indicates a female patient who complained of nausea 2 h after oral administration of ALA

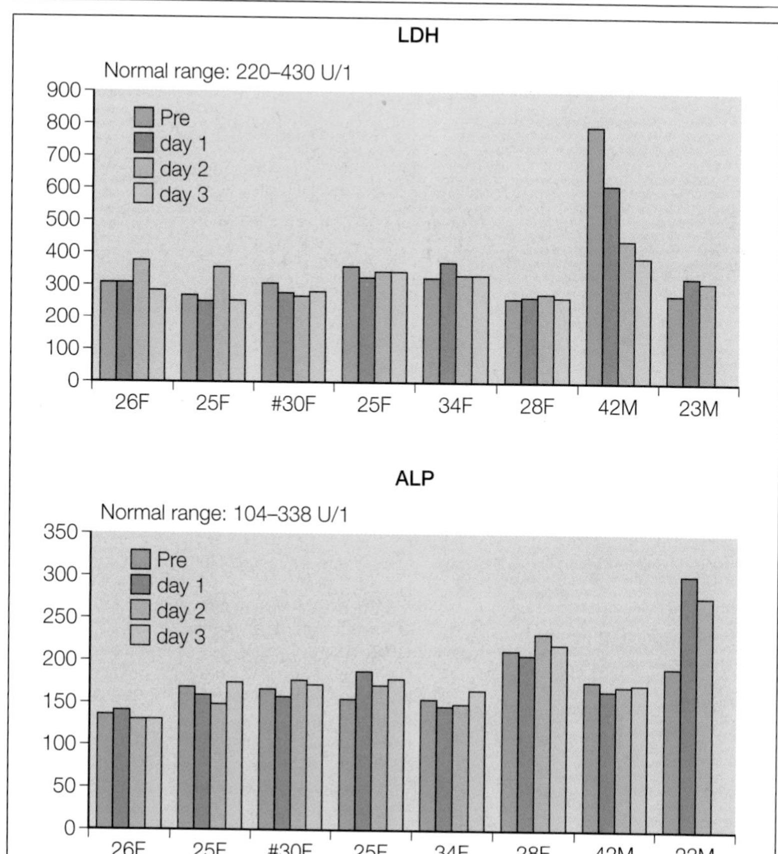

Fig. 2.18 Change over time of lactate dehydrogenase (LDH) and alkaline phosphatase (ALP) at an ALA dosage of 10 mg/kg BW for two males and six females. One male patient shows a high score of LDH; this patient had a history of drinking a large amount of alcohol on the night before the test. However, the LDH score gets closer to the normal range day by day. # as in Figure 2.17

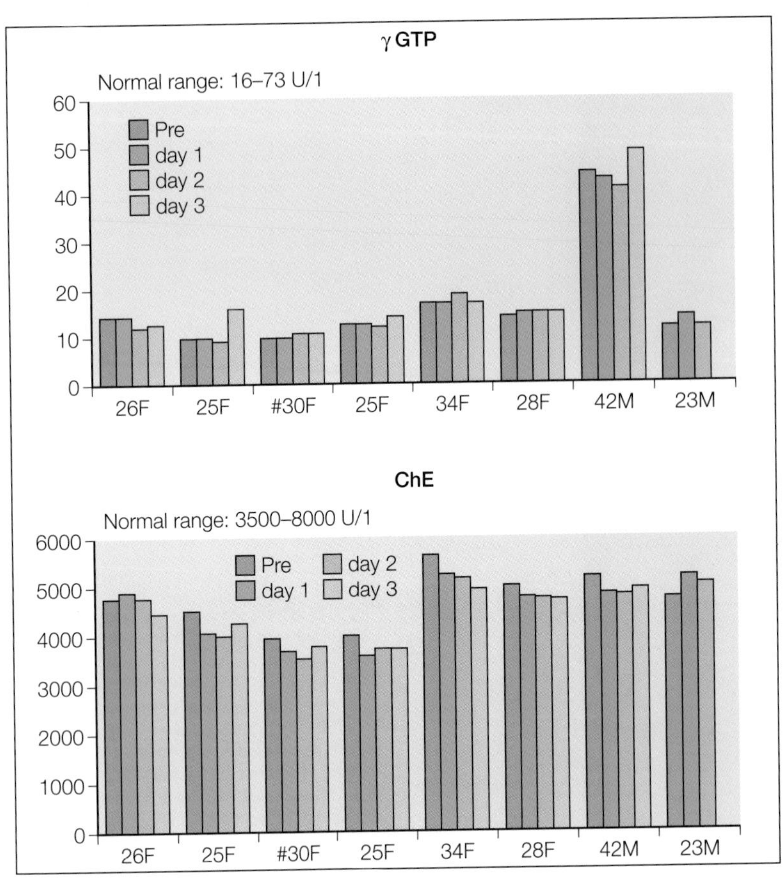

Fig. 2.19 Change over time for gamma GTP and cholinesterase at an ALA dosage of 10 mg/kg BW for two males and six females. All scores are within normal range. # as in Figure 2.17

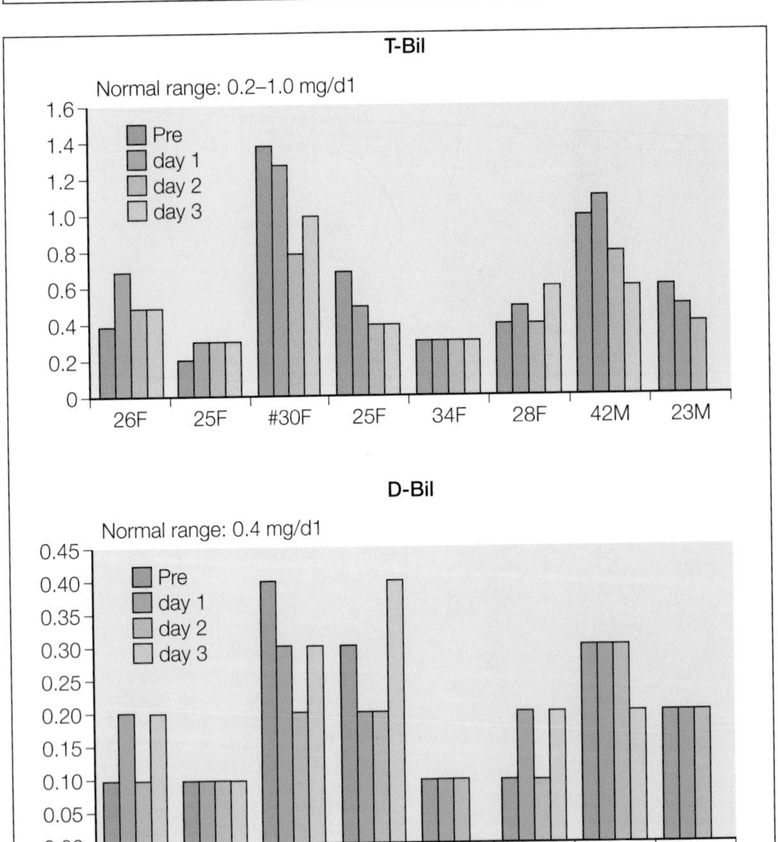

Fig. 2.20 Change over time for total and direct bilirubin at an ALA dosage of 10 mg/kg BW for two males and six females. The female patient marked #, who complained of nausea 2 h after oral administration of ALA, shows a high score of total bilirubin. However, this abnormality is already observed on the day before ALA dosage. The change after ALA dosage becomes closer to the normal range. One male patient shows a slightly high score for total bilirubin. This change after ALA dosage also becomes closer to the normal range

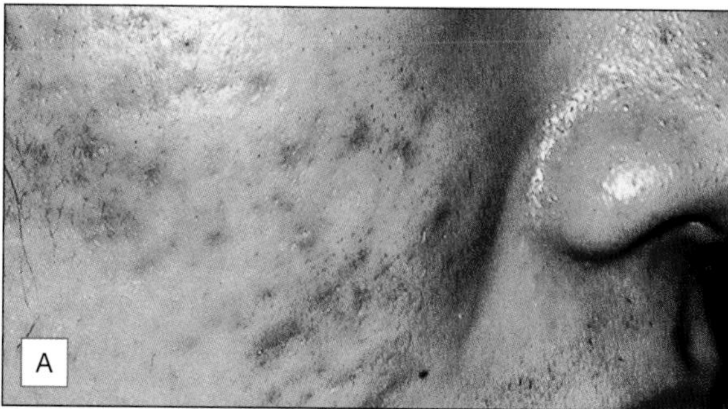

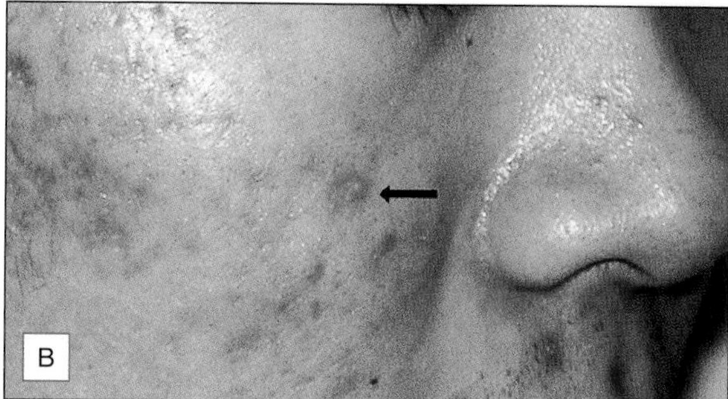

Fig. 2.21 (**A**) Red acne scar 1 week after one PDT series. There is no elective lesion. (**B**) One month later, one acne papule (arrow) is seen. This hair follicle showed a red acne scar in (**A**). The same hair follicle had a tendency to repeat papulopustular lesions

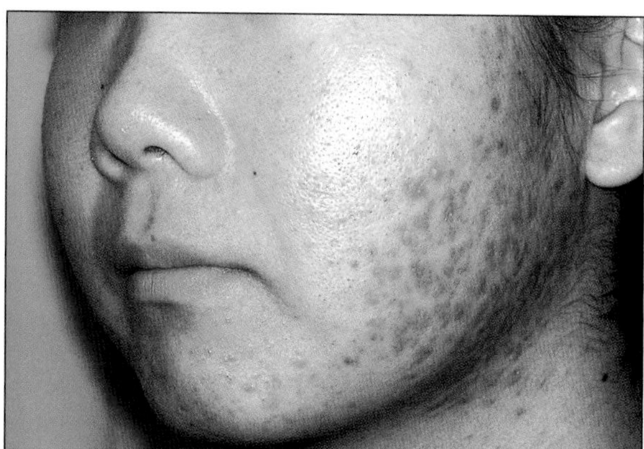

Fig. 2.22 Acne patient of grade V on the Burton scale

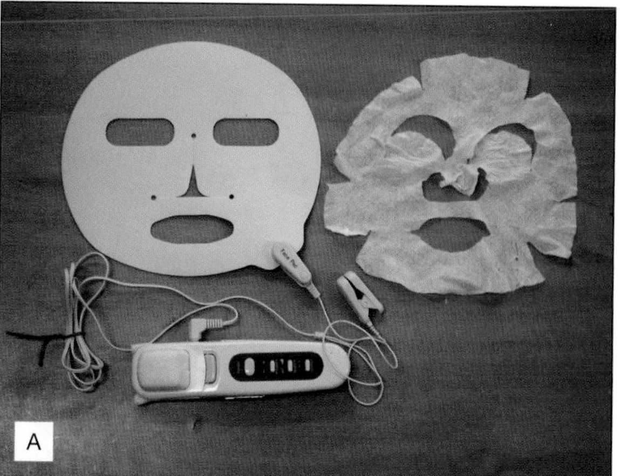

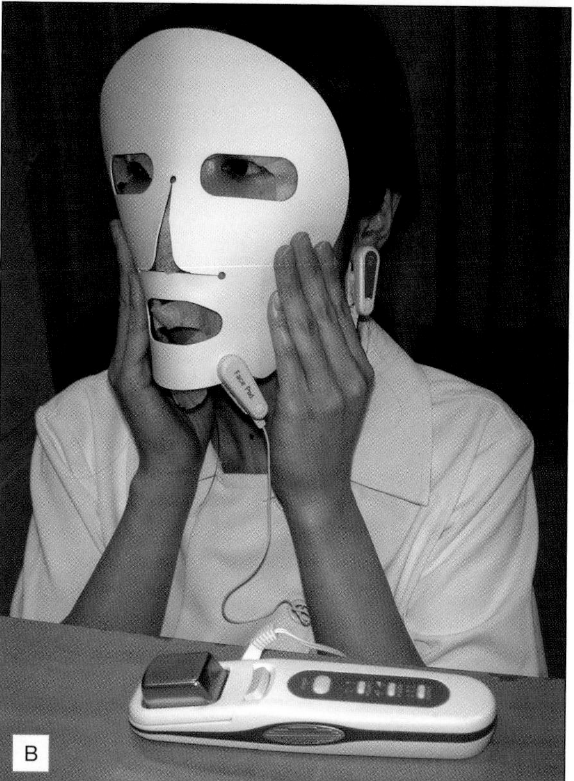

Fig. 2.23 (**A,B**) Iontophoretic device with a face-shaped wide electrode. The disposable cotton sheet contains 5% magnesium L-ascorbyl-2-phosphate solution

this time until the start of irradiation, patients should stay indoors. No specific sun shielding should be prescribed, but it is preferable that dark clothing is worn on the treatment day.

It is not necessary to use anesthesia during irradiation but the eyes, conjunctiva, lips, and mucosa must be thoroughly protected from irradiation. The total energy dose in the first PDT session with polychromatic visible light for facial acne is routinely approximately 25 J/cm^2. Dosages for the second, third, and fourth PDT sessions are 30, 35, and 40 J/cm^2, respectively. However, for serious facial acne, the first PDT session may entail only 15 J/cm^2, as in this condition excessive erythema, swelling, and reactive acne are often seen and can produce severe and persistent cutaneous effects, including scar formation. For body acne, the first, second, and third PDT sessions are usually at 50, 60, and 70 J/cm^2, respectively.

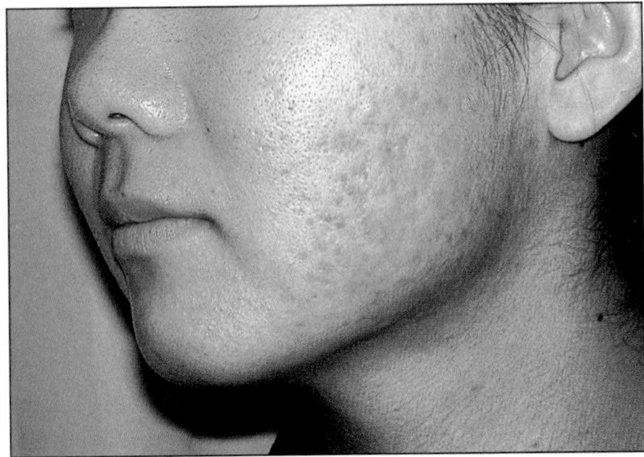

Fig. 2.24 One week after one PDT series (four PDT sessions with 2-week intervals), the affected area in the patient in Figure 2.22 shows no papulopustular lesions. The red acne scar with dimple is remarkable. The patient continues daily iontophoresis of 5% magnesium L-ascorbyl-2-phosphate solution

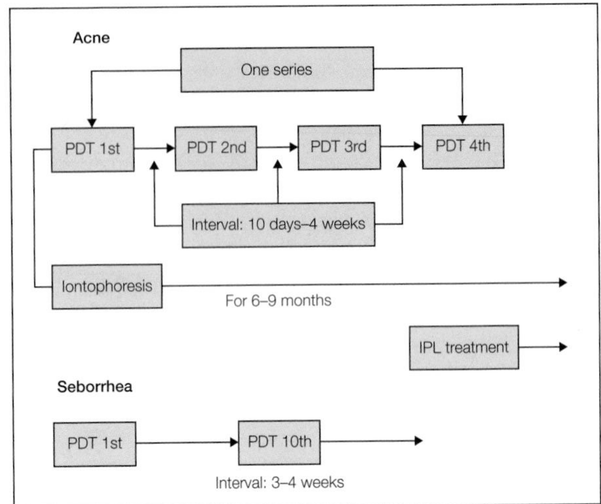

Fig. 2.27 PDT treatments for acne and seborrhea

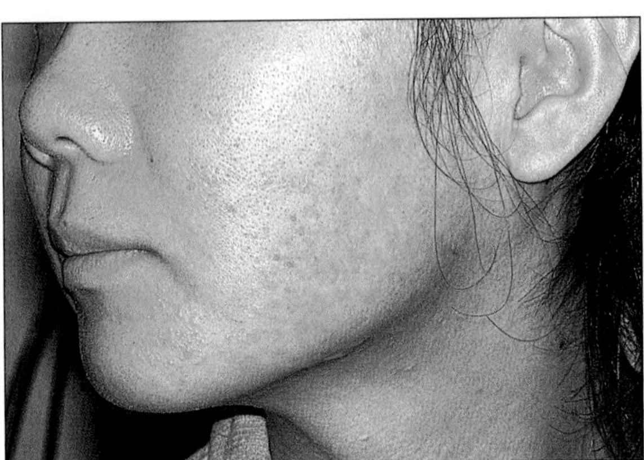

Fig. 2.25 Three months after the PDT series in the patient in Figure 2.22, discoloration of the red acne scar developed

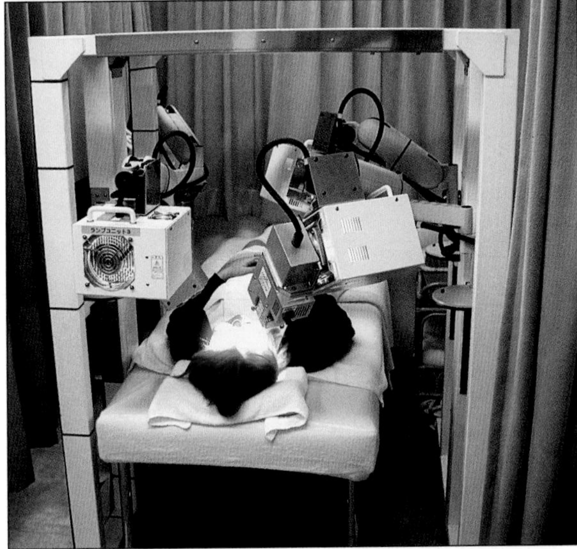

Fig. 2.28 Polychromatic visible light source with a four-lamp box by a metal halide lamp. As the movable region of each lamp box is free, it is easy to correspond the light to uneven regions

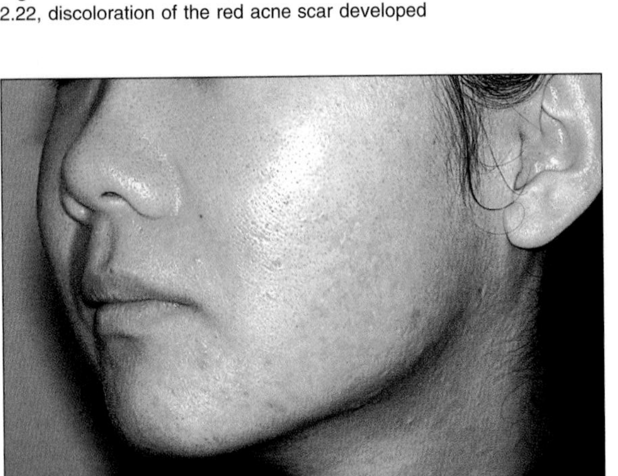

Fig. 2.26 Six months after the PDT series, the affected area in the patient in Figure 2.22 is close to normal skin appearance by daily iontophoresis. This skin condition is thought to be free from repeated recalcitrant acne. The dimple shown in Figure 2.22 is noted to have become flat. Compared with the old dimple, the dimple with redness is relatively easy to improve

Overlap irradiation should be avoided as it causes severe reactive acne. To perform precise irradiation, the irradiated area may be divided into several parts, e.g. cheek, nose, and forehead.

During irradiation, most patients feel a burning sensation. If there is no such sensation, the energy density of the irradiation may be too low. If patients complain of discomfort, the energy density of the irradiation can be decreased. However, if the energy density is changed, the total energy dosage must be kept as previously scheduled. Immediately after PDT, the affected lesions show slight erythema. If there is no erythema, the energy dosage

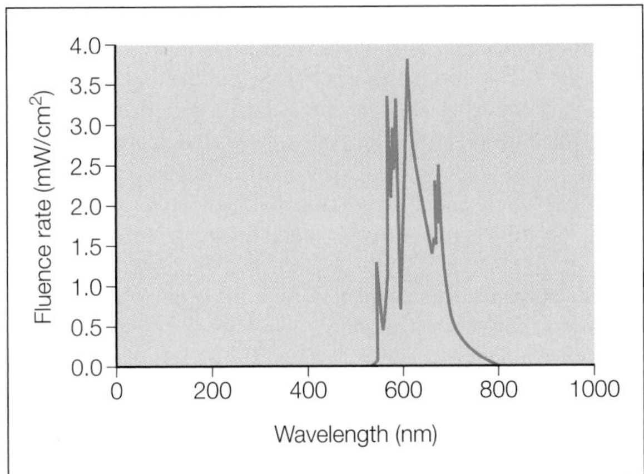

Fig. 2.29 Spectrum output of the light source in Figure 2.28. Although the highest peak is 610 nm, the wavelength efficiently covers 545, 580, 630, and 670 nm. The wavelengths of 545, 580, and 630 nm are absorbed to PpIX. As photosensitizing photoproducts with 670 nm are produced during ALA-PDT, its excitation is also advantageous

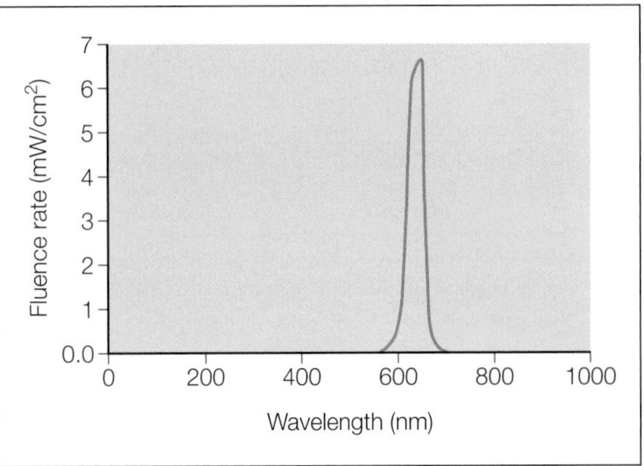

Fig. 2.31 Spectrum output of the red light in the LED light source (Omnilux). It presents a narrow band, centering on 630 nm, with high power

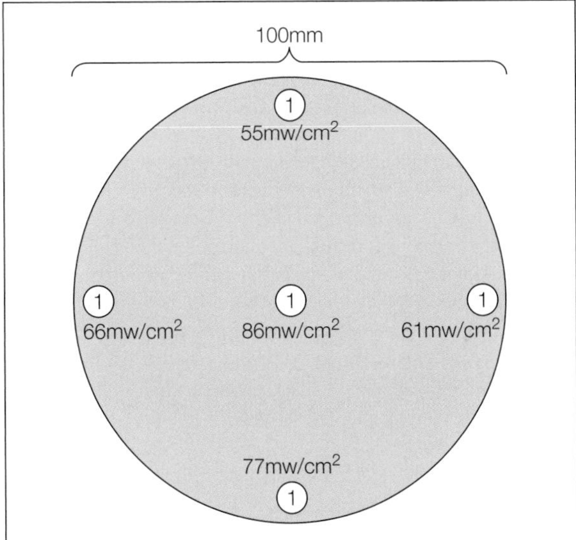

Fig. 2.30 Energy density of the light in Figure 2.28. The distance between the lamp and the affected surface is 13 cm. The average fluence rate and the energy-density uniformity of the light are 69.2 mW/cm² and an accidental error of ± 11.5% on the circle area with a diameter of 10 cm, respectively

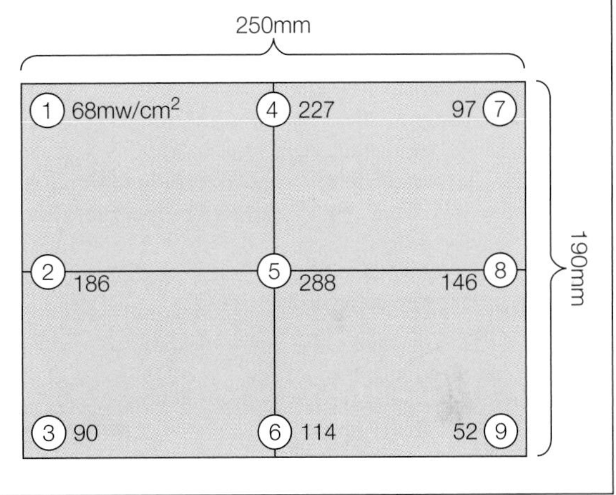

Fig. 2.32 Energy density of the light in Figure 2.31. The distance between the lamp and the affected surface is 20 cm. An accidental error of the energy-density uniformity is too large

used may have been insufficient and may need to be increased.

There is almost no acne which is not affected by PDT; especially among younger patients, treatment resistance is rare. If there is a fast or slower metabolizer of ALA, the starting time for irradiation will need to be changed. Usually, irradiation is started 4 h after the oral administration of ALA. The starting time may be brought forward to 3 h after ALA dosage in younger patients. To calculate the most suitable starting time of irradiation, it is useful to take ultraviolet pictures.

After irradiation, the affected lesions are cooled for about 10 min. Cooling may be continued when the patient goes home. Sufficient cooling will decrease erythema and swelling, improving the therapeutic effects. However, cooling does not decrease the occurrence of reactive acne. After PDT, make-up can be used and sun shielding on the treatment day is desirable. For 3 days after PDT, anti-oxidizing agents, including vitamins C and E, should be stopped. We prefer to use daily iontophoresis of vitamin C derivatives beginning on the fourth day after PDT.

SIDE EFFECTS AND COMPLICATIONS

Side effects and complications are summarized in Box 2.2. After the oral administration of ALA, nausea is frequently observed. When this occurs an antiemetic and a nausea stop are prescribed for the patient. Nausea is limited to the PDT treatment day.

During irradiation, discomfort, burning, and stinging are observed. If patients do not tolerate the light irradiation, decreasing the energy density of irradiation may solve this problem.

Almost all patients develop erythema immediately after PDT treatment. Although erythema and swelling are not usually worrisome, if strong reactive acne does occur, cooling immediately after facial PDT is important and results in a decrease in erythema and swelling. Excessive reactive acne can lead to an acne scar. To avoid this problem, an energy density that is too strong and energy dosage that is too large should be avoided. The PDT operator has to pay attention to the degree of erythema, burning, and stinging during irradiation, and should change the intensity if needed.

Daily iontophoresis with vitamin C derivatives may be effective for treating excessive reactive acne and swelling, and for postinflammatory pigmentation. Furthermore, an oral corticosteroid can be tried.

Although the irradiated light does not contain ultraviolet frequencies, immunosuppression induced by the light may cause herpes simplex. Iontophoresis with vitamin C has been reported to be effective for recovery of immunoactivity.

• Iontophoresis with vitamin C

The ALA-PDT technique is fairly certain to eradicate etiologic bacteria and for a time can also prevent new papulopustular lesions developing. However, in the absence of the return of acne-associated hair follicles to their normal state, papulopustular acne lesions will recur (see Fig. 2.21), and patients can never be free from chronic acne. Red acne scars may persist in their inflammatory state for a long time. The redness in acne scars has to be treated after the bacteria have been eradicated. To return the hair follicle to a normal undiseased state, we prefer to use vitamin C iontophoresis (see Figs 2.22–2.26).

L-ascorbic acid (vitamin C) modulates collagen synthesis and plays an essential role in wound healing. Moreover, it also acts as an antioxidant, suppresses melanogenesis, and reduces immunosuppression. These actions may help with skin healing after the suppression of acne by PDT by diminishing redness and dimpling associated with acne scars. L-ascorbic acid is very unstable and is easily oxidized even though its molecular weight is adequate for transcutaneous penetration. Recently, some ascorbic acid derivatives have been introduced that are stable over a long period of time. We use magnesium L-ascorbyl-2-phosphate, which becomes attached to lipid, but the beneficial effects of this treatment appear to be limited.

Transcutaneous iontophoresis is a technique that facilitates the transport of permeants across the skin by using an electromotive force. The underlying principles of transcutaneous iontophoresis involve the placement of two oppositely charged electrodes at appropriate sites on the skin. The drug in its ionic form is placed under the electrode bearing the same charge as the drug, and the voltage source most often supplies a constant electric current that is converted to an ionic current by oxidation–reduction reactions at the electrodes. As the ions carry this current through the skin barrier, charged molecules are repelled from the active electrode into the skin and then into the systemic circulation. This has been extensively explored as a potential means for the delivery of hydrophilic agents (Fig. 2.33).

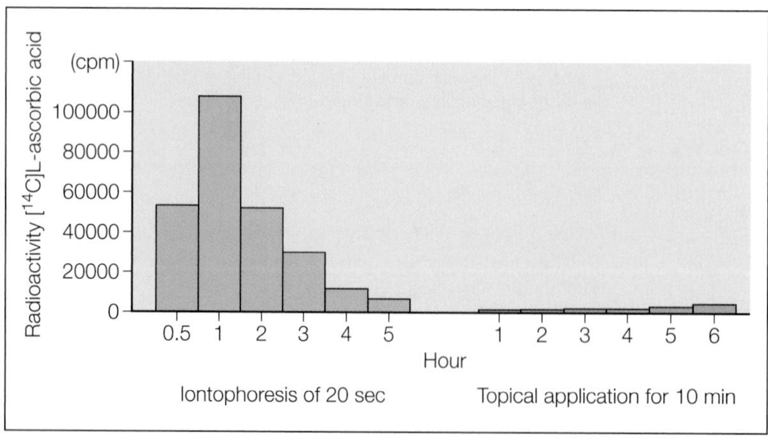

Fig. 2.33 Effect of iontophoresis on percutaneous absorption of [^{14}C]-ascorbic acid in rat skin. Swabs were wetted with radioactive ascorbic acid and placed on the back skin. The iontophoretic device was immediately placed on the swabs and electric current was passed through the skin for 20 s. Swabs and electric device were removed, and then remaining radioactive ascorbic acid on the skin surface was washed exhaustively. The skins were biopsied at 0.5, 1, 2, 3, 4, and 5 h after application of ascorbic acid. The dermal layers were obtained by disperse digestion and their radioactivities were counted. For control assays, swabs were simply placed on the skin surface for 10 min instead of iontophoresis for 20 s and the skins were biopsied at 0.5, 1, 2, 3, 4, and 5 h after application of ascorbic acid. The difference between the two methods is apparent

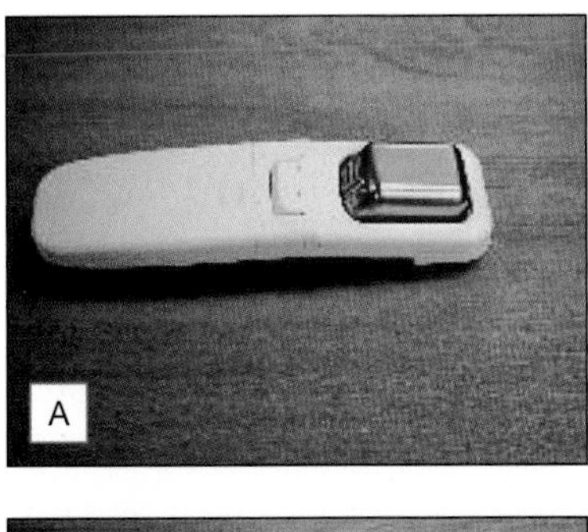

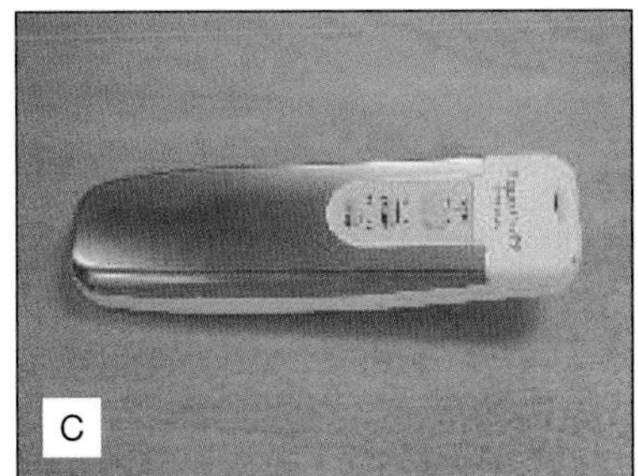

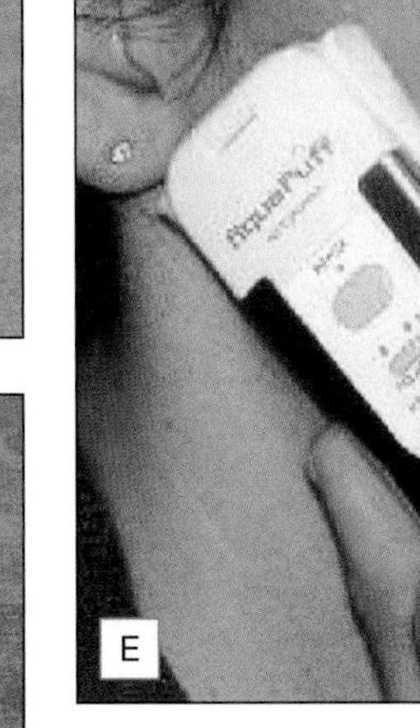

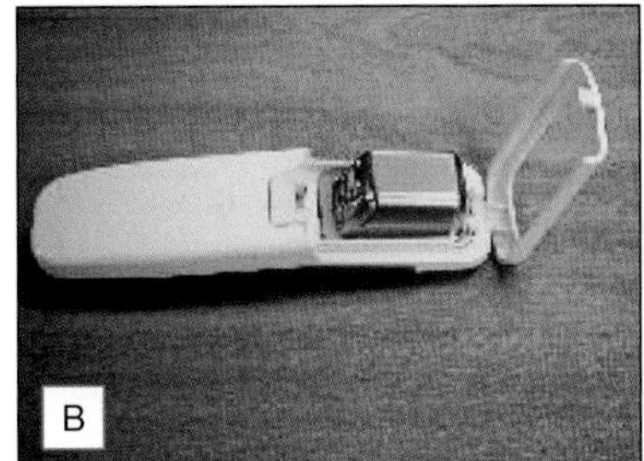

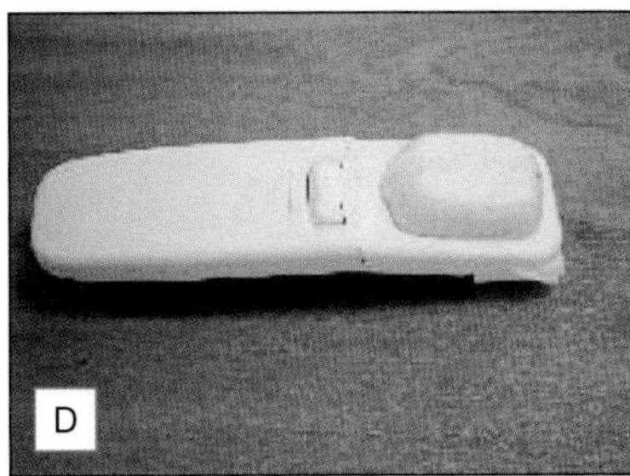

Fig. 2.34 **(A–E)** Handy iontophoretic device. The disposable cotton piece contains 5% magnesium L-ascorbyl-2-phosphate solution. Two electrodes are set up to the face and hand

For daily iontophoresis, patients use a handy iontophoretic device (Aquapuff, Toshiba Medical Supply Co, Tokyo, Japan; Fig. 2.34). The author believes this is of value for patients with persistent acne receiving PDT treatment.

FURTHER READING

Cunliffe WJ, Goulden V 2000 Phototherapy and acne vulgaris. British Journal of Dermatology 142:855–856

Ebihara M, Akiyama M, Ohnishi Y et al 2003 Iontophoresis promotes percutaneous absorption of L-ascorbic acid in rat skin. Journal of Dermatologic Science 32:217–222

Hongcharu W, Taylor CR, Chang Y et al 2000 Topical ALA-photodynamic therapy for the treatment of acne vulgaris. Journal of Investigative Dermatology 15:183–192

Itoh Y, Ninomiya Y, Tajima S, Ishibashi A 2000 Photodynamic therapy for acne vulgaris with topical 5-aminolevulinic acid. Archives of Dermatology 136:1093–1095

Itoh Y, Ninomiya Y, Tajima S, Ishibashi A 2001 Photodynamic therapy of acne vulgaris with topical delta-aminolevulinic acid and incoherent light in Japanese patients. British Journal of Dermatology 144:575–579

Nair V, Pillai O, Poduri R, Panchagnula R 1999 Transdermal iontophoresis. Part I: basic principles and considerations. Methods and Findings in Experimental and Clinical Pharmacology 21:139–151

Papageorgiou P, Katsambas A, Chu A 2000 Phototherapy with blue (415 nm) and red (660 nm) light in the treatment of acne vulgaris. British Journal of Dermatology 142:973 978

Tokuoka Y, Kosobe T, Kimura M et al 2003 Photodynamic therapy for cancer cells using metal-halide lamps. Optical Review 10:116–119

3 Treatment of Acne with Topical Photodynamic Therapy

Macrene Alexiades-Armenakas

INTRODUCTION

Acne is the most prevalent skin disease, affecting 80% of the population at some time during their lifetime, and is often recalcitrant to treatment. Conventional acne treatments include topical and oral antibiotics, benzoyl peroxides, sulfur compounds, retinoids, and oral hormonal agents, such as oral contraceptives or antiandrogens. When acne patients fail to respond to conventional treatments, oral isotretinoin, a highly effective drug with significant side effects, has been prescribed; however, it has been difficult to obtain under the recent Food and Drug Administration (FDA) regulatory status. Laser and light treatments are alternatives, including the FDA-approved blue light and diode laser, both of which have modest efficacy. A safe and effective treatment is needed, and photodynamic therapy (PDT) is emerging as a practical and effective treatment option for recalcitrant acne patients.

ENDOGENOUS PORPHYRINS AND LIGHT TREATMENT

The scientific basis for treating acne with PDT originated with the finding that porphyrins, mainly coproporphyrin III, are produced by *Propionibacterium acnes*, the anaerobic bacterium that proliferates and incites inflammation in obstructed sebaceous follicles. The endogenous porphyrins act as photophores and mediate a PDT response following exposure to light, particularly blue light. This reaction has been shown to generate singlet oxygen and to mediate bacterial destruction.

The treatment of acne with blue light has been only mildly-to-moderately effective in clinical trials, presumably due to the poor skin penetration by blue light. In one study, blue light once weekly for 2 weeks demonstrated only 25% improvement in acne severity. In another study, blue light for 15 min daily resulted after 4 weeks in a 30% and 15% mean lesional reduction for inflammatory and comedonal acne, respectively, with a final mean improvement after 12 weeks of 63% and 45%, respectively.

Although red light is less effective than blue light at porphyrin photoactivation, it penetrates deeper. When red light (635 nm) was combined with blue light (415 nm) for 15 min daily, it was found to increase effectiveness with a mean lesional reduction of approximately 50% for inflammatory and 25% for comedonal acne after 4 weeks, and 76% and 58%, respectively, after 12 weeks. Another protocol of blue light once weekly for 4 weeks yielded a 43% reduction. Thus, the application of light alone to trigger PDT in the treatment of acne has been encumbered by a low efficacy rate per treatment, thus requiring numerous treatments to achieve adequate efficacy.

SYSTEMIC AMINOLEVULINIC ACID

The application of exogenous aminolevulinic acid (ALA) to enhance the efficacy of PDT in the treatment of acne was based upon the findings that endogenous *P. acnes* porphyrins are present only in small quantities and exogenous ALA concentrates in sebaceous units (see Ch2). Intraperitoneal injection of ALA was found to result in the accumulation of photosensitive protoporphyrin IX (PpIX) in the sebaceous glands of normal skin in albino mice and light of the appropriate wavelength then destroyed the sebaceous glands. Thus, exogenous application of ALA enhanced the PDT reaction in sebaceous glands.

TOPICAL AMINOLEVULINIC ACID

• With red wavelengths

In a hallmark study, the topical application of ALA was shown to result in PpIX fluorescence that was greater in acne lesions than in surrounding normal skin, and subsequent exposure to red light was effective in diminishing sebaceous gland size. Since that initial finding, ALA-PDT combined with red light and lasers has been shown to be effective for the treatment of acne, but has the disadvantage of significant side effects. Red broadband light (550–700 nm) in conjunction with ALA incubated for 3 h under occlusion resulted in a significant improvement in acne counts, but with side effects of blistering, erythema, edema, and dyspigmentation. Another study of topical ALA incubated for 3 h followed by red diode laser at 635 nm for the treatment of back acne demonstrated similar efficacy and side effects. In a comparison of blue

(415 nm) and red (630 nm) light without ALA there was a mean improvement in acne counts of approximately 50% at 1 month after a single treatment with red and blue light combined, as opposed to 30% with blue light alone. Longer red wavelengths yielded higher efficacy rates, presumably due to deeper penetration. Similarly, in two studies of patients treated with topical ALA incubated for 4 h followed by a 635-nm laser or a polychromatic (600–700 nm) light, improvement in acne counts was reported, but there were significant side effects of crusting and hyperpigmentation with both light sources. In most studies employing red wavelengths for PDT, pain, erythema, blistering, crusting, and dyspigmentation have been reported.

• With blue light

Topical ALA and blue light (peak emission 417 nm) has yielded modest efficacy rates in reported studies which may be explained by the shallow penetration of blue light but this awaits confirmation by larger trials. In one study, blue light therapy once a week for 2 weeks resulted in 25% lesional improvement when light alone was used, versus 32% when ALA was applied before illumination. ALA incubated for 30–60 min followed by blue light once a week for 4 weeks resulted in a response rate of approximately 60%, as opposed to 43% for blue light alone. In another 18-patient study comparing short-incubation ALA-PDT with activation by blue light or intense pulsed light (IPL), superior improvement was seen in the IPL-PDT group. A recent study comparing topical ALA with long pulsed-dye laser (LP PDL) or blue light, lower effectiveness was found in the ALA-blue light group. Recent phase IIa FDA trials of topical ALA and blue light failed to demonstrate higher efficacy relative to blue light alone, excepting subgroup analysis. Phase IIb trials comparing topical ALA with blue light or LP-PDL to controls will help explain these findings.

• With the LP-PDL

During the course of investigating alternative light sources for PDT, we analyzed the absorption spectrum of PpIX: among the Q bands, a peak at 575 nm was noted. In a prior study, the PDL at 585 nm was used in conjunction with topical 20% ALA-PDT for the treatment of actinic keratoses (AKs) and showed clearance rates of 79% at 1-month follow-up, but with purpura and crusting. As the 595-nm wavelength is present on the side of this Q band for PpIX, the LP-PDL (595 nm) was selected as an alternative light source for use in conjunction with ALA-PDT. This laser possessed the advantages of variable pulse duration in the nonpurpuric range; a longer wavelength with greater penetration depth as compared to blue light; dynamic cooling spray to minimize discomfort; large 10-mm spot size, and fast treatment with a firing speed of 1 Hz. For the treatment of AK, the side effects of PDT were diminished without compromising efficacy by employing the LP-PDL with topical ALA.

During the course of this study, a reduction in sebaceous hyperplasia was serendipitously observed, a finding which was subsequently reproduced. On the basis of these observations and the results of the aforementioned studies, the use of topical ALA in conjunction with LP-PDL and PDL was assessed in a pilot study. Acne patients received a single treatment with 1-month follow-up. The patient mean percent lesional clearance rates were 69% for LP-PDL- and 59% for PDL-mediated PDT. Importantly, side effects were minimal, consisting of mild erythema lasting 1–2 days.

Recently, a trial assessing ALA-PDT with activation by LP-PDL 595-nm laser energy combined with topical therapy demonstrated effectiveness in the treatment of recalcitrant acne of various types and levels of severity. The patients in this study had failed multiple conventional therapies, including isotretinoin, and exhibited mild-to-severe comedonal, inflammatory, and cystic acne. The mean percent lesional clearance rate per treatment for the LP-PDL-mediated PDT group was 77%, although all patients, including controls, were maintained on topical therapy. Complete clearance was achieved in 100% of patients following a mean of 2.9 treatments (range 1–6) and maintained for a mean follow-up interval of 6.4 months (range 1–13). Side effects were minimal, consisting of mild erythema resolving within 1–2 days. Those treated with LP-PDL-mediated PDT achieved clearance at a rate per treatment superior to control patients maintained on topical therapy and treated with either conventional medical therapies (20%) or laser energy without ALA (32%), and the clearance was sustained during the long-term follow-up interval. These findings indicate that LP-PDL-mediated PDT may provide a highly effective and easily tolerated alternative to isotretinoin for recalcitrant acne patients, although the findings of the upcoming phase IIb FDA trial are pending. An example of a patient prior to and following LP-PDL-mediated PDT is shown in Figure 3.1.

The LP-PDL alone demonstrated comparable or higher efficacy than conventional treatment, suggesting the anti-acne efficacy of LP-PDL is achieved through a PDT response or another mechanism. The mean lesional clearance rate per treatment for LP-PDL without exogenous ALA was 32% as opposed to 20% for the topical control, although this comparison was limited by sample size. This efficacy is likely fluence-dependent, requiring fluences of 7–7.5 J/cm^2. A previous report had suggested efficacy of PDL (585 nm) in treating acne vulgaris, which was contradicted by another study employing low fluences of 3 J/cm^2 and short pulse durations of 350–550 μs. It is possible that use of LP-PDL at higher fluences and pulse durations may augment the photodynamic activation of porphyrins and photothermal effects on vascular targets, without exceeding the purpura threshold. The mechanisms of acne clearance by LP-PDL alone may include the targeting of blood vessels and a resultant anti-inflammatory effect, as described in the treatment of scars by PDL (see below). Additionally, LP-PDL may photoactivate endogenous

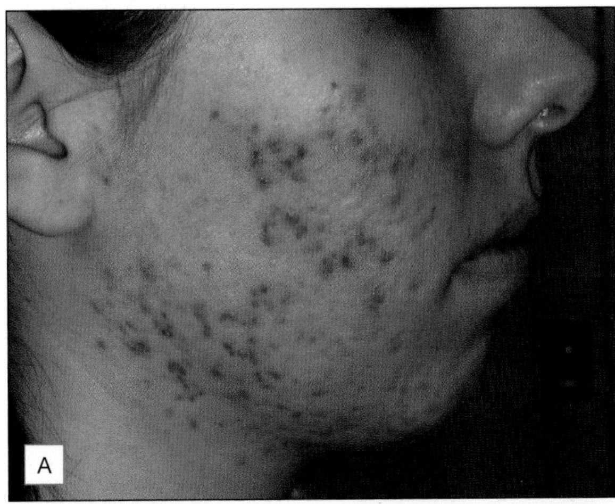

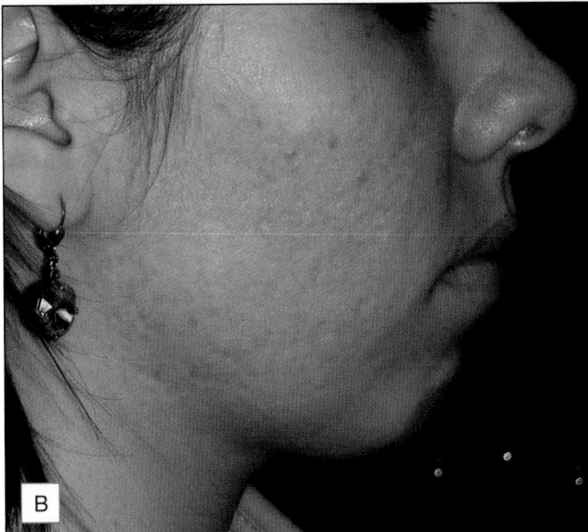

Fig. 3.1 Severe cystic and recalcitrant acne responds to LP-PDL-mediated PDT. A patient (**A**) before and (**B**) following two treatment sessions of topical ALA 1-h incubation and LP-PDL at a fluence of 7.5 J/cm^2, 10-ms pulse duration, 10-mm spot size, and dynamic cooling spray of 30 ms with a 30-ms delay. Both the cystic lesions and active erythematous scars improved dramatically following treatment. This patient has remained clear to 1-year follow-up

porphyrins produced by *P. acnes* in the sebaceous follicle, potentially inducing sebaceous gland shrinkage and decreased bacterial counts, as shown for blue and red light.

An additional significant advantage of employing the LP-PDL for PDT of acne is the dramatic improvement in erythematous scars. The laser alone, namely PDL and LP-PDL, has been shown to effectively treat active erythematous scars, hypertrophic scars, and keloids in particular. This effect may be explained by the fact that ALA accumulates in papillary blood vessels and may mediate photodynamic and photothermal injury to blood vessels. PDT has been employed for the treatment of vascular malformations and port wine stains (see Ch10 and Ch14). Lichen sclerosus et atrophicus, a scarring dermatosis with dilated blood vessels in the dermis, was successfully treated by LP-PDL-mediated PDT with a 2-year disease-free follow-up. Thus, enhanced resolution of erythematous scars may be achieved with ALA and LP-PDL.

The efficacy rate of ALA-PDT with LP-PDL combined with topical therapy suggests the LP-PDL may be superior to other light sources employed in the past. Previous studies of ALA-PDT employing blue and red light, lasers or IPL demonstrated lesional clearance rates of 32–75% after multiple treatments. LP-PDL-mediated PDT combined with topical therapy resulted in a mean lesional clearance rate of 77% per treatment and was the first PDT regimen to achieve complete clearance for up to 13 months follow-up. LP-PDL-mediated PDT is performed at monthly intervals, which is more practical than the more frequent intervals used in other protocols. Examples of patients treated with this protocol are shown in Figures 3.1 and 3.2.

• With intense pulsed light

Topical ALA combined with IPL has been used to treat moderate-to-severe acne. In one study, the use of IPL (430–1100 nm) following 1-h incubation with ALA demonstrated a response in 12 of 15 patients. Lesion counts were reduced by 50.1%, 68.5%, and 71.8% at the end of the 4-week period of once-weekly treatments, 4 weeks after the final treatment, and 12 weeks after the final treatment, respectively. Treatments were well tolerated and no treated lesion returned during the follow-up period. In another study of 18 patients, ALA-PDT with activation by blue light or a combination of optical and radiofrequency energy was evaluated. In this protocol, ALA was incubated for 15–30 min, and patients received two to four treatment sessions during a 4–8-week period or over a 4-week period, and salicylic acid peels. Among the 12 patients who responded, 11 demonstrated a 50% response and five showed a 75% response. Thus, early studies suggest IPL-mediated PDT with short-incubation ALA may be an effective, well-tolerated acne treatment, and larger, controlled studies are warranted. An example of a patient treated with ALA and IPL is shown in Figure 3.3.

MECHANISM OF PDT IN ACNE

PDT appears to target sebaceous gland activity, as is the case for many effective acne treatments. Although hormones are the main driving force in acne, the target of hormones is the pilosebaceous unit. This activation results in hypercornification, sebum production, and proliferation of *P. acnes*. Serum levels of dihydrotestosterone, dehydroepiandrosterone sulfate, and insulin-like growth factor 1 correlate with acne lesion counts. Androgens influence the sebocyte activity in sebaceous follicles, which express androgen receptors. As aforementioned, exogenous ALA results in PpIX fluorescence in acne lesions and preferential accumulation of porphyrins in *P. acnes*. PDT targeting

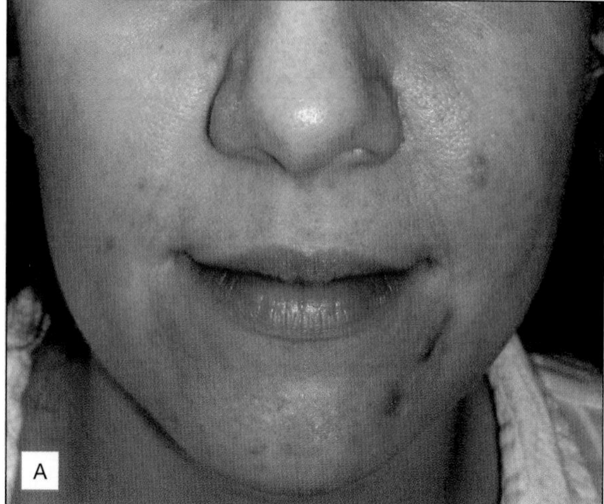

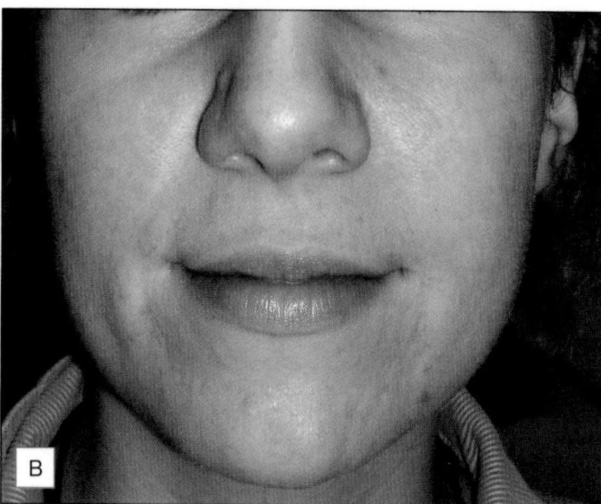

Fig. 3.2 Cystic acne cleared with ALA and LP-PDL. A patient (**A**) before and (**B**) following five monthly treatments with topical ALA 1-h incubation and LP-PDL at a fluence of 7.5 J/cm^2, 10-ms pulse duration, 10-mm spot size, and dynamic cooling spray of 30 ms with 30-ms delay. This patient has been maintained on topical therapy without recurrence to 18 months follow-up

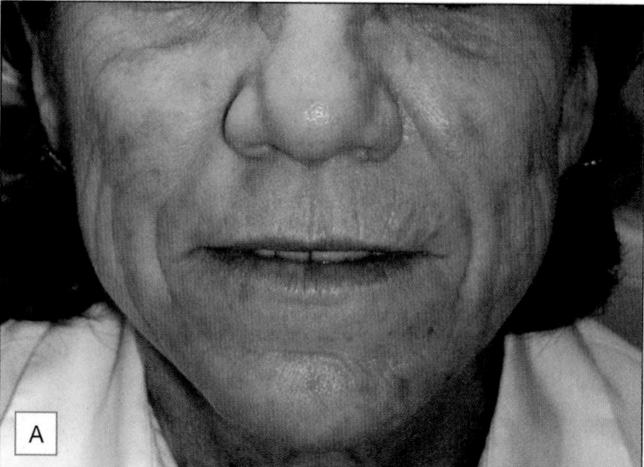

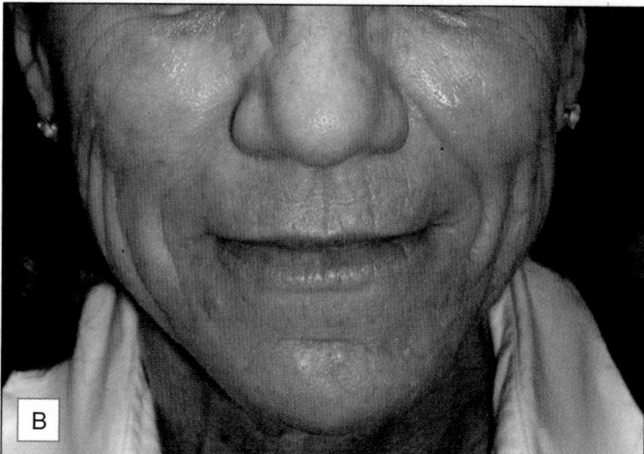

Fig. 3.3 Cystic acne in an adult following treatment with ALA and IPL. A patient (**A**) before and (**B**) following a single treatment with ALA 1-h incubation and two passes of IPL (Aurora, Syneron) at optical fluence of 16 J/cm^2, radiofrequency fluence of 18 J/cm^2, and long pulse mode

of the sebaceous gland has been demonstrated by decreased sebaceous gland size and vacuolization of sebocytes after PDT. The mechanism of PDT in acne treatment may involve direct thermal injury to the sebaceous glands, destruction of *P. acnes*, or manipulation of keratinocyte turnover in the infundibulum. The number of treatments required to achieve complete clearance may be determined by the degree of hormonal stimulation and the level of sebaceous activity at baseline.

COST-EFFECTIVENESS OF PDT FOR ACNE

Although larger trials are pending, PDT may serve as a safe and effective alternative to isotretinoin in patients who are recalcitrant to conventional acne treatments, and may also be a cost-effective one, depending upon the comparative need for retreatment. Analysis of costs indicates that three ALA-PDT sessions with the LP-PDL ($1800, or $600 per session) is higher than the cost of 5 months of isotretinoin therapy at $1200. However, in addition to the isotretinoin costs, the cost must be added of six sets of blood pregnancy tests, oral contraceptives, and office visits to an obstetrics and gynecology specialist and to a dermatologist. Costs related to the potential toxicity of isotretinoin must also be computed. The overall cost of three ALA-PDT sessions is then less than that of a 5-month isotretinoin regimen. The cost of frequency of retreatment is an important comparison that cannot be made until further data are collected. Longer follow-up intervals beyond 13 months are necessary to further assess whether the long-term cost of LP-PDL-mediated ALA-PDT remains less than that of a course of isotretinoin.

Table 3.1 ALA-PDT sample protocols for the treatment of acne			
	Incubation time (min)	**Treatment time or passes**	**Treatment intervals**
ALA and blue light[a]	45–60	500–1000 s	Varies weekly to monthly
ALA and LP-PDL[b]	45–60	One pass over entire face; two passes over distinct lesions	1–6 treatments at monthly intervals
ALA and IPL[c]	45–60	Single pass	Varies weekly to monthly

[a]Blu-U: 10 W/cm^2
[b]LP-PDL (595 nm): 7–7.5 J/cm^2, 10-ms pulse duration, 10-mm spot size, dynamic cooling spray of 30 ms with 30-ms delay
[c]IPL: photorejuvenation settings, vary with device

CONCLUSION

ALA-PDT with activation by various light sources, including the LP-PDL, blue and red wavelengths, and IPL has been shown to be efficacious in the treatment of acne. Table 3.1 presents ALA-PDT sample protocols employing the most commonly used light sources. ALA with red wavelengths has been very effective, though side effects were an early consideration. ALA combined with blue light has yielded variable efficacy and awaits further study. Currently, ALA with activation by the LP-PDL has been shown to be a safe and highly effective treatment in acne of all types and levels of severity with minimal side effects. It may provide an alternative to isotretinoin in the treatment and clearance of resistant acne. ALA with the LP-PDL and combined with topical therapy is cosmetically well-accepted, and is the first PDT modality to achieve complete clearance among patients with long-term follow-up as compared to controls. The results of a randomized, vehicle-controlled, double-blinded study of ALA-PDT in the treatment of acne will further direct the use of this effective regimen in our armamentarium for treating this highly prevalent condition.

FURTHER READING

Alexiades-Armenakas MR 2004 Laser-mediated photodynamic therapy of lichen sclerosus. Journal of Drugs in Dermatology 3(6 Suppl):S25–S27

Alexiades-Armenakas MR 2006 Laser-mediated photodynamic therapy. Clinics in Dermatology 24:16–25

Alexiades-Armenakas MR 2006 Long pulsed dye laser-mediated photodynamic therapy combined with topical therapy for mild-to-severe comedonal, inflammatory and cystic acne. Journal of Drugs in Dermatology 5:45–55

Alexiades-Armenakas MR, Geronemus G 2003 Laser-mediated photodynamic therapy of actinic keratoses. Archives of Dermatology 139:1313–1320

Alexiades-Armenakas MR, Bernstein L, Chen J, Jacobson L, Geronemus R 2003 Laser-assisted photodynamic therapy of acne vulgaris and related conditions. American Society of Laser Surgery Medical Abstracts, Anaheim, April 2003

Alster T 2003 Laser scar revision: comparison study of 585-nm pulsed dye laser with and without intralesional corticosteroids. Dermatologic Surgery 29:25–29

Alster TS, Tanzi EL 2003 Photodynamic therapy with topical aminolevulinic acid and pulsed dye laser irradiation for sebaceous hyperplasia. Journal of Drugs in Dermatology 2:501–504

Arakane K, Rya A, Hayashi C et al 1996 Singlet oxygen (1 delta g) generation from coproporphyrin in *Propionibacterium acnes* on irradiation. Biochemical and Biophysical Research Communications 223:578–582

Cappel M, Mauger D, Thiboutot D 2005 Correlation between serum levels of insulin-like growth factor 1, dehydroepiandrosterone sulfate, and dihydrotestosterone and acne lesion counts in adult women. Archives of Dermatology 141:333–338

Divaris DX, Kennedy JC, Pottier RH 1990 Phototoxic damage to sebaceous glands and hair follicles of mice after systemic administration of 5-aminolevulinic acid correlates with localized protoporphyrin IX fluorescence. American Journal of Pathology 136:891–897

Evans AV, Robson A, Barlow RJ, Kurwa HA 2005 Treatment of port wine stains with photodynamic therapy, using pulsed dye laser as a light source, compared with pulsed dye laser alone: a pilot study. Lasers in Surgery and Medicine 36:202–205

Gold MH 2003 The utilization of ALA-PDT and a new photoclearing device for the treatment of severe inflammatory acne vulgaris—results of an initial clinical trial. Journal of Lasers in Surgery and Medicine 15(Suppl):46

Gold MH, Bradshaw VL, Boring MM, Bridges TM, Biron JA, Carter LN 2004 The use of a novel intense pulsed light and heat source and ALA-PDT in the treatment of moderate to severe inflammatory acne vulgaris. Journal of Drugs in Dermatology 3(Suppl 6):S15–S19

Goldman MP, Boyce S 2003 A single-center study of aminolevulinic acid and 417 nm photodynamic therapy in the treatment of moderate to severe acne vulgaris. Journal of Drugs in Dermatology 2:393–396

Hongcharu W, Taylor CR, Chang Y, Aghassi D, Suthamjariya K, Anderson RR 2000 Topical ALA-photodynamic therapy for the treatment of acne vulgaris. Journal of Investigative Dermatology 115:183–192

Itami S, Kurata S, Sonoda T, Takayasu S 1995 Interaction between dermal papilla cells and follicular epithelial cells in vitro: effect of androgen. British Journal of Dermatology 132:527

Itoh Y, Ninomiya Y, Tajima S, Ishibashi A 2000 Photodynamic therapy for acne vulgaris with topical 5-aminolevulinic acid. Archives of Dermatology 136:1093–1095

Itoh Y, Ninomiya Y, Tajima S, Ishibashi A 2001 Photodynamic therapy of acne vulgaris with topical delta aminolevulinic acid and incoherent light in Japanese patients. British Journal of Dermatology 144:575–579

Karrer S, Baumler W, Abels C et al 1999 Long-pulse dye laser for photodynamic therapy: investigations in vitro and in vivo. Lasers in Surgery and Medicine 25:51–59

Kelly KM, Kimel S, Smith T et al 2004 Combined photodynamic and photothermal induced injury enhances damage to in vivo model blood vessels. Lasers in Surgery and Medicine 34:407–413

Kennedy JC, Marcus SL, Pottier RH 1996 Photodynamic therapy and photodiagnosis using endogenous photosensitization induced by 5-aminolevulinic acid: mechanisms and clinical results. Journal of Clinical Laser Medicine and Surgery 14:289–304

Kono T, Ercocen AR, Nakazawa H, Nozaki M 2005 Treatment of hypertrophic scars using a long-pulsed dye laser with cryogen-spray cooling. Annals of Plastic Surgery 54:487–493

Kuo YR, Jeng SF, Wang FS et al 2004 Flashlamp pulsed dye laser (PDL) suppression of keloid proliferation through down-regulation of TGF-beta1 expression and extracellular matrix expression. Lasers in Surgery and Medicine 34:104–108

Kuo YR, Wu WS, Jeng SF et al 2005 Activation of ERK and p38 kinase mediated keloid fibroblast apoptosis after flashlamp pulsed-dye laser treatment. Lasers in Surgery and Medicine 36:38–42

Lee WL, Shalita AR, Poh-Fitzpatrick MB 1978 Comparative studies of porphyrin production in *Propionibacterium acnes* and *Propionibacterium granulosum*. Journal of Bacteriology 133:811–815

Orringer JS, Kang S, Hamilton T et al 2004 Treatment of acne vulgaris with a pulsed dye laser: a randomized controlled trial. JAMA 291:2834–2839

Papageorgiou P, Katsambas A, Chu A 2000 Phototherapy with blue (415 nm) and red (660 nm) light in the treatment of acne vulgaris. British Journal of Dermatology 142:973–978

Pollock B, Turner D, Stringer MR et al Topical aminolaevulinic acid-photodynamic therapy for the treatment of acne vulgaris: a study of clinical efficacy and mechanism of action. British Journal of Dermatology 151:616–622

Pottier RH, Chow YFA, LaPlante J-P, Truscott TG, Kennedy JC, Beiner LA 1986 Non-invasive technique for obtaining fluorescence excitation and emission spectra in vivo. Photochemistry and Photobiology 44:679–687

Ramstad S, Futsaether CM, Johnsson A 1997 Porphyrin sensitization and intracellular calcium changes in the prokaryote *Propionibacterium acnes*. Journal of Photochemistry and Photobiology B 40:141–148

Seaton ED, Charakida A, Mouser PE, Grace I, Clement RM, Chu AC 2003 Pulsed-dye laser treatment for inflammatory acne vulgaris: randomized controlled trial. Lancet 362:1342

Taub AF 2004 Photodynamic therapy for the treatment of acne: a pilot study. Journal of Drugs in Dermatology 3(Suppl 6):S10–S14

Wood AJJ 1997 Therapy for acne vulgaris. New England Journal of Medicine 336:1156–1162

Zouboulis CC, Akamatsu H, Stephanek K, Orfanos CE 1994 Androgens affect the activity of human sebocytes in a manner dependent on the localization of the sebaceous glands and their effect is antagonized by spironolactone. Skin Pharmacology 7:33

4 Treatment of Hidradenitis Suppurativa

Michael H. Gold

INTRODUCTION

Hidradenitis suppurativa (HS) is a chronic suppurative disorder which has been shown to be associated with the apocrine glands. There appears to be great uncertainty associated with HS, from its diagnoses to its incidence and, more specifically, relating to the various treatment options now available. This chapter reviews HS, focusing on treatment and introducing the use of topical 20% 5-aminolevulinic acid (ALA) photodynamic therapy (PDT) as a therapeutic option for this difficult skin condition.

HISTORY, ETIOLOGY, AND PREVELANCE

The history of HS dates back to the first descriptions of human sweat glands in 1833 by Purkinje, and the first description in the medical literature of HS by Valpeau in 1839. In 1845 Robin described the structure and function of apocrine glands and in 1854 Verneuil associated HS with abnormalities in these glands. Verneuil originally called the disorder "hydrosadenite phlegmoneuse", which then became known simply as HS. Research on HS was not active for many years following these original descriptions. It was Shelley and Kahn, in 1955, who described HS pathology as keratinous plugging and dilation of the apocrine glands, with an inflammatory infiltrate surrounding these glands. It was not until the 1990s that researchers were able to show that HS is an acne vulgaris-like disorder, with histology showing follicular occlusion and the apocrine glands playing a prominent role in the associated perifollicular inflammatory response.

How many people are afflicted with HS? This question has baffled clinical investigators and epidemiologists for many years. Prevalence rates for this chronic disorder vary between 1:100 and 1:600 individuals. This equates to upwards of 100 000 affected individuals in the UK and approximately 600 000 in the USA. Further epidemiologic studies have suggested that upwards of 1% of the US population may be at risk for the development of HS, raising the prevalence rates to upwards of 2 million. Reasons given for the uncertainty in determining how many individuals suffer from HS include the fact that clinicians often misdiagnose HS as another acne-like disorder, and many individuals with HS do not present to physicians for diagnosis and/or treatment.

HS has been described as a genetic disorder, with both autosomal dominant and autosomal recessive properties having been described. Reports have shown that 13–38% of patients with HS have positive family histories for HS. HS is more prominent in females, with reports noting a 4:1 ratio in favor of females. HS flares are often associated with menses. Other factors shown to be associated with HS include stress, heat, sweating, and friction. Smoking also appears to be associated; over 70% of patients with HS smoke, a higher percentage than that among the population without HS.

The Dermatologic Life Quality Index (DLQI), a measurement of impairment potential from dermatologic disorders, ranks HS at a higher impairment rating in comparison to many other dermatologic disorders, such as acne vulgaris, eczema, and psoriasis.

HS is typically described as a primary skin condition, without obvious cause. However, a variety of other diseases, including Crohn's disease and irritable bowel syndrome, Down's syndrome, certain forms of arthritis, Grave's disease and Hashimoto thyroiditis, Sjögren's syndrome, hyperandrogenism, herpes simplex, and acanthosis nigricans have been associated with HS.

The clinical presentation of HS has been extensively described. Most typically, patients present with inflammatory cystic lesions in apocrine-gland bearing skin, most commonly the axillary and inguinal regions of the body, but also the inframammary folds of the breasts, periumbilical region, perineum and buttock regions, scrotum, mons pubis, and abdominal folds in overweight individuals.

On presentation painful, tender, and firm nodular lesions are seen, which on occasion open and drain a serosanguinous fluid spontaneously. These nodules heal slowly, with or without scarring, usually in about 10–30 days. The nodules typically recur several times a year and it is not unusual for new nodular lesions to form as older lesions begin to heal. On occasion, and one of the major concerns for patients with HS, is abscess formation, leading to the formation of epithelial-lined intradermal or subcutaneous sinus tracts. These sinus tracts are a continual source of the associated inflammatory infiltrate. HS may remain

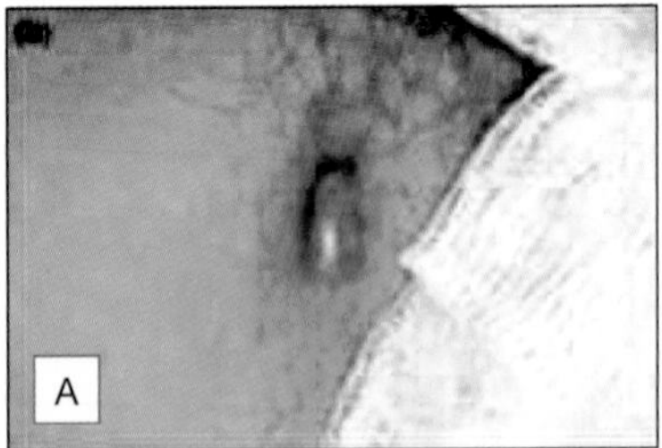

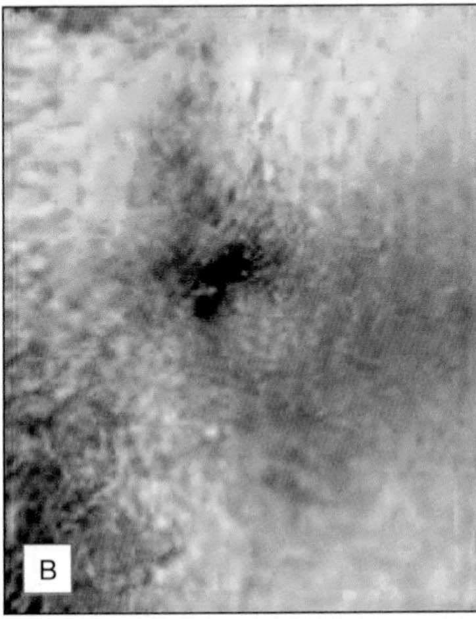

Fig. 4.1 (**A,B**) Clinical examples of phases I and II 2 HS (Reproduced with permission from Gold, MH. ALA-PDT for Hidradenitis Suppurativa. In Dermatologic Clinics (editor), 25:67–73, 2007.)

active for months at a time but spontaneous remissions, sometimes lasting months to years, is also reported. One recent HS study found that patients suffered, on average, 4.8 inflammatory lesions per month and most had disease activity for upwards of 20 years.

CLINICAL SIGNS OR PHASES

Most researchers separate HS lesions into three distinct phases. Phase I, or the primary stage, is the original phase of inflammatory nodular formation, typically described by patients as "boils". These nodules are usually separate and, on occasion, precursor inflammatory lesions are seen. Phase II, or the secondary stage, typically shows sinus tract formation linking inflammatory nodules together; scarring is also seen during this stage. Phase III, or the tertiary stage, is associated with coalescing of the nodular lesions and extensive scarring; sinus tract development dominates at this stage, with continued inflammation and chronic discharge apparent. Clinical examples of the phases (stages) and the histologic findings associated with these phases are shown in Figures 4.1–4.3.

TREATMENT

The treatment of HS remains as frustrating as the diagnosis of HS, both to the patient and, at times, the physician.

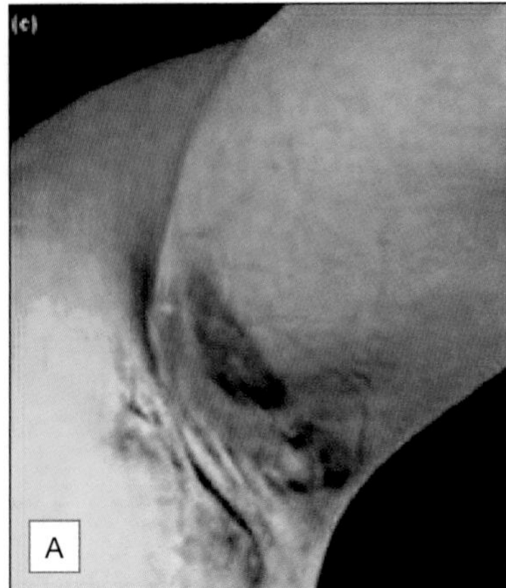

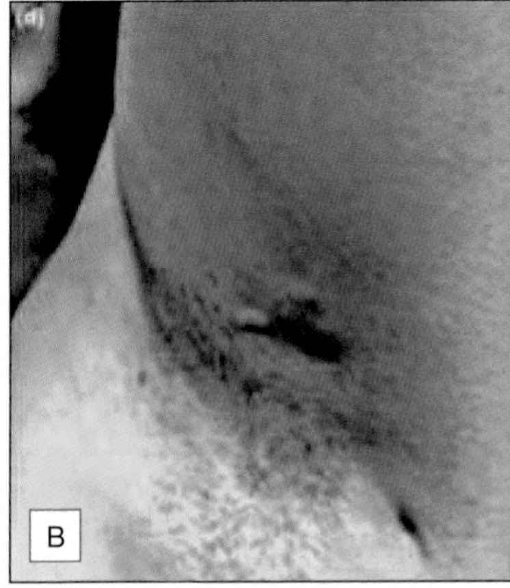

Fig. 4.2 (**A,B**) Clinical examples of phase III HS (Reproduced with permission from Gold, MH. ALA-PDT for Hidradenitis Suppurativa. In Dermatologic Clinics (editor), 25:67–73, 2007.)

Physicians who care for patients with HS must be aware that management of this disorder must focus on two separate but distinct fronts: the management of acute flares of the disease and the long-term management of the disease. It is beyond the scope of this chapter to review the entire medical literature with regards to the management of HS.

Acute flares in HS are typically treated medically or surgically, and at times a combination is used. Medical management typically involves the use of systemic and topical antibiotics, as well as systemic and intralesional corticosteroids. Hormonal therapy, on occasion, has been used, with mixed results. Although the efficacies of all these first-line therapies are disputed by many, most dermatologists feel fairly comfortable utilizing these modalities as first-line medical therapies. Systemic isotretinoin has also been used by many in the management of HS, again with mixed results. Several of the newer antitumor necrosis factor medications, commonly used for Crohn's disease, rheumatoid arthritis, as well as psoriasis vulgaris, are also showing promise in some individuals with HS. Clinical trials with these medications, including inflix-

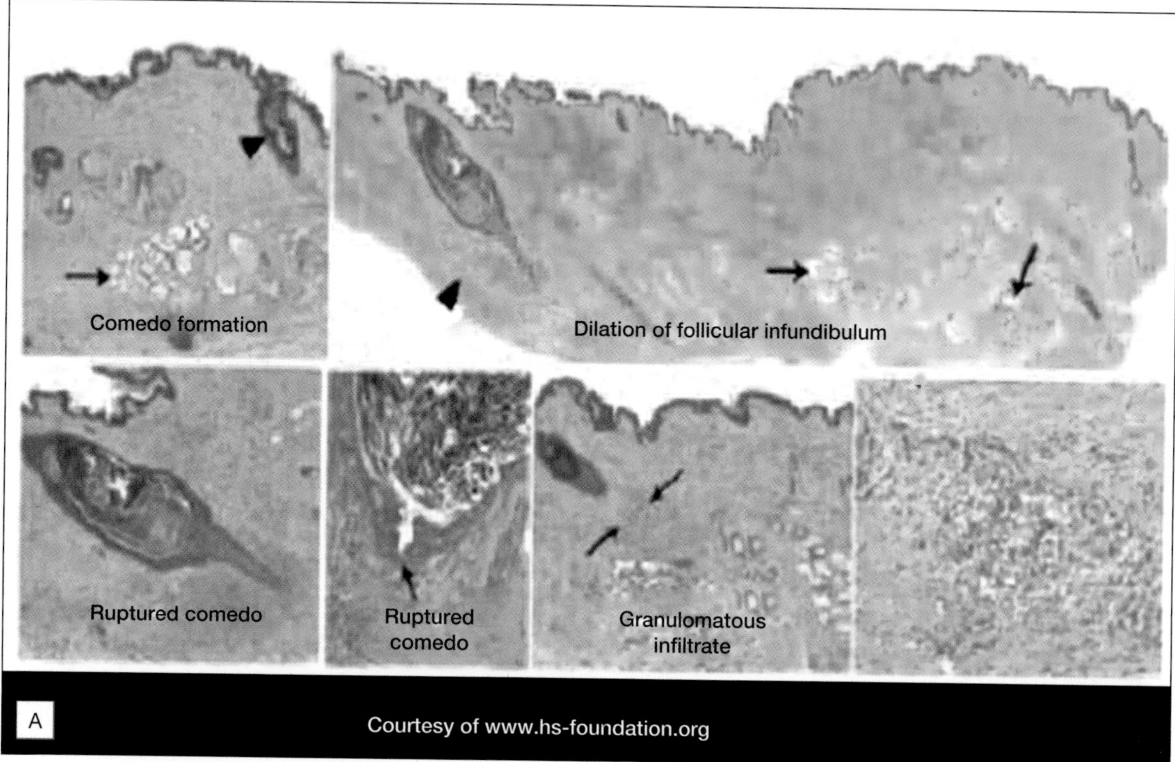

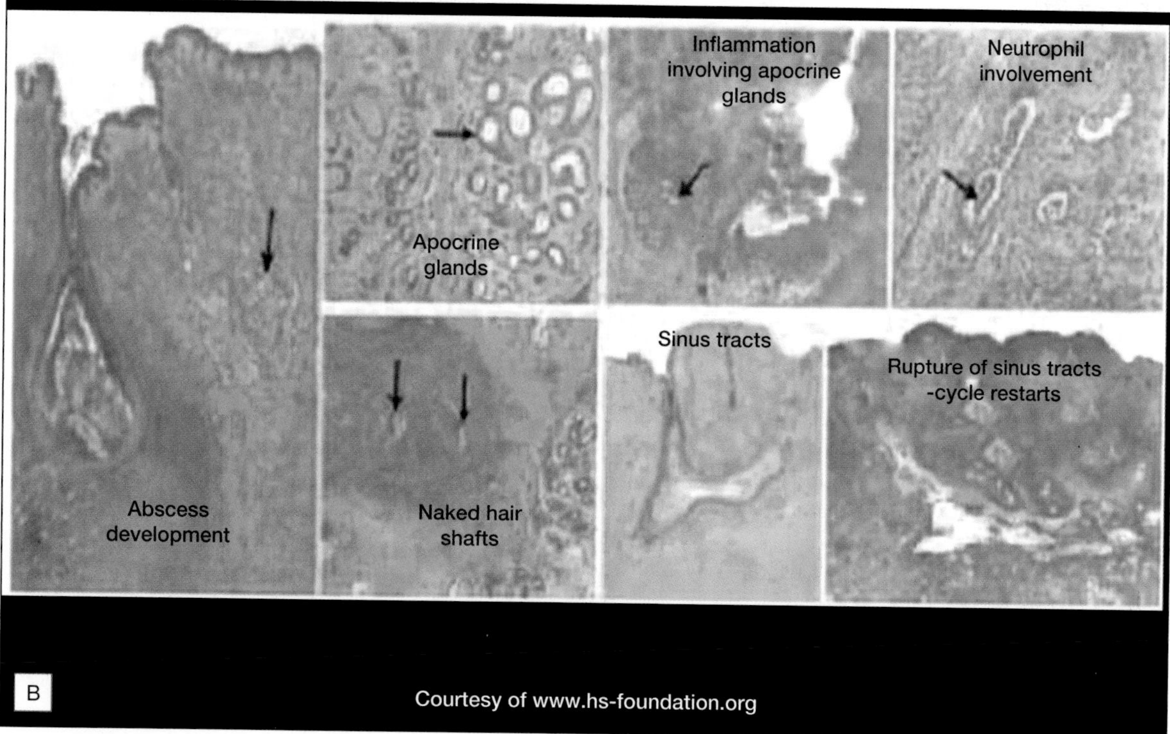

Fig. 4.3 (**A,B**) Histologic findings (Reproduced with permission from Gold, MH. ALA-PDT for Hidradenitis Suppurativa. In Dermatologic Clinics (editor), 25:67–73, 2007.)

imab, etanercept, and efalizumab, are ongoing to assess their efficacy in suppressing HS lesions for both the acute phases of HS and the long-term suppression of HS.

Are surgical modalities a better way to manage HS? Many surgeons advocate surgical management of all patients with HS. Incision and drainage of individual lesions of HS is a common mainstay of HS therapy used by many clinicians. Although many HS patients receive immediate relief with incision and drainage, there is growing evidence that this procedure actually hastens the development of further inflammation to the area, perhaps worsening the overall disease process. Excisional surgery of small areas of HS disease activity has been performed but most surgeons would argue that radical, wide surgical excision may be the only true way to control the disease, both in the short and the long term. Most dermatologists would counter that they have seen HS patients who have had these kinds of surgical procedures but they have done little, if anything, to halt the continued disease progression, and may reduce the success with other future therapeutic modalities. Lasers, specifically the CO_2 laser, have been used in many patients with HS, again with mixed results.

• Newer therapies

Recently, there has been interest in the use of topical 20% ALA-PDT as a potential therapeutic option in individuals suffering from HS. PDT has gained in popularity in recent years and is finding many new uses in the dermatologic arena. PDT, in its simplest form, utilizes a photosensitizer, oxygen, and an appropriate light source to selectively destroy certain cells in the body, including actinically damaged skin cells, nonmelanoma skin cells, and sebaceous glands. Currently, two photosensitizers are available for use with PDT in the skin: Levulan® (20% 5-ALA, DUSA Pharmaceuticals, Wilmington, MA) and Metvix®/ Metvixia® (methyl ester of 20% 5-ALA [MAL], PhotoCure ASA, Norway; Galderma, Fort Worth, TX). At the time of the writing, only Levulan® is available in the USA; it is FDA approved for the treatment of nonhyperkeratotic actinic keratoses (AKs) of the face and scalp, utilizing a blue light source after a drug incubation of 14–18 h. Metvix®, available for use in Europe, has European Union clearance for the treatment of nonhyperkeratotic AKs and superficial basal cell carcinomas unsuitable for conventional therapy. In the USA, Metvixia® is cleared for the treatment of nonhyperkeratotic AKs and will be available at some point in the near future. It is recommended that the MAL cream is applied for 3 h under occlusion after gentle curetting of the affected lesion, and then exposed to a red light source. Both of the currently available medications have been utilized in the treatment of HS, although ALA-PDT for the treatment of HS is an off-label use and this needs to be made clear to patients receiving this type of therapy.

CLINICAL STUDIES

We have reported on our experiences with ALA-PDT in the management of four patients with recalcitrant HS. Patients received short-contact ALA for 15–30 min and then exposure to a blue light source for 18 min. They were treated at 1–2-week intervals and received three to four treatments in total. This was not an Investigational Review Board (IRB) controlled clinical trial but a retrospective analysis of clinic patients in a very active dermatology practice where PDT treatments are routinely performed for a variety of clinical conditions. Patients were followed for 3 months in the published report and 75–100% clearance was noted in these patients. Further analysis has shown clearance in three of the patients for upwards of 2 years; the fourth patient has required routine maintenance PDT therapy at 6-month intervals to control the HS. Clinical examples of treated HS patients are shown in Figure 4.4.

As HS is an apocrine disorder and PDT affects sebaceous gland disease processes, a reasonable explanation of how PDT might work in HS is not readily apparent. Most consider that because there is a PDT reaction in the nearby sebaceous glands of these patients, an inflamma-

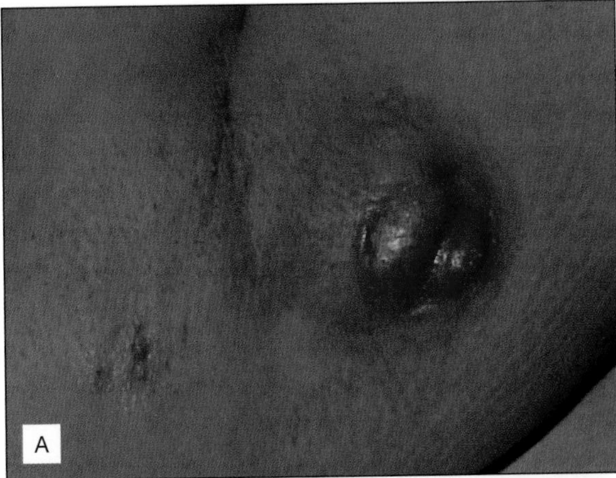

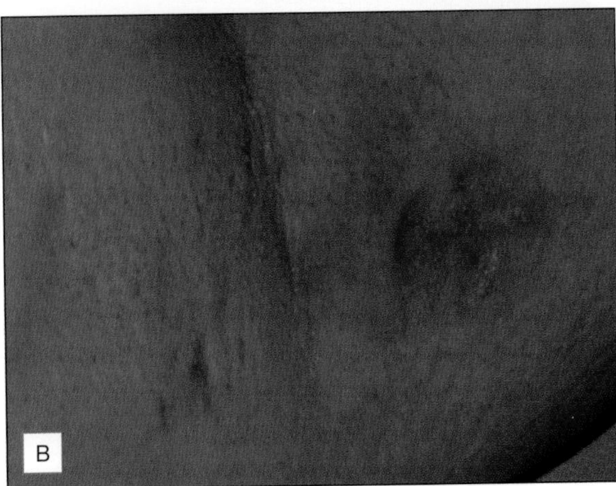

Fig. 4.4 **(A,B)** Clinical examples of HS treatments (Reproduced with permission from Gold MH, Bridges TM, Bradshaw VL, Boring M 2004 ALA/PDT and blue light therapy for hidradenitis suppurativa. Journal of Drugs in Dermatology 3:S32–39)

tory response affecting the apocrine glands may result in a positive response for these patients. Further research is required to determine how PDT may work in cases of recalcitrant HS.

Another study by Strauss et al in 2005, using MAL, did not show as promising results as the above study. Four patients received 4 h of MAL drug incubation and a local anesthesia prior to light therapy. A Ceramoptic (633 nm) diode laser was utilized in three of the cases and a broadband light source (570–640 nm) was used in the fourth case. The protocol called for three weekly treatments and an 8-week follow-up period. The one patient who received all three treatments showed improved disease activity; the two patients who received two treatments showed worsening of the disease process. The remaining patient did not complete the study because of severe adverse events (excessive burning and stinging). The authors concluded that PDT with MAL was not useful in HS patients.

A third study, by Rivard and Ozog in 2006, reported on their experiences with two patients with HS, one treated with a blue light source and the other with a long pulsed-dye laser (PDL). Both patients had shrinkage of their HS lesions during their observation period.

Table 4.1 Other dermatologic disorders treated with PDT

Disorders treated with PDT	Reference	Number of patients	Efficacy
Disseminated superficial actinic porokeratosis (DSAP)	Nayeemuddin et al (2002)	3	Poor response
	Taub (2006)	3	Successful response with ALA and pre-treatment of lesions
Psoriasis vulgaris	Robinson et al (1999)	10	8–10 clinical response; 1–45 sites cleared fully; ALA with broadband visible radiation at 8 J/cm^2
	Fransson & Ros (2005)	12	Significant improvement; pain high; ALA 20% solution with red light at 10–30 J/cm^2
	Radakovic-Fijan et al (2005)	29	Decrease in PSI in > 95% of patients; slow, pain; 1% ALA after keratolytic treatment and 5, 10 or 20 J/cm^2 of a filtered metal halide light (600–740 nm)
	Smits et al (2006)	8	Positive response and cytologic marker changes noted; 10% ALA ointment under occlusion for 4 h; fractionated broadband light (650–700 nm)
Lichen planus (LP)	Aghahosseini et al 92006)	26 lesions oral LP	16 positive responses; patients gargled 5% methylene blue; irradiation with 632 nm at 120 J/cm^2
Scleroderma	Szeimies et al (2002)		Localized disease responded well
Cutaneous T-cell lymphoma (CTCL)	Eich et al (1999)	2	Positive responses
	Orenstein et al (2000)	2	Positive responses
	Leman et al (2002)	1 (2 lesions)	Positive response
	Paech et al (2002)	CTCL in HIV-positive individual	Positive response
	Edstrom et al (2001)	10	7–10 complete responses; 20% ALA, 6-h incubation; red light

The study by Strauss et al raises some interesting issues which may explain why their patients had difficulty with this therapy. The use of MAL under occlusion for 4 h and exposure to a red light source is a painful procedure and has been associated with a PDT effect, or downtime with healing, in the majority of patients receiving this form of PDT. Also, pain associated with this long drug incubation and light exposure is well documented. The theory behind the long drug incubation is that this is required for the medicine to penetrate deep enough for a proper PDT response to occur. If the mechanism is, as is postulated, an inflammatory response leading to disease regression, then this type of drug incubation may not be required and the associated pain seen with this therapy could be avoided.

CONCLUSION

ALA-PDT, and perhaps MAL-PDT, may have a role in the management of patients with recalcitrant HS, but further clinical studies are required. These studies should be multicentered, placebo-controlled, and utilize a variety of lasers and light sources to determine which might work best with ALA-PDT in HS. Also, utilizing tagged ALA or performing histologic examination might provide further insights into how ALA-PDT affects those suffering from this disease process, both on a short- and a longer-term basis.

For further information on HS, clinicians are encouraged to visit and support the HS Foundation at www.hs-foundation.org.

A variety of other dermatologic disorders have also been described as being successfully treated with PDT. Although the majority of dermatologists would not recommend utilizing PDT as a primary treatment modality in these settings, it is interesting to note the versatility of PDT and its increasing usage throughout the world. The entities and supporting clinical studies are listed in Table 4.1.

FURTHER READING

Aghahosseini F, Arbabi-Kalati F, Fashtami LA et al 2006 Methylene blue-mediated photodynamic therapy: a possible alternative treatment for oral lichen planus. Lasers in Surgery and Medicine 38:33–38

Attanoos RL, Appleton MA, Douglas-Jones AG 1995 The pathogenesis of hidradenitis suppurativa: a closer look at apocrine and apoeccrine glands. British Journal of Dermatology 133:254–258

Breitkopf C et al 1995 Pyoderma fistulans sinifica (akne inversa) und eauchgewohnheiten. Z Haut 70:332–334

Edstrom DW, Porwit A, Ros AM 2001 Photodynamic therapy with topical 5-aminolevulinic acid for mycosis fungoides: clinical and histological response. Acta Dermato-Venerologica 81:184–188

Eich D, Eich HT, Otte HG et al 1999 [Photodynamic therapy of cutaneous T-cell lymphoma at special sites] [Article in German] Hautarzt 50:109–114

Fitzsimmons JS, Guilbert PR 1985 A family study of hidradenitis suppurativa. Journal of Medical Genetics 22:367–373

Fransson J, Ros AM 2005 Clinical and immunohistochemical evaluation of psoriatic plaques treated with topical 5-aminolaevulinic acid photodynamic therapy. Photodermatology, Photoimmunology & Photomedicine 21:326–332

Galen WK, Cohen I, Roger M et al 1996 Bacterial infections In: Schachner LA, Hansen RC (eds) Pediatric dermatology, 2nd ed. New York. Churchill Livingstone, 1206–1207

Gold MH, Goldman MP 2004 5-Aminolevulinic acid photodynamic therapy: where we have been and where we are going. Dermatologic Surgery 30:1077–1084

Gold MH, Bridges TM, Bradshaw VL et al 2004 ALA-PDT and blue light therapy for hidradenitis suppurativa. Journal of Drugs in Dermatology 3 (Suppl):32–39

Gordon SW 1978 Hidradenitis suppurativa: a closer look. Journal of the National Medical Association 70:339–343

Harrison BJ, Mudge M, Hughes LE 1991 The prevalence of hidradenitis suppurativa in South Wales. In: Marks R, Plewig G (eds) Acne and related disorders. London. Martin Dunitz, 365–366

Jemec GB, Hansen U 1996 Histology of hidradenitis suppurativa. Journal of the American Academy of Dermatology 34:994–999

Layton AM, Pace D, Cunliffe WJ et al 1995 A perspective histological study of acute hidradenitis suppurativa. British Journal of Dermatology 131:38–39

Leman JA, Dick DC, Morton CA 2002 Topical 5-ALA photodynamic therapy for the treatment of cutaneous T-cell lymphoma. Clinical and Experimental Dermatology 27:516–518

Nayeemuddin FA, Wong M, Yell J et al 2002 Topical photodynamic therapy in disseminated superficial actinic porokeratosis. Clinical and Experimental Dermatology 27:703–706

Orenstein A, Haik J, Tamir J et al 2000 Photodynamic therapy of cutaneous lymphoma using 5-aminolevulinic acid topical application. Dermatologic Surgery 26:765–769; discussion 769–770

Paech V, Lorenzen T, Stoehr A et al 2002 Remission of cutaneous *Mycosis fungoides* after topical 5-ALA sensitization and photodynamic therapy in a patient with advanced HIV-infection. European Journal of Medical Research 7:477–479

Radakovic-Fijan S, Blecha-Thalhammer U, Schleyer V et al 2005 Topical aminolaevulinic acid-based photodynamic therapy as a treatment option for psoriasis? Results of a randomized, observer-blinded study. British Journal of Dermatology 152:279–283

Rivard J, Ozog D 2006 Henry Ford Hospital dermatology experience with Levulan Kerastick and blue light photodynamic therapy. Journal of Drugs in Dermatology 5:556–561

Robinson DJ, Collins P, Stringer MR et al 1999 Improved response of plaque psoriasis after multiple treatments with topical 5-aminolaevulinic acid photodynamic therapy. Acta Dermato-Venerologica 79:451–455

Smits T, Kleinpenning MM, van Erp PE et al 2006 A placebo-controlled randomized study on the clinical effectiveness, immunohistochemical changes and protoporphyrin IX accumulation in fractionated 5-aminolaevulinic acid-photodynamic therapy in patients with psoriasis. British Journal of Dermatology 155:429–436

Strauss RM, Pollock B, Stables GI et al 2005 Photodynamic therapy using aminolaevulinic acid does not lead to improvement in hidradenitis suppurativa. British Journal of Dermatology 152:803–804

Szeimies RM, Landthaler M, Karrer S 2002 Non-oncologic indications for ALA-PDT. Journal of Dermatologic Treatment 13 (Suppl 1):S13–18

Taub AF 2007 Photodynamic therapy: other uses. Dermatol Clin 25:101–109

Von der Werth JM, Jemec GB 2001 Morbidity in patients with hidradenitis suppurativa. British Journal of Dermatology 144:809–813

Von der Werth JM, Williams HC 2000 The natural history of hidradenitis suppurativa. Journal of the European Academy of Dermatology and Venereology 14:389–392

Von der Werth JM, Williams HC, Raeburn JA 2000 The clinical genetics of hidradenitis suppurativa revisited. British Journal of Dermatology142:947–957

Wiltz O, Schoetz DJ Jr, Murray JJ et al 1990 Perianal hidradenitis suppurativa. The Lahey Clinic experience. Diseases of the Colon and Rectum 33:731–734

Yu CC, Cook MG 1990 Hidradenitis suppurativa: a disease of follicular epithelium, rather than apocrine glands. British Journal of Dermatology 122:763–769

5 Treatment of Sebaceous Hyperplasia

Dore J. Gilbert

INTRODUCTION

Sebaceous hyperplasia (SH) is a benign condition found most commonly among adults and the aged. Lesions appear singly or in groups as raised, yellowish papules with central umbilication. When diagnosing SH, care must be taken to differentiate the lesions from those of basal cell carcinoma, molluscum contagiosum, xanthoma, dermal nevi, sebaceous adenoma, and sebaceous epithelioma. SH lesions are distinguished by their location in the facial region and their umbilicated nature. If there is doubt in diagnosing a lesion, a biopsy should be performed.

PATIENT SELECTION FOR PHOTODYNAMIC THERAPY

Candidates for photodynamic therapy (PDT) with 5-aminolevulinic acid (ALA) exhibit multiple lesions and express a wish to avoid the risk of scarring and blemishing associated with surgical excision. Other eligibility criteria include failure or negligible results obtained with other therapies, reluctance to submit to CO_2 or erbium laser treatments, and a desire to avoid extended recovery time.

In our opinion, ideal patients for ALA-PDT have multiple lesions, preferably 10 or more. They do not wish to undergo laser or electrocautery surgery. Patients with actinic keratosis (AK) lesions or acne vulgaris in addition to SH are also ideal because ALA-PDT has proven effectiveness in treating both conditions.

Patients aged 28–61 years have been successfully treated with ALA-PDT. This therapy should not be applied to women who are pregnant or lactating, those with a history of porphyria or other condition that causes photosensitivity, and those taking photosensitizing drugs or cyclosporine. Patients allergic to ALA should also not be considered.

PRE-TREATMENT PATIENT EDUCATION

During the initial consultation it is important to make patients aware of potential issues with ALA-PDT. For example, the exposure to the light or laser may be painful, pain medications may be required, and the treatment carries no guarantee of results. Side effects include redness or tenderness of skin, swelling or bruising, scabbing, scarring, crusting, the possibility of burning, and hypo- or hyper-pigmentation. Four treatments may be necessary to achieve satisfactory results and maintenance treatments may be needed to prevent recurrence. Finally, it should be made clear that ALA-PDT is Food and Drug Administration (FDA) cleared in the USA only for the treatment of AK of the face and scalp; it is not cleared for the treatment of SH. While ALA-PDT is safe, its effectiveness in the treatment of SH has not been fully evaluated.

MEDICAL HISTORY

Clinicians should determine whether patients have received previous treatments for SH and what results they expect from ALA-PDT. They should note current over-the-counter (OTC), prescription (oral and topical), and herbal medications, as well as permanent make-up. Pregnancy, diabetes, bleeding disorders, allergies, herpes simplex, pigmentation problems, formation of keloid scars, photosensitivity, and drug-induced photodermatitis should also be determined, as well as skin type, skin condition (dry, seborrheic, normal), and tanning history.

EXPECTED BENEFITS

Table 5.1 summarizes the results of five studies of the use of ALA-PDT for the treatment of SH. Treatment variables include ALA incubation time, light source, number of treatments, time intervals between treatments, and follow-up time. All studies resulted in the regression or elimination of SH lesions to varying degrees.

In 2003, Horio and colleagues reported the first successful treatment of SH with ALA-PDT. A 61-year-old Japanese man presented with multiple facial SH lesions (1.5–4.0 mm) that had exhibited slow enlargement over a 10-year period. Wishing to avoid the risk of scarring associated with surgical treatment, the patient gave informed consent and received PDT with 20% ALA in an oil-in-water emulsion. ALA was applied to the lesions which were then exposed to light from a red-filtered halogen bulb. While the patient experienced a mild

Table 5.1 Treatment parameters and results of studies of the treatment of SH by ALA-PDT

Reference	Hours of ALA incubation (number of treatments, intervals in weeks)	Light source	Number of lesions treated	Efficacy	Adverse effects	Recurrence	Follow-up time (months)
Horio et al (2003)	4 (4,1)	300-W halogen bulb (> 620 nm)	8	Lesions regressed; decreased sizes persisted for 12 months	Some burning, erythema, edema, hyperpigmentation (10 days)	None	12
Alster and Tanzi (2003)	1 (1–2,6)	PDL (595 nm)	Multiple	Total clearing of lesions after 1 or 2 treatments	Some burning, focal edema and crusting in 70% of patients (2–5 days)	None	1,3
Goldman (2003)	0.25 (2–4,1)	IPL (560 nm), Violet–blue light (410 nm)	Multiple	Relative clearing of acne (75%) after 2–4 treatments	Some photosensitivity	None	None
Richey and Hopson (2004)	0.75–1 (3–6,1)	Blue light (410 nm)	Multiple	70% clearance of lesions	Some burning, erythema, edema, hyperpigmentation (10–21 days), crusting (4–7 days)	10–20% recurrence in 3–4 months	6
Gold et al (2004)	0.5–1 (4,4)	IPL (550 nm), blue light(405–420 nm)	Multiple	IPL: 53.4% reduction in lesions; blue light: 55.3% reduction	Mild erythema	None	1,3

IPL = intense pulsed light; PDL = pulsed-dye laser
Adapted from Nestor MS, Gold MH, Kauvar AN et al 2006 The use of photodynamic therapy in dermatology: results of a consensus conference. Journal of Drugs in Dermatology 5:140–154

burning sensation during treatment and post-treatment erythema, edema, scaling, and hyperpigmentation were noted in the treated area, small papules had nearly disappeared and large papules were notably reduced in size after three sessions. The lesions did not recur for the next 12 months.

Alster and Tanzi obtained total clearance of SH lesions in 7 of 10 patients (skin types I–IV, aged 28–56 years) after a single ALA-PDT session with 595-nm pulsed-dye laser (PDL) activation. The remaining three patients experienced total clearance after a second treatment session 6 weeks later. All patients had at least three lesions, 3–8 mm in diameter; matched lesions were used as controls and were left untreated or treated with PDL alone. Individual lesion improvements were measured on a remnant scale of 0–4 (0 = < 25% of lesion remaining; 4 = > 75% remaining). Lesions treated with ALA-PDT scored a mean of 0.3 after a single treatment, far better than the 1.8 for PDL alone or 4.0 for untreated controls. These results indicated that formation of protoporphyrin IX (PpIX) in sebocytes from ALA application enhances the efficacy of PDL treatment. As a result, fewer treatment sessions and less pulse stacking are required than with PDL alone. While mild pain during treatment, edema, and focal crusting were reported, hyperpigmentation was not observed in any patient.

Goldman reported encouraging results by using ALA-PDT with blue light or intense pulsed light (IPL) to treat acne vulgaris and SH. ALA was applied to the entire face to allow treatment of sebaceous glands that could develop into acne as well as active acne lesions. Relative clearance of acne lesions was obtained after two to four weekly treatments. Patients reported no pain or discomfort, and post-treatment photosensitivity was ameliorated by application of a sunscreen with a sun protection factor (SPF) greater than 45.

Richey and Hopson also used blue light to treat 10 patients (aged 30–60 years, skin type II–V), each with 10–50 SH lesions 1–3 mm in diameter. ALA was applied to the entire facial area and allowed to incubate for 45–65 min. Patients received an average of four treatments and were followed for 6 months. Lesions whose size was reduced by less than 50% were considered nonresponsive, while those with at least 50% reduction in size were considered partially responsive. Complete response indicated disappearance of the lesion at the treatment site. Complete response was obtained in 70% of lesions. Some lesions did not begin to clear until after a second or third treatment; continuous improvement was noted thereafter. Reported side effects were similar to those of Horio and colleagues.

Richey and Hopson hypothesized that recurrence of SH lesions in their study was due to (1) decreased time of ALA incubation as compared to the study by Horio and colleagues, and (2) shallower penetration of the lesions by the light source as compared to the study by Alster and Tanzi. The former factor reduced the amount of ALA that could be absorbed by the skin for conversion to PpIX. The latter factor may have prevented the light source from destroying enough sebocytes to completely eliminate a lesion.

In the study of Gold and colleagues, 12 patients (aged 42–61 years) received once-monthly ALA-PDT for SH over 4 months with either blue light or IPL activation. Lesion count reduction was substantial with both light sources (Table 5.1), slightly higher for blue light than IPL. Recurrence was not reported with the use of either light source during the 3-month follow-up.

The first case report of the use of PDT for the treatment of SH in an organ transplant recipient has been published. The patient had more than 100 SH lesions on the face 3 years after renal transplantation. After cryotherapy, 40% trichloroacetic acid, CO_2 laser treatment, and 1450-nm laser treatments had resulted in post-treatment hypopigmentation, the decision was made to try PDT. Two sessions of PDT with methyl aminolevulinate under occlusion for 3 h and photoactivation with noncoherent red light (633 nm) removed or reduced all lesions 1 month after the second treatment. The improvement persisted for 6 months. The patient considered the cosmetic result superior to that of earlier treatments.

In the author's experience, 80% of patients who receive ALA-PDT for SH respond positively. Post-treatment scarring has not been observed. Redness and scaling last between 4 and 7 days. Most treated lesions recur over a 3–12-month period. No patient has required long-term courses of medication in conjunction with treatment.

TREATMENT TECHNIQUES

Horio and colleagues (Table 5.1) treated their patient with light from a 300-W halogen bulb after 4 h of ALA incubation. ALA-treated lesions were exposed to red-filtered light at a distance of 5 cm for 15–20 min. The patient received four treatments at 1-week intervals.

Alster and Tanzi used a 595-nm PDL (Vbeam, Candela Laser Corp) to activate ALA-induced PpIX. PDL settings were 7.0 J/cm^2 fluence and 6-ms pulse duration, and the 7-mm spots were double-stacked. Lesions were cleansed with soap and water before ALA application. Results were evaluated by pre- and post-treatment digital photography.

Goldman used three light sources with ALA-PDT: two 410-nm light sources and one IPL source with a 560-nm cut-off filter. ALA was applied to the entire face and allowed to incubate for 15 min. The treated area was exposed to one of the three light sources for 15 min. For IPL treatment the author used a double-pulse technique of 3–6-ms pulses with a 10-ms delay and 35-J/cm^2 fluence.

In the Richey and Hopson study, patients were treated with ALA-PDT and ALA-induced PpIX was activated with a 410-nm blue light (BLU-U, DUSA Pharmaceuticals, Wilmington, MA) source. Patients received an average of four sessions weekly. The areas to be treated were cleansed with acetone before full-face application of ALA. After ALA had been in contact with skin for 45–65 min, patients were exposed to a blue light source for 8–12 min. Patients were instructed to use SPF 45 sunblock daily for 1 week after treatment.

Gold and colleagues activated ALA-induced PpIX with either 405–420-nm blue light (ClearLight™ PhotoClearing System, Curelight™, Lumenis) or (500–1200 nm) IPL (Vasculight™, Lumenis, Inc). Participants received treatments once per month for 4 months. Topical ALA was applied to the entire face and incubated for 30–60 min before 15-min exposure to blue light. The IPL source was set to 3.5 ms/3.5 ms pulse duration with a 20-ms pulse delay time and 32 J/cm^2 fluence. Lesions were counted at each visit and results were further evaluated by photographic analysis at each treatment session and during follow-up 4 and 12 months after the final treatment.

ALA-PDT PARAMETERS FOR SEBACEOUS HYPERPLASIA

Our pre-treatment protocol is shown in Box 5.1.

IPL treatment parameters for various skin types are presented in Table 5.2. Activation of ALA-induced PpIX is successful only with cut-off filters of 640 nm or lower. To optimize outcome after IPL treatment, we expose the IPL-treated areas to blue light for 4–10 min. When the 595-nm PDL is used, we recommend pulse stacking with 6 J/cm^2 fluence and 10–20-ms pulse duration for maximum efficacy.

If the initial treatment is ineffective, the practitioner may modify treatment parameters at the next treatment session. Fluence may be increased, pulses may be stacked, or light or laser treatment time may be increased to a maximum of 15 min. To increase penetration of ALA, we recommend light electrodessication of the lesion approxi-

Box 5.1 ALA-PDT pre-treatment protocol

1. Photograph the patient with both digital and Polaroid cameras. Place photographs on the patient's chart
2. Instruct patient to continue topical or systemic medications
3. Wash the target area with soap and water or alcohol
4. Perform single-pass microdermabrasion and/or acetone scrub to remove the keratin layer and increase ALA penetration. In teenaged patients, scrub to the patient's comfort level
5. Gently crush ALA ampules with the fingers and shake the Kerastick for approximately 3 min, keeping the sponge end up
6. Apply ALA liberally to the skin, using extra pressure to the target lesions. Spread the solution uniformly with gloved fingertips. Avoid mucous membranes
7. Allow ALA to incubate for at least 30–60 min
8. Remove ALA with soap and water only if using large amounts of gel during IPL treatment. Otherwise, leave ALA on the skin
9. Wash the patient's face after treatment is completed

Adapted from Gilbert DJ 2007 Incorporating PDT into a medical and cosmetic dermatology practice. In: Gold MH (ed) Photodynamic Therapy. Dermatologic Clinics. Philadelphia: WB Saunders

Table 5.2 IPL* settings for the treatment of SH in skin types I–IV†

Skin type (hyperpig. color), treatment number	Pulses Mode	Pulses Duration (ms)	Pulses Delay (ms)	Fluence (J/cm^2)	Cut-off filter wavelength (nm)
I–III (Mild)					
1	Double	3.8/3.8	20	34	590
2	Double	2.4/4.0	20	30	560
I–III (Dark)					
1	Double	5.0/5.0	40	30	640
2	Double	3.8/3.8	20	34	590
3–5	Double	2.4/5.0	20	30	560
IV (Lighter)					
1	Double	5.0/5.0	40	37	640
2–5	Double	3.8/3.8	30	34	590
IV (Darker)					
1	Double	5.0/5.0	50	30	640
2	Double	4.5/4.5	40	34	615
3–5	Triple	4.0/4.0/4.0	40	36	590

*VascuLight SR, Lumenis, Inc., Santa Clara, CA
†Patient must be treated with blue light after IPL treatment
Adapted from Gilbert DJ 2007 Intense pulsed light in cosmetic dermatology. In: Hanke W (ed) The Cosmetic Dermatology Procedure Manual for Dermatology Residents and Practicing Dermatologists. New York: Physicians Continuing Education Corporation

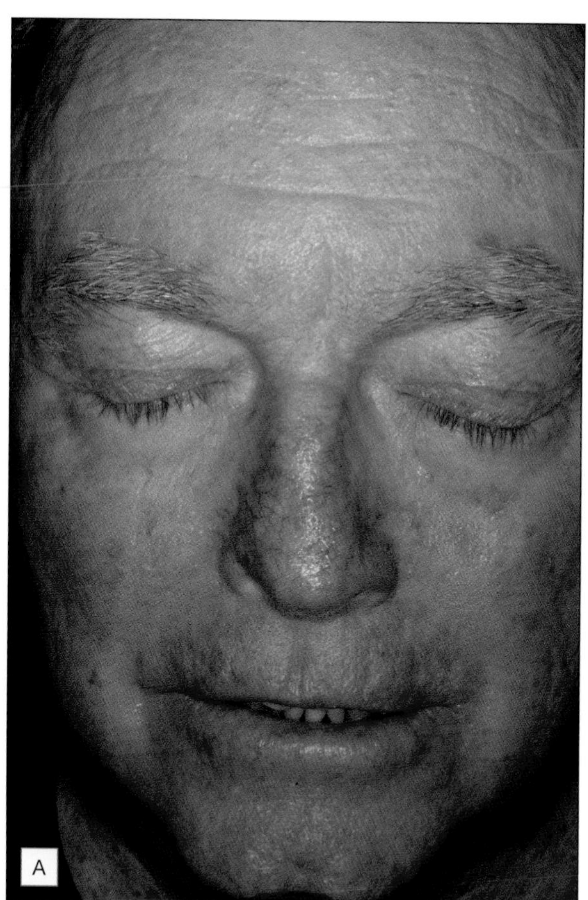

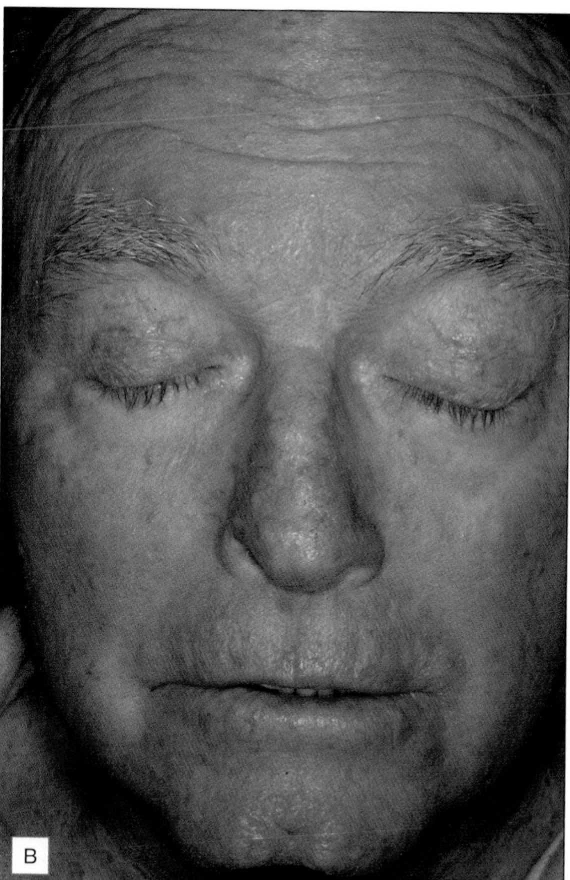

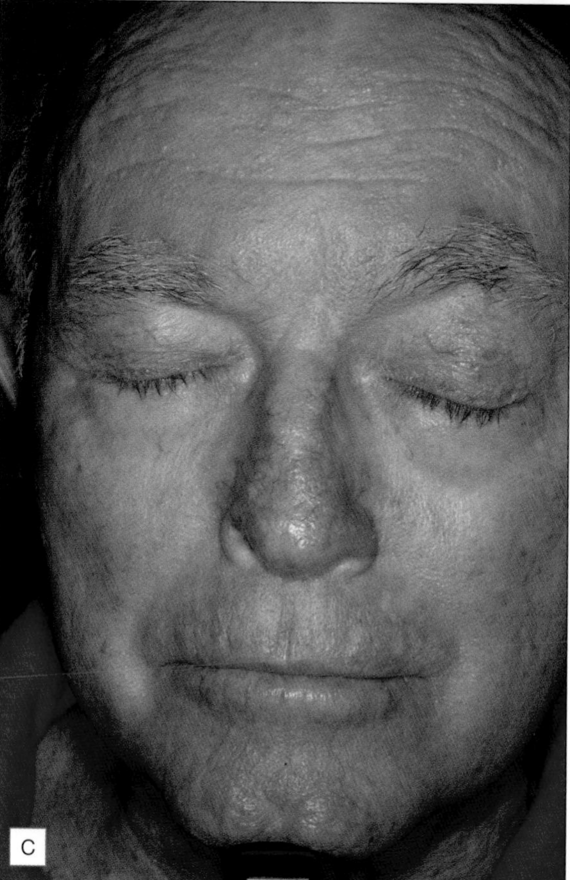

Fig. 5.1 A 79-year-old man with SH (**A**) before treatment, (**B**) 1 month, and (**C**) 6 months after a single treatment with ALA-PDT. ALA remained in contact with skin for 1 h before activation with a PDL device at 12-mm spot size and 40-ms pulse duration. The entire face received a single pass at 4 J/cm^2 fluence and the nose received a second pass at 6.8 J/cm^2. Note improvement in the nose and forehead after 6 months

mately 2 weeks before the first ALA-PDT session. Three to 4 weeks between treatments allows both physician and patient to correctly evaluate the effectiveness of earlier treatments. The total number of treatments depends on the amount of improvement with successive treatments as well as patient expectations (which must be carefully managed by the physician). Clinical examples are shown in Figures 5.1–5.3.

Our protocol for post-treatment care is shown in Box 5.2.

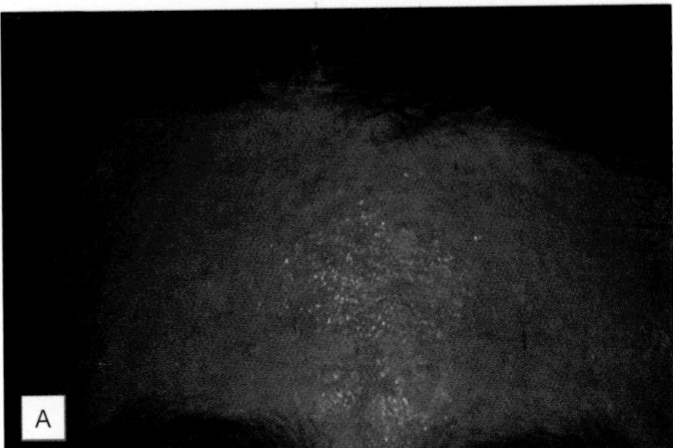

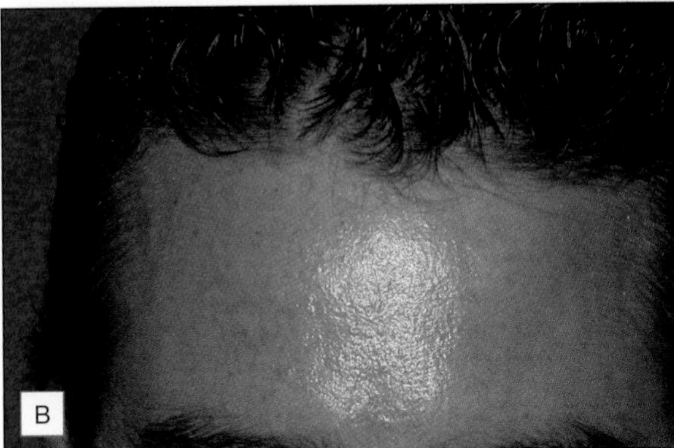

Fig. 5.2 (**A**) A 33-year-old man with multiple SH lesions on the forehead and glabella and (**B**) after four treatments with ALA-PDT. ALA remained in contact with skin for 30 min before 8-min exposure to blue light. Oiliness is nearly absent and lesions are barely visible. (Photograph courtesy of Donald F. Richey, MD, and Brent Hopson, PA-C, MMSc. Reproduced with permission from Hopson B 2006 Dermatology diagnosis: Asymptomatic erythematous facial papules. Case #3. The Clinical Advisor 95;99–100)

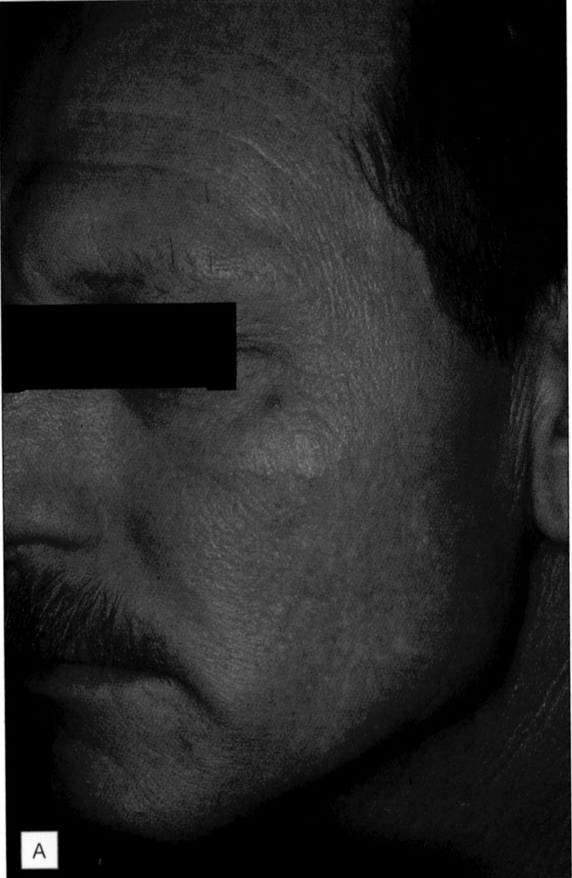

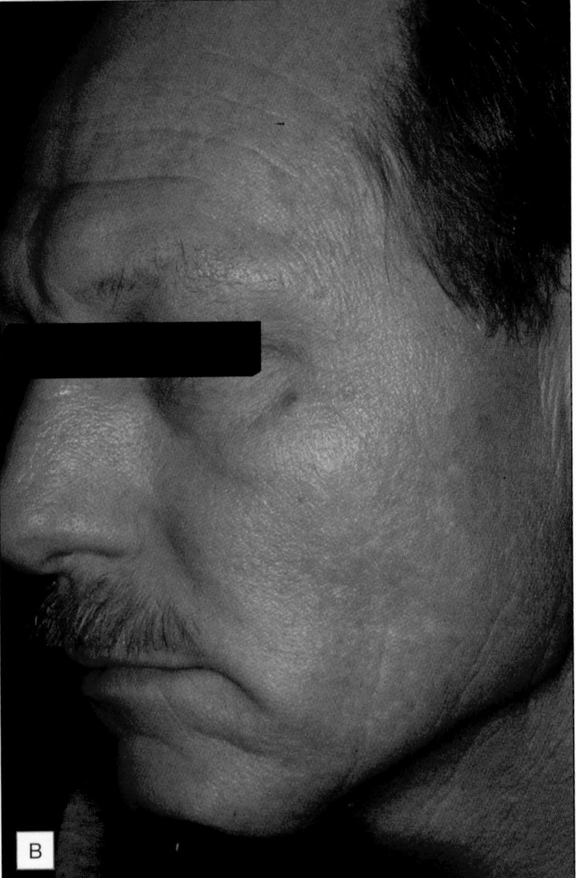

Fig. 5.3 Patient with SH lesions on the cheek (**A**) before and (**B**) 3 months after the final of four treatments with ALA-PDT and IPL activation (Photograph courtesy of Michael H. Gold, MD. Reproduced with permission from Gold MH, Bradshaw VL, Boring MM, Bridges TM, Biron JA, Lewis TL 2004 Treatment of sebaceous gland hyperplasia by photodynamic therapy with 5-aminolevulinic acid and a blue light source or intense pulsed light source. Journal of Drugs in Dermatology 3(6 Suppl):6–9)

Box 5.2 Post-treatment home care after PDT

Day of ALA-PDT

Apply ice packs to treated areas

- Take pain medication as needed
- Avoid sun exposure for 24 h
    - Stay indoors
    - Apply sunscreen (to all exposed skin, not just treated area)
    - Wear a hat
- Apply hydrocortisone (1%) ointment to treated area
- Take a shower if desired

Days 2–7

- Continue pain medication and ice packs as needed
- Protect treated area from sun exposure
- If blisters develop:
    1. Soak in white vinegar solution (1 tsp vinegar in 1 cup cold water)
    2. Apply ice over vinegar-soaked areas for 20 min
    3. Pat areas dry
    4. Apply petrolatum or hydrocortisone (1%) ointment
    5. Repeat steps 1–4 at 4–6-h intervals during waking hours
    6. Apply petrolatum (Aquaphor) or hydrocortisone (1%) ointment twice daily as needed

Day 7

- Apply make-up if healing is complete, use moisturizer before applying make-up
- Protect treated area from sun exposure (for 2 weeks total after treatment)
- Apply sun block (at least SPF 30) to treated area during sun exposure for 2 weeks after treatment
- If treated area is red after crusting has subsided, apply green-based cover up to hide redness

Adapted from Gilbert DJ 2006 Post-treatment care for photodynamic therapy with topical 5-aminolevulinic acid. US Dermatology. London: Touch Briefings, 85–87

FURTHER READING

Alster TS, Tanzi EL 2003 Photodynamic therapy with topical aminolevulinic acid and pulsed dye laser irradiation for sebaceous hyperplasia. Journal of Drugs in Dermatology 2:501–504

Horio T, Horio O, Miyauchi-Hashimoto H, Ohnuki M, Isei T 2003 Photodynamic therapy of sebaceous hyperplasia with topical 5-aminolaevulinic acid and slide projector. British Journal of Dermatology 148:1274–1276

Goldman MP 2003 Using 5-aminolevulinic acid to treat acne and sebaceous hyperplasia. Cosmetic Dermatology 16:57–58

Gold MH, Bradshaw VL, Boring MM, Bridges TM, Biron JA, Lewis TL 2004 Treatment of sebaceous gland hyperplasia by photodynamic therapy with 5-aminolevulinic acid and a blue light source or intense pulsed light source. Journal of Drugs in Dermatology 3 (6 Suppl):6–9

Perrett CM, McGregor J, Barlow RJ, Karran P, Proby C, Harwood CA 2006 Topical photodynamic therapy with methyl aminolevulinate to treated sebaceous hyperplasia in an organ transplant recipient. Archives of Dermatology 142:781–782

Richey DF, Hopson B 2004 Treatment of sebaceous hyperplasia by photodynamic therapy. Cosmetic Dermatology 17:525–529

6 Treatment of Skin Cancer Precursors

Sari M. Fien, James Ralston, Joyce B. Farah, Nathalie C. Zeitouni, Allan R. Oseroff

INTRODUCTION

This chapter will discuss topical photodynamic therapy (PDT) for actinic keratoses (AKs). Therapeutic approaches for both thin and hyperkeratotic AK will be described, including 5-aminolevulinic acid (ALA) application times, skin preparation techniques, and light sources.

AKs are common premalignant lesions occurring predominantly in individuals with Fitzpatrick skin types I–III (Table 6.1). High-risk individuals have significant histories of sun exposure. They may perform outdoor professional or recreational activities, or reside in sunny climates at low latitudes where UV exposure is significant. The estimated prevalence of AKs is less than 10% in the third decade, increasing to approximately 80% by the seventh decade. Although rare, young individuals in their 20s and 30s can present with clinically typical lesions, and 60% of predisposed individuals 40 years old and older have at least one AK. Patients who have received solid organ transplants or who are chronically immunosuppressed are also at greater risk for developing AK.

Although traditionally considered precancerous, AKs represent points on a continuum of histologic and biologic change towards squamous cell carcinoma (SCC). It is estimated that approximately one in 20 lesions will progress to invasive carcinoma. Individuals with more than 10 AKs have about a 14% probability of developing an SCC within 5 years. Because of the difficulty of predicting which lesions will become invasive, the general consensus is that all AKs should be treated.

Table 6.1 Fitzpatrick skin types

Skin type	History of sun exposure
I	Never tans and always burns
II	Tans minimally and always burns
III	Tans gradually after burning initially
IV	Tans well and burns minimally
V	Tans darkly and rarely burns
VI	Tans black and never burns

CLINICAL PRESENTATION

The clinical presentation of AK ranges from a slightly erythematous scaly papule to a firm hyperkeratotic plaque. Occasionally, AK may be pigmented. Occurring on chronically sun-exposed skin, the lesions are predominantly located on the scalp, face, dorsal hands, lower extremities, and dorsa of the feet. Patients may find them asymptomatic, or may complain of burning, pruritus, tenderness or

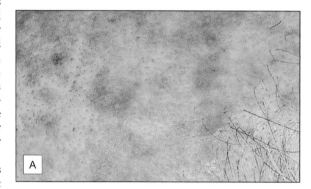

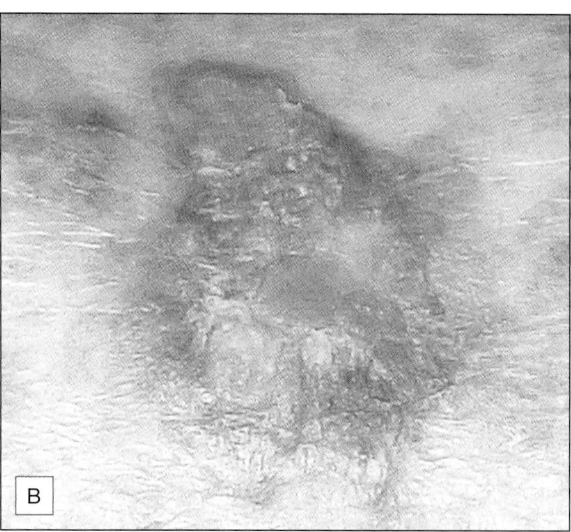

Fig. 6.1 (**A**) Thin AK on the scalp, with erythema and minimal scaling. (**B**) Hyperkeratotic and hypertrophic AK on the lower leg, with thick scaling overlying an erythematous base

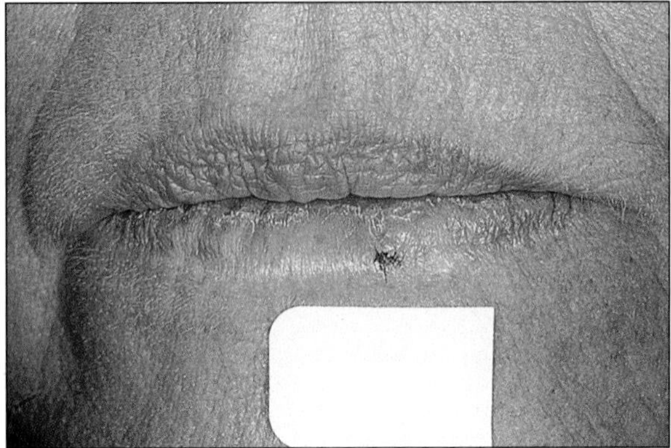

Fig. 6.2 Actinic cheilitis of the lower lip at the time of biopsy

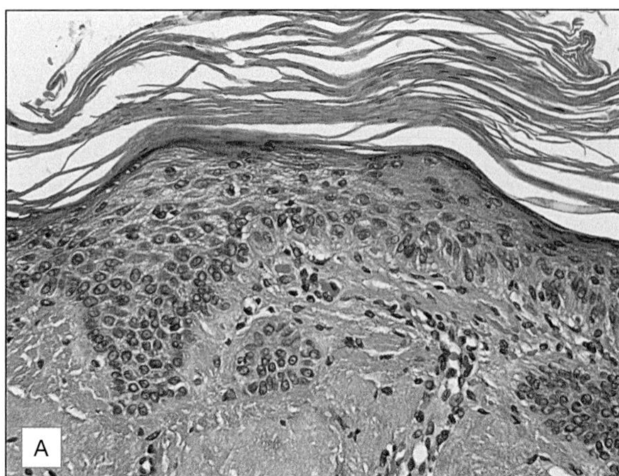

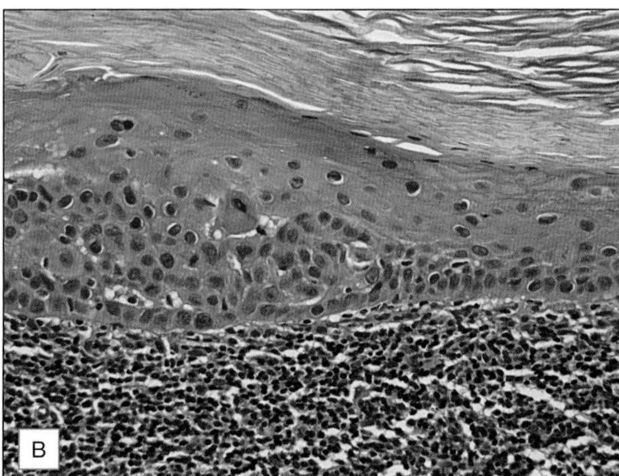

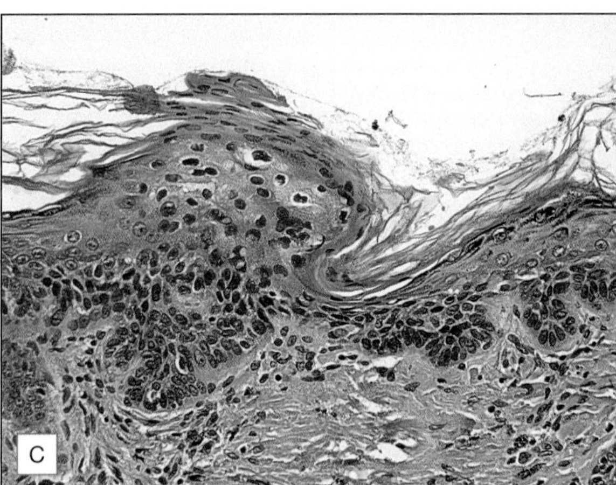

Fig. 6.3 (A) AK with focal parakeratosis overlying a zone of epithelial dysplasia with a diminished granular cell zone. The dermis exhibits severe elastosis (H&E, 200×). (B) Pigmented AK, with focal parakeratosis associated with epithelial dysplasia, prominent pigmentation of the basal cell zone, and dermal pigment incontinence (H&E, 200×). (C) Lichenoid AK, with focal parakeratosis, epithelial dysplasia, and single cell dyskeratosis associated with a dense dermal lichenoid mononuclear cell infiltrate (H&E, 200×) (Courtesy of Richard Cheney, MD, Roswell Park Cancer Institute)

bleeding. A change in lesion character, such as an increase in size, thickness or erythema, or development of ulceration, is an indication for biopsy (Fig. 6.1).

AKs may also present as cutaneous horns, actinic cheilitis, or lichen planus-like keratosis. In addition to occurring on AKs, an estimated 16% of cutaneous horns overlie SCCs; they can also occur on a seborrheic keratosis, inverted follicular keratosis, tricholemmoma or verruca. Since it is often difficult clinically to distinguish what is underlying the cutaneous horn, a biopsy generally is required for definitive diagnoses. Actinic cheilitis most commonly involves the lower lip. Clinically, there is scaling, fissuring, and/or swelling (Fig. 6.2). Painful erosions also may occur. A biopsy should be performed on any thickened area that does not heal to rule out a more invasive process. Lichen planus-like keratoses or benign lichenoid keratoses present as erythematous to violaceous discrete lesions with a thin overlying scale.

HISTOPATHOLOGY

Focal parakeratosis, hypogranulosis, and atypical keratinocytes are confined to the lower third of the epidermis. The epidermis can be acanthotic or atrophic. The rete ridges often form irregular downward buds (a "budding down" appearance). Dermal changes include solar elastosis. There are thickened, serpiginous fibers that appear basophilic on hematoxylin and eosin (H&E) sections, or clumps of elastotic material in which the outline of individual fibers is lost. There is typically a mild, chronic inflammatory cell infiltrate in the upper dermis. Pigmented AKs have all the features of common AKs with excess melanin in both the keratinocytes and melanocytes; melanophages may also be present in the dermis. Actinic cheilitis features are those of an AK, although plasma cells usually are more prominent due to the involvement of the mucous membranes. Lichen planus-like keratosis has a brisk lichenoid reaction pattern with numerous Civatte bodies in the basal layer and accompanying mild vacuolar alteration. The inflammation is quite dense and mostly lymphocytic but can have plasma cells and a number of eosinophils (Fig. 6.3).

RATIONALE FOR ALA-PDT TREATMENT

• Background

The basic principles of ALA-PDT are covered in Chapter 1. In brief, topical ALA-PDT involves the penetration of the prodrug ALA through the stratum corneum layer of the epidermis to the viable target cells, the in situ biosynthesis of the photosensitizer protoporphyrin IX (PpIX), and the subsequent photoactivation of PpIX to cause therapeutic phototoxicity by the conversion of molecular oxygen into singlet oxygen.

• PpIX concentration

Since PpIX is biosynthesized from ALA, its concentration depends on the penetration of ALA through the stratum corneum to the viable epidermal cells. ALA penetration is affected by the thickness and integrity of the stratum corneum, and can be manipulated by measures taken to modify the stratum corneum. Additionally, PpIX levels increase with longer ALA application times.

• Light dose

The effective light dose depends on the amount of light absorbed by the photosensitizer, and thus depends on the delivered light dose and the extent that its wavelengths are absorbed by PpIX. The major light sources in the US are the BLU-U (417 ± 5 nm) (DUSA Pharmaceuticals, Wilmington, MA), the ClearLight (405–420 nm) (CureLight, Gladstone, NY), the VersaClear (420 or 630 nm + blue light) (TheraLight, Carlsbad, CA), the pulsed-dye laser (PDL), and the intense pulsed light (IPL). A broadband (570–670 or 590–690 nm) or narrow band (630 ± 15 nm) red light is commonly used in Europe for AK, and narrow-band LED sources centered at 630–635 nm recently have become available. As shown in Figure 6.4, significant PpIX absorption bands are around 410, 505, 540, 580, and 635 nm. The Soret band absorption, at 410 nm, with 80% of its absorption extending from 358–435 nm, is up to 15–30-fold stronger than the longer wavelength "Q bands". Thus, for thin epidermal lesions the most effective light sources are the BLU-U, the ClearLight, and the blue VersaClear, because their output is matched to the PpIX Soret band. These sources are somewhat less effective for hyperkeratotic lesions (because short-wavelength light is strongly scattered), or for pigmented lesions or pigmented skin (because of increased melanin absorption). For the same delivered light dose, longer wavelength light targeting the Q bands is less efficient because it is less well absorbed; 10 J/cm^2 at 410 nm is equivalent to 200–300 J/cm^2 at 580 or 635 nm. However, red light has better penetration into thick or pigmented lesions. The 630-nm fluorescent lamp in the VersaClear also has significant mercury line emissions in the blue and green (near 406, 434, 546, and 578 nm), possibly making it effective for both thin and thicker lesions.

A laser, narrow-band lamp or LED source at 630–635 nm may have 100% of its output absorbed by PpIX. Babilas et al found ALA-PDT with the LED system to be as efficacious as an incoherent lamp in killing cultured cells and in treating AK. There was no significant difference between the light sources in pain during light treatment, patient satisfaction, or cosmesis following therapy. At a 6-week follow-up, the LED system achieved complete remission rates of 84.3%.

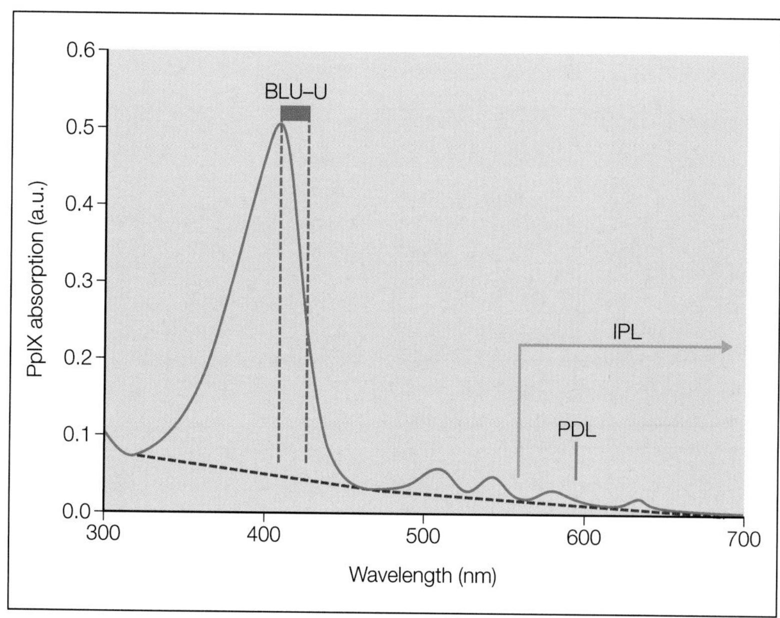

Fig. 6.4 Absorption spectrum of PpIX in a biologic environment. The wavelengths produced by the BLU-U®, the IPL (560-nm filter), and the 595-nm PDL are indicated (The brown dashed line represents nonspecific light scattering; the PpIX absorbance is above this line)

• PDT dosimetry

The concepts of PDT dose and PDT dose rate are critical to understanding the different approaches to therapy. PDT depends on the production of singlet oxygen, and the amount of singlet oxygen and other reactive species produced in and around the lesion principally determines the outcome of the therapy. If there are adequate tissue levels of molecular oxygen, the *PDT dose* is proportional to the product of (the local concentration of PpIX)×(the fraction of delivered light that is absorbed by the PpIX). Because PpIX is eventually destroyed (photobleached) during PDT, there is an upper limit on the maximum PDT dose that can be achieved with any PpIX concentration, and a limit to the amount of useful light that can be delivered. In the simplest approximation, the *PDT dose rate*, or the rate of formation of singlet oxygen, is proportional to the product of the (absorbed light dose rate [irradiance])×(PpIX concentration).

A particular PDT dose can be achieved with high PpIX concentrations and relatively low light doses, or vice versa, or with moderate levels of each component. Efficiently absorbed blue light is effective even with small amounts of photosensitizer. In contrast, light from a 595-nm PDL (e.g. Candela Vbeam laser) does not lie on a PpIX absorption band and is relatively weakly absorbed. When using the Vbeam, higher levels of PpIX may be desirable. The IPL, when operated with a 560-nm short wavelength cut-off filter, emits light from 560 to 1200 nm, with about 70% of the energy below 700 nm. Therefore, only about 10–15% of the IPL output is utilized by the 580- and 635-nm PpIX absorption bands, and higher levels of PpIX may be necessary to get an effective PDT dose. A 570–670-nm red lamp (e.g. Photocure CureLamp or Waldmann 1200) may have about 40–50% of its output utilized for PpIX absorption.

An example of the effect of ALA application time in a patient spot-treated for thin AK on the face is shown in Figure 6.5. He had a 1-h Levulan® application to one side and a 24-h Levulan application to the contralateral side, followed by Vbeam therapy at a subpurpuric light dose of 7.5 J/cm^2 in a single 6-ms pulse, using a 10-mm spot size.

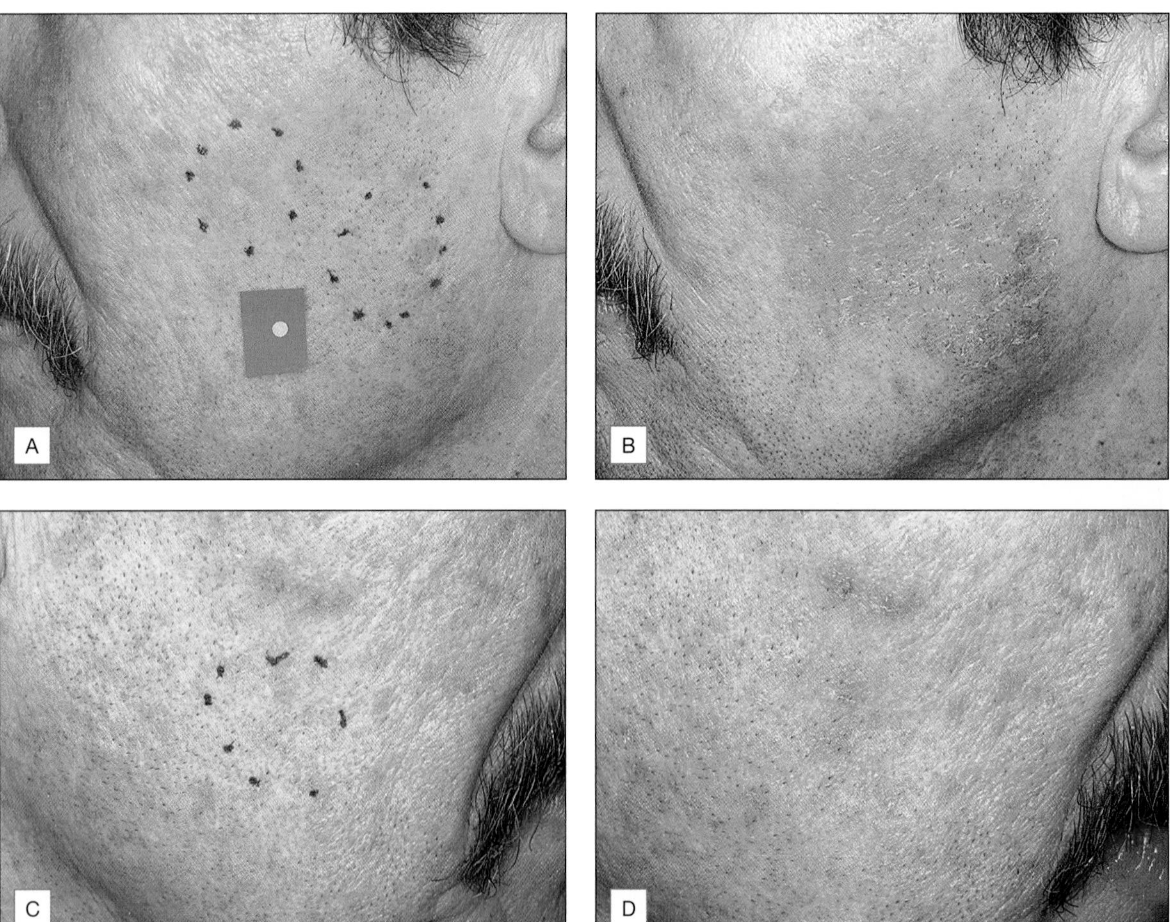

Fig. 6.5 A 57-year-old man with Levulan® applied to individual AK for 1 h or 24 h followed by Vbeam® treatment, with the clinical reactions 4 days later. (**A**) Left side before PDT. (**B**) Reaction to 24-h ALA application. (**C**) Right side before PDT. (**D**) Minimal reaction to 1-h ALA application. The dashed circles indicate treatment areas

As can be seen at the 4-day follow-up, there is a more vigorous reaction with erythema and desquamation at the 24-h application site.

The FDA-approved PDT treatment of AK using 20% ALA in an alcohol–water solution (Levulan® Kerastick®, DUSA Pharmaceuticals, Wilmington, MA) applies ALA without occlusion to nonhypertrophic AK of the face and scalp for 14–18 h. The prolonged application time leads to high levels of PpIX. Illumination is with the BLU-U Blue Light Photodynamic Therapy Illuminator, which has an intensity of 10 mW/cm^2 and delivers a high absorbed light dose of 10 J/cm^2 over the prescribed 16 min and 40-s treatment time. Thus, with both high levels of PpIX and absorbed light, the approved treatment delivers a large PDT dose at a rapid rate. Although the treatment conditions are efficacious, they also can cause discomfort. Pain from ALA-PDT is proportional to the PDT dose rate more than the PDT dose, and is probably due to direct photodynamic injury to cutaneous nerves. Pain is also proportional to the surface area treated. With the FDA-approved treatment conditions, PDT-induced discomfort generally limits treatment to individual AKs, rather than to the whole face or scalp.

It has become evident that AK can respond to relatively low PDT doses, in contrast to the treatment of skin cancers, where high PDT doses appear necessary for a durable complete response. The PDT dose can be reduced by decreasing either the PpIX level or the absorbed light, or both. As of yet, there is no clear consensus either on the best approach or on the minimum dose. For instance, if the dose is too low, multiple treatments become necessary, but in some circumstances this may be desirable as it reduces the morbidity of each treatment.

PATIENT SELECTION

Patients of either sex with multiple, thin AKs on the face and scalp respond best to ALA-PDT. Individuals who have failed or are intolerant of other therapies should be considered for treatment. Immunosuppressed patients or individuals with genodermatoses such as xeroderma pigmentosum also may benefit, since large areas can be treated repeatedly with minimal morbidity such as scarring or infection. Although durable clinical clearance rates are lower in immunosuppressed patients when matched to immunocompetent controls, ALA-PDT can be an effective maintenance therapy. A recent study by Dragieva et al of transplant recipients found good tolerability of ALA-PDT with minimal morbidity and excellent cosmesis. There were no reported cases of infection. Overall pooled complete clearance rates (CCRs) for all anatomic areas treated were 86% at 1 month, 68% at 3 months, 55% at 4 months, and 48% at 1 year. As expected, hyperkeratotic lesions did not respond as well.

Patients with type IV–V skin should be treated with caution due to the increased risk of developing post-inflammatory hyperpigmentation. Patients who recently have received other topical therapies should not be treated with ALA-PDT until the erythema and inflammation have subsided. Exclusion criteria include porphyria or known hypersensitivity to porphyrins, known photosensitivity diseases, concurrent use of photosensitizer drugs, or women who are pregnant or lactating. Patients who are suntanned must have treatment with ALA-PDT delayed until the tan fades to avoid blistering, hypopigmentation, and decreased efficacy (Table 6.2).

EXPECTED BENEFITS

The efficacy of treatment is assessed by the number and/or percent of AKs cleared, both as a fraction of the total AKs in all patients in a study, or as the percent of patients who achieve some benchmark such as 75–100% clearance. The response of an AK to ALA-PDT will depend on the thickness, size, and location of the lesion. Complete clearance rates on the face and scalp are higher than on the extremities; the larger and more keratotic the lesion, the less likely it will completely clear with a single treatment. Outcomes also depend on the treatment parameters; more aggressive treatments usually give better outcomes, while also increasing side effects. In general, the response rates for individual lesions and for all AKs on a patient may range from 50 to 100%. Many patients require at least two treatments for complete resolution. The durability of the response over time is also a measure of efficacy. The more effective the treatment, the longer the area will

Table 6.2 Patient selection and exclusion criteria

Selection criteria	Exclusion criteria
Patients with multiple AKs from chronic sun exposure, immunosuppression or organ transplant, or xeroderma pigmentosum	Patients with photosensitivity diseases, porphyria or known hypersensitivity to porphyrins, or current use of photosensitizing drugs
Patients with thin lesions will respond better than those with hyperkeratotic lesions	Pregnant or lactating patients
Patients with large or multiple AKs who have failed other therapies or are intolerant to topical chemotherapeutic agents	Patients treated with other topical therapies until the erythema and inflammation have subsided
	Patients with suntans until the tan fades, or with type IV–V skin

Table 6.3 Results using different application times and light sources for AK treatment

Application time	Light source	Reference	Sites	Average AK complete response rate (%)	Number of treatments	Length of follow-up (months)
14–18 h	Blu-U	Jeffes et al (2001) (ALA)	Face or scalp	85	1–2	4
14–18 h	Blu-U	Piacquadio et al (2004) (ALA)	Face or scalp	83/91 lesions; 60/73 patients	1/2	3
14–18 h	PDL 1–4 pulses	Alexiades-Armenakas et al (2003) (ALA)	Face or scalp	92	1	4
14–18 h	PDL 1–2 pulses	Oseroff et al (unpublished) (ALA)	Face or scalp	85	1	4
3–4 h	PDL 1–4 pulses	Alexiades-Armenakas et al (2003) (ALA)	Face or scalp	84	1	4
3 h	570–670-nm lamp	Szeimis et al (2002) (Metvix)	Face, scalp, other	69	1	3
3 h	570–670-nm lamp	Pariser et al (2003) (Metvix)	Face or scalp	89	2	3
3 h	570–670-nm lamp	Freeman et al (2004) (Metvix)	Face or scalp	91	1	3
1–3 h	Blu-U	Touma et al (2004) (ALA)	Face or scalp	93 (1 hr) 84 (2 h) 90 (3 h)	1	1
1 h	Blu-U	Smith et al (2003) (ALA)	Face or scalp	80	2	1
1 h	PDL 2 pulses	Smith et al (2003) (ALA)	Face or scalp	50	2	1
1 h	IPL	Avram et al (2004) (ALA)	Face	68%	1	3
1 h	Chemolum patch 431–515 nm 1.7 J/cm^2	Zelickson et al (2005) (ALA)	Face, scalp, hand	36–100% (range of patient responses)	1	3
30–60 min	IPL	Gold et al (2006) (ALA)	Face	78	3	3
3 h	600–730-nm lamp	Draviega et al (2004) (Metvix)	Face, scalp, neck, extremities	90	2	4

stay clear. Two months is probably the minimum follow-up interval to assess durability. A summary of results for ALA-PDT using different treatment conditions is given in Table 6.3.

In 1997, DUSA completed two multicenter Levulan-PDT phase III studies on over 1500 AK lesions in 243 patients treated with Levulan or a placebo, plus blue light. Patients whose lesions did not clear completely were retreated after 8 weeks. In one of the studies (117 patients), 86% of the AK lesions responded completely after a single treatment with Levulan-PDT, with 94% clearance after two treatments, compared with 32% clearance after two treatments with placebo and light. In the other study (126 patients), 81% of the AK lesions responded completely after a single treatment with Levulan-PDT, with 90% clearance after two treatments, compared with 20% clearance after two treatments with placebo and light. When the results of the two studies were combined, over 90% of the lesions had cleared after one or two Levulan-PDT treatments, compared to 25% in control groups. All of these results were statistically significant ($P < 0.001$). Piacquadio et al, in a multicenter investigator-blinded study using topical ALA and a BLU-U light source, found 77% of patients had a 75% response rate at 8 weeks (i.e. 75% of AKs cleared). Patients who did not achieve a 75% response rate at 8 weeks were retreated; and at 12 weeks, 89% of patients had a 75% response rate. An example of overnight ALA and BLU-U treatment is shown in Figure 6.6. The treatment was well tolerated with excellent cosmetic results; the complete clinical response was durable at 1-year follow-up.

Much of the current use of Levulan involves lower PDT doses, from shorter application times and/or pulsed light sources. Lower doses have made it feasible to treat entire anatomic areas such as the face, rather than individual AKs. In a large, single-center study, Alexiades-Armenakas et al used the 595-nm PDL (one to four pulses) and both 14–18 h and 3-h ALA application times. The 3-h ALA application was occluded to increase uptake, and hyperkeratotic lesions were covered with surgical lubricant jelly prior to laser treatment to reduce light scattering. At 4 months, the average clearance rates were 93% head, 71% extremities, and 65% trunk. The 14–18-h applications were somewhat more effective than the 3-h applications, with about an 8% greater response rate on the face and a 16% greater response rate on the extremities; however, the number of patients treated with the shorter application time was small. The lesions that did not respond tended to be greater than 2 mm and hyperkeratotic. All nonresponding lesions were biopsied and 69% were SCCs.

At our institution, 18–24-h Levulan application was used followed by multiple spot or confluent treatment with a 595-nm PDL (Candela Vbeam) in 14 patients with 46 different anatomic areas affected. Hypertrophic lesions were pre-treated with gentle abrasion with 3M Red Dot EKG tape. The entire anatomic area was single pulsed, and hypertrophic lesions were double pulsed. For a single treatment with 18–24-h application, on a response per patient basis, we found an 80% overall CCR rate (range 60–100%) for the face and scalp, a 65% overall CCR rate (range 60–70%) for the upper extremities, and a 55% CCR rate (range 30–70%) for the lower extremities. On a response per lesion basis, the face and scalp had an 85% CCR rate (Table 6.3). There was no significant pain, and mild erythema and edema typically resolved within a week. We also use 4-h ALA applications, but find this regimen less effective except on the lip or mucosal surfaces. Figure 6.7A shows a 45-year-old woman with type I skin at initial evaluation. Marked erythema and some edema are apparent immediately after spot treatment with 24-h Levulan and Vbeam irradiation, despite premedication with diphenhydramine (Fig. 6.7B). The treatment reaction has largely resolved 1 week later (Fig. 6.7C).

Several other studies have investigated short application times. Using the BLU-U in 18 patients, Touma et al found 1-, 2-, and 3-h ALA application times as efficacious in clearing AKs as 14–18-h application times. At a 1- and 5-month follow-up, they achieved an average 90% lesion CCR rate. An "acid mantle" cream was applied to the skin for 45 min before light treatment, which may have increased the ALA uptake. Smith et al investigated the efficacy of 1-h application PDT using both the BLU-U and a 595-nm PDL, compared to treatment with 5-fluorouracil (5-FU). Patients were treated twice at 30-day intervals. Hyperkeratotic lesions were excluded. The patients were assessed at 1 month post-treatment and the cumulative clearance rate or individual AK lesion response rate was found to be 79%, 80%, and 60% for 5-FU, BLU-U, and PDL-PDT, respectively. The 5-FU and BLU-U groups experienced enhanced improvements in tactile roughness, whereas the 5-FU and PDL groups had better response in terms of pigmentation. Avram and Goldman studied the

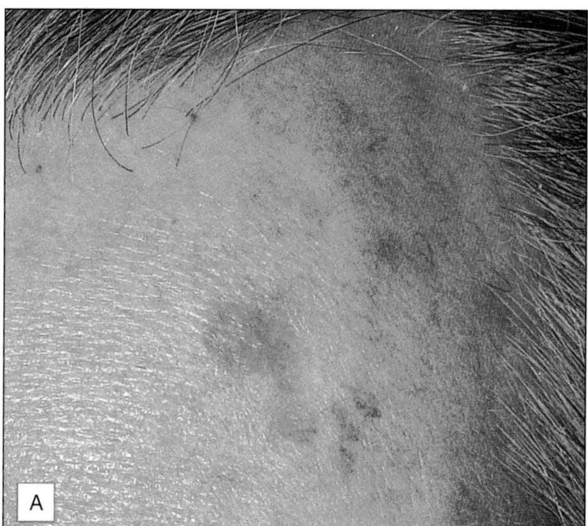

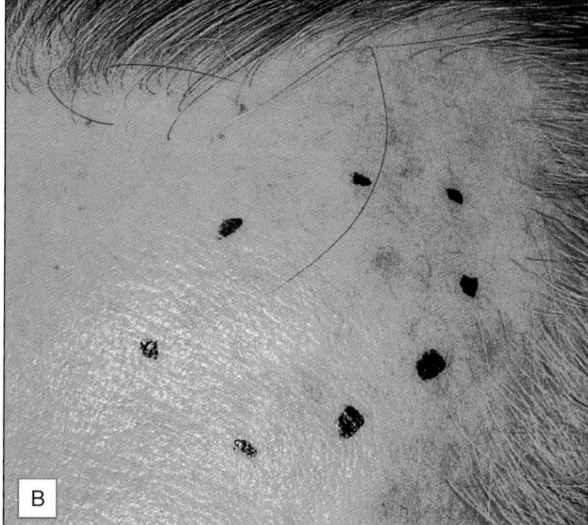

Fig. 6.6 (**A**) A 63-year-old man with an AK on the forehead. (**B**) Appearance 1 year after Levulan® BLU-U® PDT

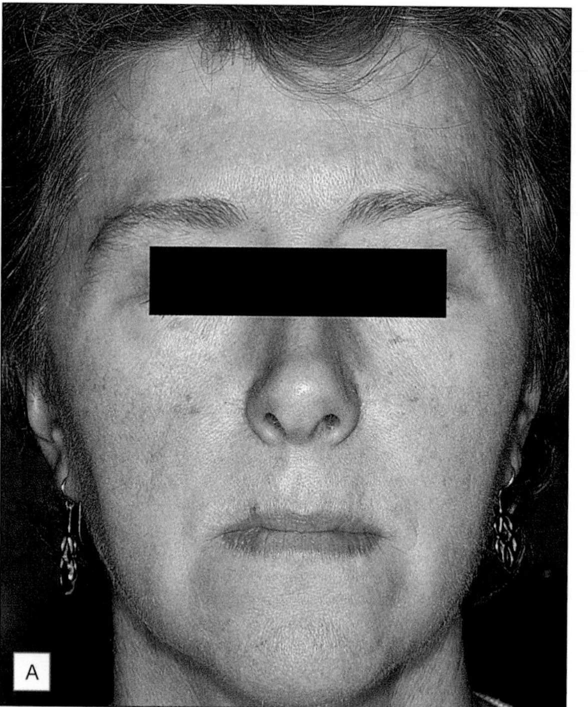

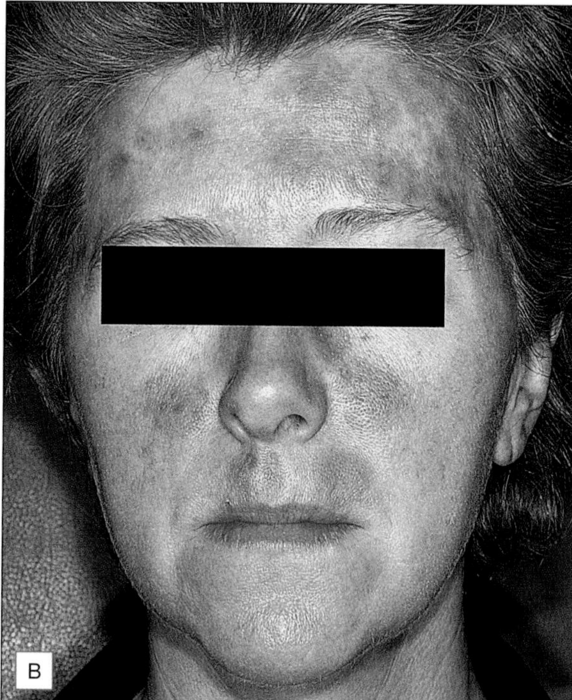

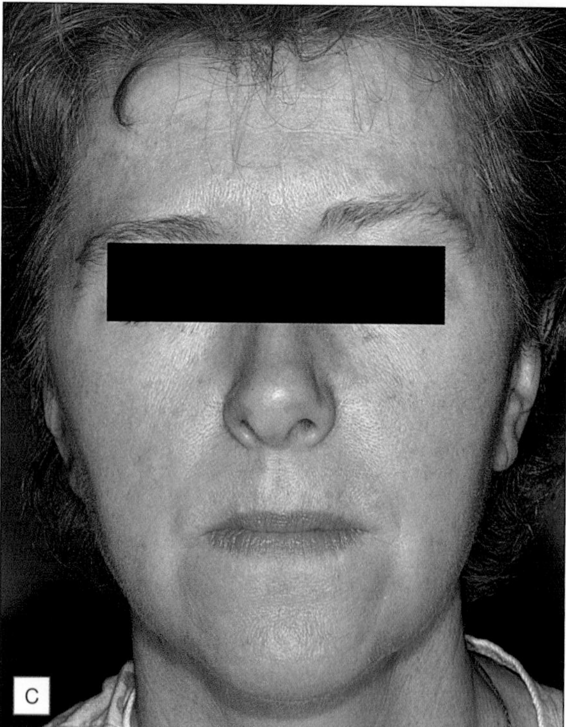

Fig. 6.7 (**A**) A 45-year-old woman with type I skin before treatment. (**B**) Immediately after 24-h Levulan® application and Vbeam® treatment. (**C**) At 1-week follow-up, with erythema resolved

efficacy of the IPL in treating both AK and photodamage. A total of 17 patients with more than three AKs and signs of photodamage on the face had Levulan applied for 1 h followed by IPL therapy using a 560-nm filter and double pulse of 3.0 ms and 6.0 ms with a 10-ms delay. Of all AKs, 68% cleared after one treatment and significant improvements were seen in photodamage scores. Gold et al obtained similar results in a split-face comparison of ALA-PDT-IPL to IPL alone for the treatment of AK and photodamage. ALA was applied to one-half of the face for 30–60 min, and then the entire face was covered with a 2–3-mm layer of coupling gel. The entire face was irradiated with the IPL using a 550–570-nm filter, at 34 J/cm^2, double pulsing with a 20-ms delay, 8 × 16-mm spot size, and 6–7 s between pulses. Three treatments were administered at 1-month intervals. At the 3-month follow-up the AK clearance rate was 78% on the side of the face treated with ALA-PDT-IPL compared to 53.6% for the IPL alone. There also was greater improvement for all photoaging parameters with ALA-PDT + IPL. In an interesting preliminary study of very low-dose PDT, Zelickson et al used 1-h ALA application with a chemoluminescent patch (5 cm in diameter) as a light source. The patch emits a broad band of blue light (peak emission 431–515 nm wavelength, 55.6 mJ/cm^2 over 20 min). For a single treatment session (> 60 min), three blue patches were applied to the treatment area, delivering a total light dose of only 1.7 J/cm^2. The percent clearances for all subjects ranged from 36 to 100%.

Combination therapies are being investigated to increase efficacy and decrease ALA-PDT side effects. Akita et al propose combining cyclooxygenase (COX)-2 inhibitors and ALA-PDT because 60% of AKs were found to be high expressers of COX-2. Another interesting approach precedes PDT with a short course of 5-FU. Gilbert applied 5-FU nightly for 5 days, and then on the sixth day administered ALA-PDT. ALA was applied for 30–45 min and an IPL light source was used. At a 1-month and 1-year follow-up, 14 of 15 patients achieved a 90% resolution of all treated AKs.

The methyl ester of ALA (MAL; Metvix, PhotoCure ASA, Oslo, Norway) is a topical photosensitizer approved in Europe for the treatment of AKs. The more hydrophobic methyl ester may have increased skin penetration, although it requires conversion to ALA by tissue esterases for activity. Pariser et al used Metvix to treat AK on the face and scalp after a 3-h application with a red light source (570–670 nm). Individual lesions were pre-treated with gentle curettage, and Metvix applied under occlusion. A response rate of 89% was found at a 3-month follow-up after two treatments; the complete response rate for placebo-PDT was 38%. Freeman et al found similar results in a study comparing Metvix-PDT with cryotherapy. In addition, Draviega et al found Metvix-PDT to be safe and effective in treating AK in transplant recipients. An overall lesion complete response rate of 90% was found at a 4-month follow-up after two treatments; the overall lesion complete response rate for placebo-PDT was 0%. In contrast, Szeimis et al found only a 69% response rate for lesions treated on the face, scalp, and other locations after one treatment at a 3-month follow-up, using Metvix with a 3-h application without pre-treatment and a 570–670-nm light. The disparity in clearance rates between the studies may be due to the number of treatments performed or the differences in pre-treatment.

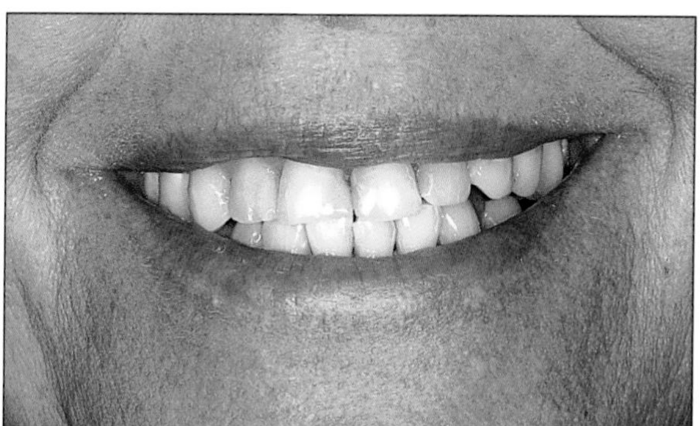

Fig. 6.8 Patient with actinic cheilitis 6 months after one treatment with Levulan® and Vbeam® laser. The pre-treatment image is Figure 6.2

Although the major clinical trials have been on AKs, case reports document efficacy in treating actinic cheilitis. The high permeability of the lip to Levulan permits short application times. Figure 6.2 shows the initial lesion of a typical patient treated by us with short application time ALA followed by PDL illumination, and Figure 6.8 shows the complete clinical resolution of the lesion 6 months after a single treatment with excellent cosmesis.

COMFORT AND CONVENIENCE

In contrast to topical chemotherapeutic agents, ALA-PDT does not require prolonged application of topical agents that can cause significant morbidity. The discomfort is limited to mild burning or pruritus with drug application, and pain during light therapy that resolves within 24 h. Erythema and desquamation generally resolves within 7–10 days, but may extend to 4 weeks. A typical response to treatment is illustrated in Figure 6.9. The patient is a 50-year-old woman with multiple AKs on the anterior chest. Figure 6.9A shows the nonhyperkeratotic lesions at the initial visit; and Figure 6.9B shows the same area after 24-h Levulan application, prior to laser therapy; some erythema is evident. Figure 6.9C shows the reaction immediately after PDL-PDT, and Figure 6.9D is the response 8 months after two treatments.

One of the major inconveniences with ALA-PDT is the delay between drug application and light delivery. Therefore, Moseley et al examined the feasibility of ambulatory PDT in a pilot study. After the application of ALA at clinic, photoactivation was accomplished by a lightweight, portable LED array light source attached to the lesion.

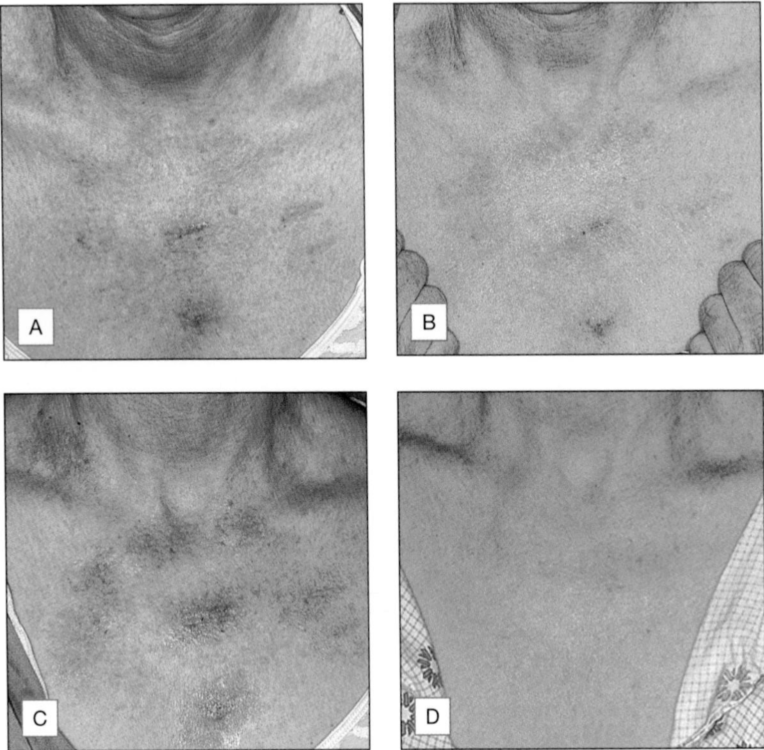

Fig. 6.9 AKs on the chest. (**A**) Before treatment. (**B**) After 24-h Levulan® application (before light). (**C**) Immediately after treatment. (**D**) At 8-month follow-up

COST AND COST/BENEFIT RATIO

In 2006, the average wholesale cost of a Levulan Kerastick is approximately $158, with a Medicare J code reimbursement of $111. One Kerastick is sufficient to cover the face, scalp, and neck, or both forearms or anterior lower legs with two passes each. Treatments often are charged per anatomic area with the cost of the Kerastick built in. Average patient charges for a face and scalp vary with geographic location, but may range from $400–700 or more per treatment. PDT requires a light source. The BLU-U is relatively inexpensive, and the PDL and IPL have multiple uses in addition to PDT. The overall cost of a Levulan-PDT treatment is similar to that of 5-FU or imiquimod. The typical cost for a 40-g tube of 5-FU in the form of Efudex is about $227, and an average treatment may require at least this amount to be applied over 2–4 weeks in addition to two or more office visits. Imiquimod costs approximately $206 for a box of 12 single-use packets. A typical treatment requires three boxes of packets applied over a 12–16-week period ($618), in addition to two to four office visits.

While the costs of the wide area AK treatments are similar, there are definite benefits associated with ALA-PDT. With PDT, complete recovery may take from less than 1 week to 2 weeks, and patients typically may resume normal activities within a few hours of treatment or the next day. By contrast, treatment time with topical chemotherapy or immunotherapy is prolonged. In addition, ALA-PDT allows more physician control of the treatment and enhanced patient compliance.

OVERVIEW OF TREATMENT STRATEGY

Topical ALA-PDT is more effective for thin AK on sun-damaged skin than for hypertrophic AK. ALA uptake and PpIX synthesis increase with longer application times. Thin lesions may respond well to short application times while hypertrophic thick lesions may be better treated with longer ALA applications. Decisions about application times also are affected by patient comorbidities and preferences, office practice considerations, and available light sources. Units that deliver higher absorbed light doses, such as the BLU-U, are more effective with shorter drug application times that result in overall lower PpIX concentrations in target cells. PDL and IPL sources delivering lower absorbed light doses may require longer times. Since our patients often have hyperkeratotic AK on their extremities and tend to prefer fewer, more aggressive treatments, we generally use 18–24-h drug application followed by 595-nm Vbeam, VersaClear or BLU-U therapy.

Box 6.1 Patient questionnaire

Extent of the problem
1. Where are your AKs located? (Face/scalp/arms/legs/body)
2. How many AKs do you have? (A few/moderate number/many)
3. Are your AKs thick or scaly? (None/some/many)

Prior therapy
4. Have you had treatment for AKs in the past? (If yes, with what?)
5. Have you had treatment in the past 2 months? (Yes/no)
6. Have you previously used 5-fluorouracil (5-FU, Efudex or Carac), or Aldara? (Yes/no)
   If so, have you had any problems with the treatment or with healing? (Yes/no)
7. Have your lesions been treated with freezing in the past? (Yes/no)
   If yes, were you pleased with the result? (Yes/no)
8. Have you ever had PDT? (Yes/no)

Lifestyle preferences
9. In addition to the treatment of your AKs, are you interested in the possibility of skin rejuvenation? (Yes/no)
10. Would you like to have your whole face treated to eliminate early AKs that are too small to see and possibly reduce photoaging, or would you prefer just treatment of the visible AKs? (Visible AKs only/whole face treated)
11. Do you prefer fewer, "stronger" treatments that may make your skin more red and take longer to heal, or a greater number of more "gentle" treatments?
12. Can you accommodate a treatment where the medication is applied in the afternoon and you are treated the next day, or do you prefer one in which the medication is applied and you are treated after a 1–4-h interval on the same day?
13. Do you use sunscreen? (Never/occasionally/frequently/every day)

Medical history
14. List your medications (prescription, nonprescription and any herbal supplements)
15. Do you have Lupus or an immune system disease? (Yes/no)
16. Have you had an organ transplant? (Yes/no)
17. Are you on immunosuppressive therapy? (Yes/no)
18. Do you have porphyria? (Yes/no)

• Treatment approach

PATIENT INTERVIEWS

Box 6.1 shows a sample patient questionnaire that can help establish suitability of ALA-PDT and the treatment plan.

LIGHT SOURCES

BLU-U

The BLU-U is the least expensive light source. The light's output is strongly absorbed by PpIX in keratinocytes above the dermal vasculature. Thus, in most patients, overnight ALA application leads to PpIX levels too high to permit full-face or scalp application; this interval generally should be reserved for spot treatments and for hyperkeratotic lesions. Shorter applications of 1–4 h allow treatment of the full face or scalp. It is often not necessary to deliver the full 10 J/cm^2 (16.6-min treatment). It may be adequate to periodically interrupt illumination and look at the skin, treating until there is mild erythema at the AK. Note that the shape of the BLU-U is optimized for facial and scalp lesions (Fig. 6.10). It can be used for the hands and feet, but is less practical for the trunk and extremities.

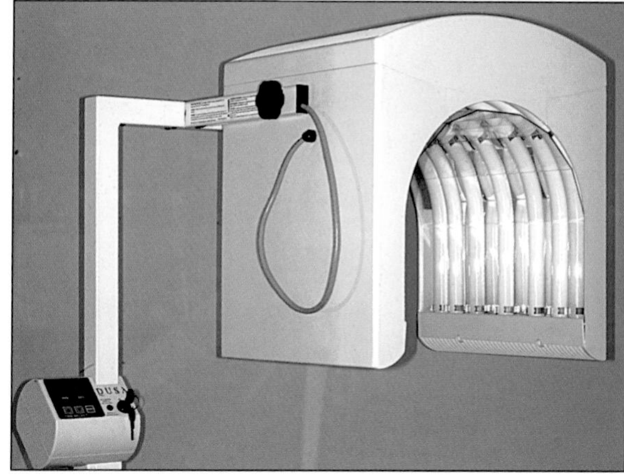

Fig. 6.10 The BLU-U® (Reproduced with permission of DUSA, Inc)

PDL and IPL

Compared to the BLU-U, the long PDL and IPL are less efficient sources for ALA-PDT of AK, but adequate efficacy can be obtained with appropriate skin preparation and ALA application time. Again, these factors may need to be adjusted for individual patients. The time required to treat an entire face can be shorter than that used with the BLU-U with a 10-J/cm^2 light dose. Both the PDL and IPL can be used for a range of ALA-PDT and non-PDT indications. There currently are no available data favoring one over the other for PDT, and a choice between them would depend on other factors, including physician preference. Figure 6.11 shows the Vbeam PDL being used to treat extensively damaged skin on a forearm.

EQUIPMENT

ALA-PDT requires a standard patient examination room with appropriate light source(s) for PpIX activation. A power table is useful, but not essential. We dispense the Levulan Kerasticks. Some practitioners have the patient obtain the drug by prescription from a pharmacy. One Kerastick usually is sufficient to cover a face and scalp, bilateral upper extremities, or bilateral lower extremities with two drug applications.

Patients having short application time treatments should be provided with a waiting area that has low levels of ambient light to avoid possible phototoxic reactions after ALA application.

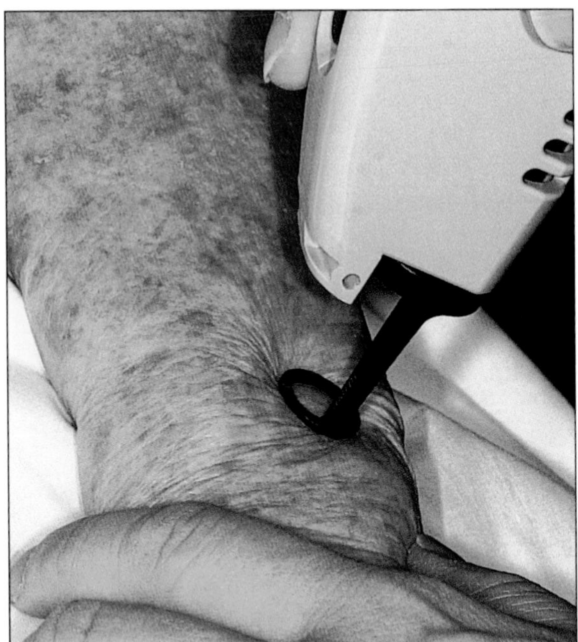

Fig. 6.11 Vbeam® laser being used to treat AKs on the forearm (Reproduced with permission of Candela Corporation)

Staffing requirements during treatment consist of a physician and a nurse or assistant. The physician generally performs the initial assessment, skin preparation, and drug application. The nurse or assistant can run the BLU-U. Depending on USA state regulations, nurses or assistants may be able to carry out the laser treatments.

• Treatment algorithm

A flow chart of treatment decisions is shown in Figure 6.12.

SKIN PREPARATION PRIOR TO DRUG APPLICATION

As previously discussed, hypertrophic lesions present a barrier to both drug and light penetration. The barrier can be decreased by removal of lipid with acetone and/or physical removal of the stratum corneum by curetting or gently sanding the lesions with 3M Red Dot EKG tape (Fig. 6.13), or by microdermabrasion. Sanding can be done on single lesions, or alternatively, entire anatomic areas can be pre-treated. Gentle pressure should be applied to avoid damage to the surrounding epidermis (Fig. 6.14). In addition, for hyperkeratotic AK, keratolytic agents such as 40% urea cream can be prescribed for use several weeks prior to drug application. According to Touma et al, these

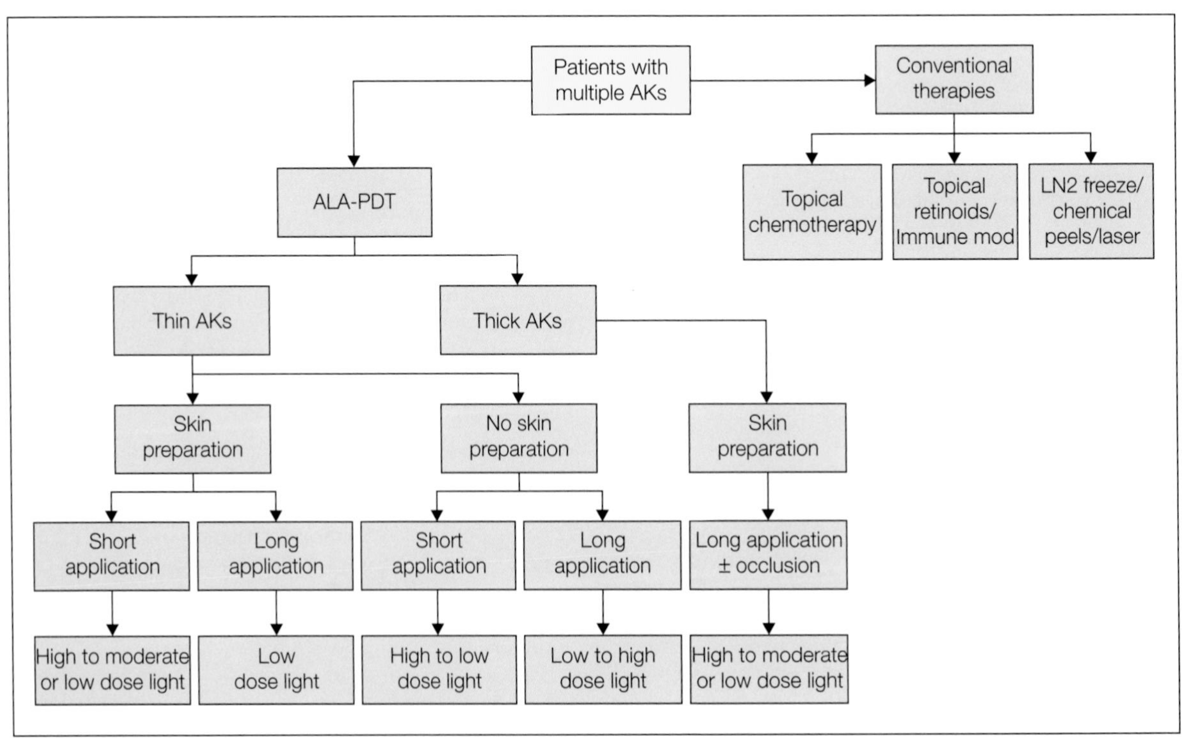

Fig. 6.12 Treatment algorithm

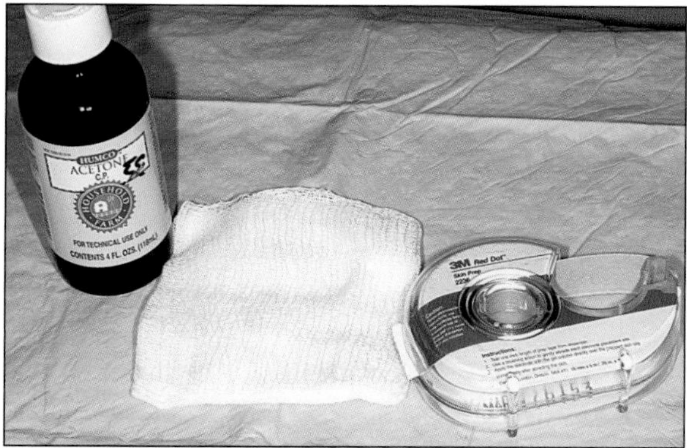

Fig. 6.13 Acetone and 3M™ RedDot™ Trace Prep 2236 tape for skin preparation (Reproduced with permission of 3M Healthcare)

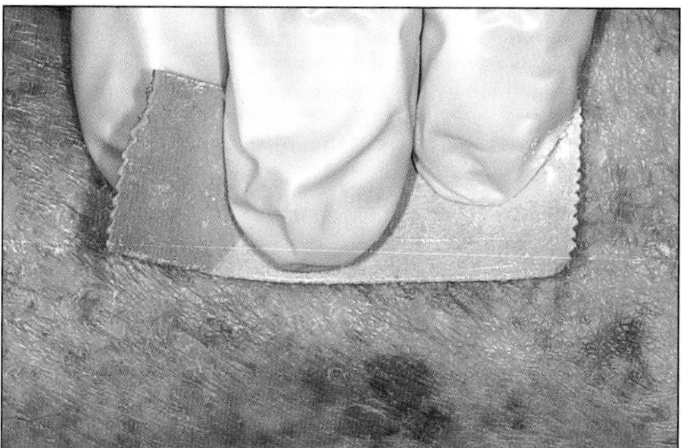

Fig. 6.14 Gentle thinning of the stratum corneum with 3M™ EKG tape

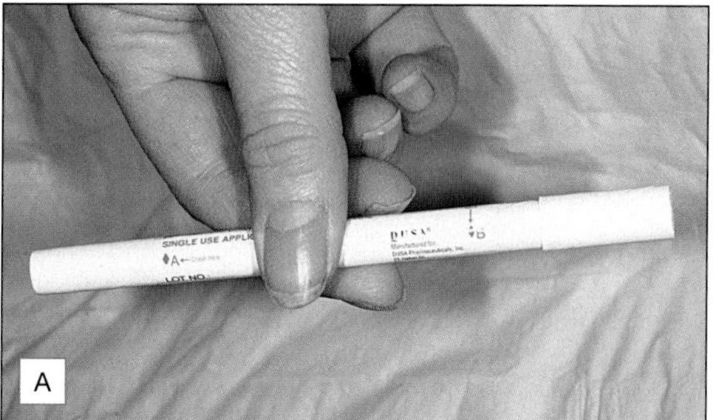

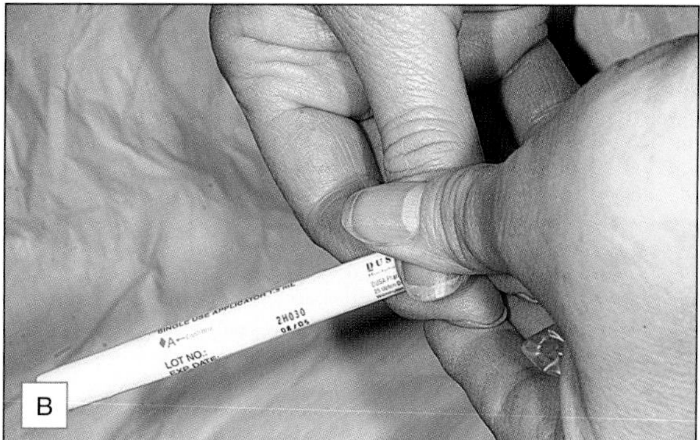

Fig. 6.15 (A) Levulan® Kerastick®. (B) Crushing the Kerastick® ampules (Reproduced with permission of DUSA, Inc)

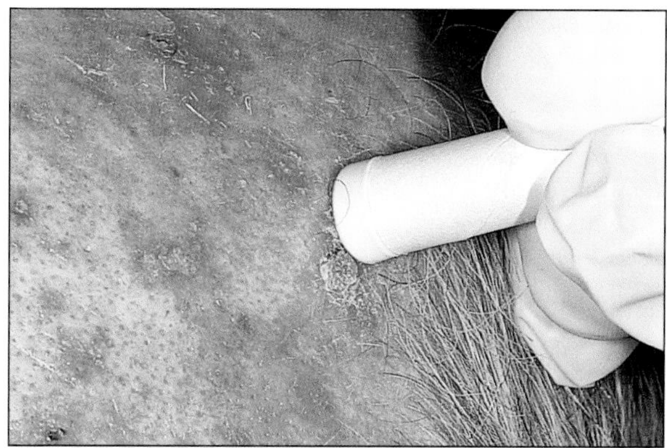

Fig. 6.16 Proper Levulan® application technique with the Kerastick® held perpendicular to the skin (Reproduced with permission of DUSA, Inc)

agents do not appear to benefit thin AK. Applying a transparent cream or gel, or mineral oil to hyperkeratotic AK prior to light treatment will reduce light scattering and increase the effective light dose.

DRUG APPLICATION TECHNIQUE

Proper application is essential for optimal target cell PpIX accumulation. The Levulan Kerastick is composed of two crushable ampules. The bottom ampule (labeled A) contains the solution vehicle and should be crushed first. Ampule B, containing the ALA, should then be crushed starting at the top and moving down toward ampule A (Fig. 6.15). The Levulan Kerastick should be held between the thumb and forefinger with the cap pointing away from the face, and shaken gently for at least 3 min to ensure complete mixing of the contents. The cap is then removed and the drug is applied to the target lesions or entire anatomic areas by gently dabbing with the applicator tip (Fig. 6.16). Once the solution has air-dried, a repeat application should be performed. For thick or resistant lesions it may be helpful to reapply the Levulan a third time. ALA is transported into the stratum corneum only until the vehicle has dried, although additional transport will occur if the site is hydrated by occlusion. The Kerastick should not be applied to the periocular area or to mucous membranes. Once activated, the Kerastick should be discarded after 2 h.

BLU-U

The Levulan Kerastick is applied to clean, dry skin either 14–18 h or 1–4 h before the patient is placed under the BLU-U, with appropriate eye protection. It takes 16 min

40 s to deliver the "standard" 10-J/cm^2 light dose, but shorter times (e.g. 8–12 min) may be adequate.

PDL AND IPL

For long application times, ALA is applied overnight for 14–24 h, and the patient returns the following day for laser therapy. For short application times, ALA is applied for 1–4 h. For the PDL, we use the Candela Vbeam laser at subpurpuric thresholds. The settings include a 10-mm spot size, 6-ms pulse duration, 7.5-J/cm^2 pulse energy, and cryogen spray settings of 30/10. Since patient skin type varies, it is suggested that a test spot be performed to ensure subpurpuric light doses. Hyperkeratotic lesions can be double or triple pulsed. With this method, either entire anatomic areas or discrete lesions can be treated. The overall approach to the IPL generally is similar to that for the PDL. Typical treatment parameters are 560-nm cut-off filter using a double pulse of 3.0 ms and 6.0 ms at 35 J/cm^2. Aggressive PDT can cause usually temporary hair loss, so the eyebrows and the beard area in men should be avoided with the pulsed sources. For both the PDL and IPL, subsequent illumination with a wide area blue light source for 5–10 min can be used to photobleach any remaining PpIX and treat areas skipped with the pulsed sources.

PATIENT PRECAUTIONS

Patients must protect the photosensitive areas from exposure to sunlight or bright indoor lighting (examination lights, tanning booths, dental examination lamps, etc.) prior to light treatment. Broad-spectrum sunscreen offers partial protection against UVA and violet light photoactivation, but will not fully protect the patient as it will not block visible light. The ambient light photoactivation reaction may lead to stinging, burning, and erythema at the drug application sites. The patient should also be cautioned not to wash the areas after drug application and prior to light treatment. After therapy, sunscreen should be applied to the treated areas in the office prior to discharge. Patients should maintain the sun and bright light precautions for the next 24–48 h to avoid phototoxic reactions from residual PpIX.

PAIN CONTROL MEASURES

Prior to therapy, patients can be given nonsteroidal anti-inflammatory drugs (NSAIDs) or acetaminophen, topical anesthetics such as EMLA cream (AstraZeneca), or cooled xylocaine gel. It should be noted that EMLA cream is pH 9 and ALA is unstable at pH greater than 4.5, so EMLA should not be applied directly after Levulan. Also, Langan et al found no significant difference in mean pain scores when comparing EMLA cream to placebo during the treatment of scalp AK. During treatment, the use of dynamic cooling devices on most lasers helps to decrease pain and epidermal damage. For lamp illuminations, a cooling fan directed at the treatment site is very effective in decreasing discomfort. Post-therapy, patients can use ice packs and NSAIDs or acetominophen as needed. PDT will degranulate mast cells, so patients with type I skin generally will benefit from an antihistamine such as diphenhydramine (Benadryl) prior to light therapy.

• Side effects, complications, and safety profile

Patients have variable skin responses to ALA-PDT. Some sense of the phototoxic reaction is evident immediately after therapy, with the maximal effect peaking at 24 h. If there is inadequate treatment response and minimal phototoxicity, the PDT dose needs to be increased by either increasing the Levulan application time and/or giving more light. More aggressive skin preparation may also help. Conversely, if an exuberant reaction occurs with a laser or the patient experiences extreme discomfort with the BLU-U, the Levulan application time or the light dose may need to be decreased.

No noncutaneous adverse events have been reported in association with ALA-PDT for the treatment of AKs. The most common side effect during treatment is a burning, stinging pain, likely due to activation of PpIX that has accumulated in cutaneous nerve endings. The pain is mild to moderate and occasionally severe, depending on the patient, area treated, and PDT dose. Pain generally is minimal with the PDL or IPL, or with the BLU-U and short ALA applications.

The pain usually subsides within 1–24 h after treatment. Because there can be damage to cutaneous nerves, some patients may notice a slight, transient decrease in sensation. In our experience, this always resolves.

The most common reaction after treatment is erythema, mild edema, and desquamation that resolves in 1–2 weeks. The reaction can be significant: Figure 6.17A shows a facial AK on a 65-year-old man before 24-h Levulan application. Figure 6.17B shows a severe erythematous edematous reaction after PDL-PDT with the Vbeam laser. Crusting purpura or scarring are very rare occurrences. Particularly after prolonged application, ALA-induced PpIX in the skin can cause phototoxic reactions from ambient light exposure before treatment, ranging from mild erythema (e.g. Fig. 6.9.B) to severe erythema and edema. If a pre-treatment phototoxic reaction occurs, it may photobleach the PpIX so there will not be a significant additional erythematous response following light treatment. This phototoxicity generally resolves within 5–10 days. In some cases, if the PDL or IPL does not fully photobleach the PpIX, ambient light may cause additional phototoxicity after treatment.

There may be damage to sebaceous glands, resulting in temporarily drier skin that can be relieved with moisturizers. With damage to the skin barrier, infection is a possible, though uncommon, complication. Routine use of either topical or oral antibiotics is not recommended. Lesions that do not respond to two treatments should be biopsied to rule out SCC.

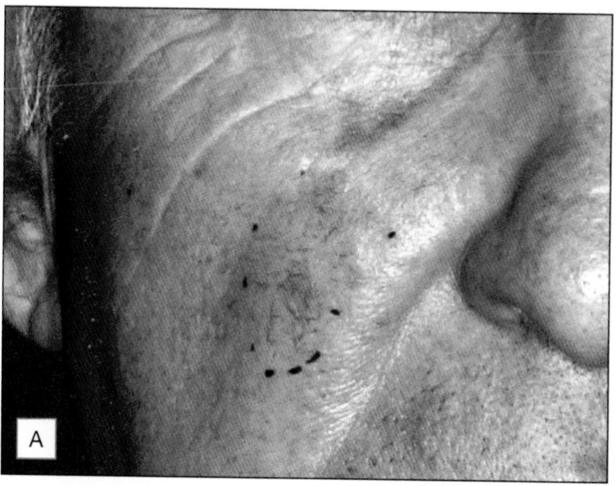

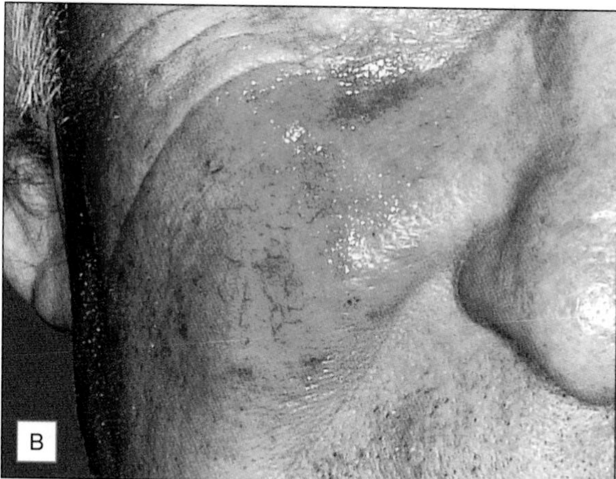

Fig. 6.17 A 65-year-old man. (**A**) Before treatment of AK on cheek. (**B**) Exuberant reaction immediately after therapy with PDL and 24-h Levulan® application

• Pitfalls

The treating physician should always be aware of the following:

- Always have a low threshold for biopsy of suspicious lesions in organ transplant recipients or immunosuppressed patients.
- Any lesion that does not heal after multiple treatments should also be biopsied.
- To avoid purpura or blistering when using the PDL or IPL, always use a test spot to confirm that you are delivering a subpurpuric light dose.
- Always consider the clinical behavior of a lesion, regardless of biopsy result. A superficial biopsy may miss a more aggressive tumor.

CONCLUSION

ALA-PDT for the treatment of pre-malignant lesions is safe and effective. It is easily accomplished in the office setting. There have been no systemic adverse events reported in association with this therapy. The added benefit of ALA-PDT is the photorejuvenation effect without adverse side effects or invasive procedures. It is cost-effective when multiple lesions and broad areas can be treated. Re-treatments may be required within intervals of months. Patient acceptance is high. More controlled clinical trials are required to elucidate the optimal drug application times and light doses using the different sources available in a clinical setting.

FURTHER READING

Akita Y, Kozaki K, Nakagawa A et al 2004 Cyclooxygenase-2 is a possible target of treatment approach in conjunction with photodynamic therapy for various disorders in skin and oral cavity. British Journal of Dermatology 151:472–480

Alexiades-Armenakas MR, Geronemus RG 2003 Laser-mediated photodynamic therapy of actinic keratoses. Archives of Dermatology 139:1313–1320

Avram DK, Goldman MP 2004 Effectiveness and safety of ALA-IPL in treating actinic keratoses and photodamage. Journal of Drugs in Dermatology 3:S36–S39

Babilas P, Kohl E, Maisch T et al 2006 In vitro and in vivo comparison of two different light sources for topical photodynamic therapy. British Journal of Dermatology 154:712–718

Cockerell CJ 2000 Histopathology of incipient intraepidermal squamous cell carcinoma ("actinic keratosis"). Journal of the American Academy of Dermatology 42:S11–S17

Dragieva G, Hafner J, Dummer R et al 2004. Topical photodynamic therapy in the treatment of actinic keratoses and Bowen's disease in transplant recipients. Transplantation 77:115–121

Draviega G, Prinz BM, Hafner J et al 2004 A randomized controlled clinical trial of topical photodynamic therapy with methyl aminolaevulinate in the treatment of actinic keratoses in transplant recipients. British Journal of Dermatology 151:196–200

Freeman M, Vinciullo C, Francis D et al 2003 A comparison of photodynamic therapy using topical methyl aminolevulinate (Metvix) with single cycle cryotherapy in patients with actinic keratosis: a prospective, randomized study. Journal of Dermatologic Treatment 14:99–106

Gilbert DJ 2005 Treatment of actinic keratoses with sequential combination of 5-fluorouracil and photodynamic therapy. Journal of Drugs in Dermatology 4:161–163

Gold MH, Bradshaw VL, Boring MM et al 2006 Split-face comparison of photodynamic therapy with 5-aminolevulinic acid and intense pulsed light versus intense pulsed light alone for photodamage. Dermatologic Surgery 32:795–801

Goldman MP, Atkin DH 2003 ALA/PDT in the treatment of actinic keratosis: spot versus confluent therapy. Journal of Cosmetic and Laser Therapy 5:107–110

Jeffes EW, McCullough JL, Weinstein GD, Kaplan R Galzer SD, Taylor JR 2001 Photodynamic therapy of actinic keratoses with topical aminolevulinic acid hydrochloride and fluorescent blue light. Journal of the American Academy of Dermatology 45:96–104

Langan SM, Collins P. 2006 Randomized, double-blind, placebo-controlled prospective study of the efficacy of topical anaesthesia with a eutectic mixture of lignocaine 2.5% and prilocaine 2.5% for topical 5-aminolaevulinic acid-photodynamic therapy for extensive scalp actinic keratoses. British Journal of Dermatology 154:146–149

Marcus SL, McIntyre WR 2002 Photodynamic therapy systems and applications. Expert Opinion on Emerging Drugs 7:331–334

Moseley H, Allen JW, Ibbotson S et al 2006 Ambulatory photodynamic therapy: a new concept in delivering photodynamic therapy. British Journal of Dermatology 154:747–750

Oseroff AR, Shieh S, Frawley NP et al 2005 Treatment of diffuse basal cell carcinomas and basaloid follicular hamartomas in nevoid basal cell carcinoma syndrome by wide area ALA-PDT. Archives of Dermatology 141:60–67

Pariser DM, Lowe NJ, Stewart DM et al 2003 Photodynamic therapy with topical methyl aminolevulinate for actinic keratosis: Results of a prospective randomized multicenter trial. Journal of the American Academy of Dermatology 48:227–232

Perry R 2004 Current concepts in the management of actinic keratosis. Journal of Drugs in Dermatology 3:S5–S16

Piacquadio DJ, Chen DM, Farber HF et al 2004 Photodynamic therapy with aminolevulinic acid topical solution and visible blue light in the treatment of multiple actinic keratoses of the face and scalp. Archives of Dermatology 140:41–46

Smith S, Piacquadio D, Morhenn V, Atkin D, Fitzpatrick R 2003 Short incubation PDT versus 5-FU in treating actinic keratoses. Journal of Drugs in Dermatology 6:629–635

Szeimis RM, Karrer S, Radakovic-Fijan et al 2002 Photodynamic therapy using topical methyl 5-aminolevulinate compared with cryotherapy for actinic keratoses: a prospective randomized study. Journal of the American Academy of Dermatology 47:258–262

Touma D, Yaar M, Whitehead SM, Konnikow N, Glichrest BA 2004 A trial of short incubation, broad-area photodynamic therapy for facial actinic keratoses and diffuse photodamage. Archives of Dermatology 140:33–40

Zelickson B, Counters J, Coles C, Selim M 2005 Light patch: Preliminary report of a novel form of blue light delivery for the treatment of actinic keratoses. Dermatologic Surgery 31:375–378

7 Treatment of Skin Cancer

Sigrid Karrer, Rolf-Markus Szeimies

INTRODUCTION

Photodynamic therapy (PDT) is a treatment modality with unique properties that make it an appealing procedure for the treatment of nonmelanoma skin cancer. Topical PDT using 5-aminolevulinic acid (ALA) or the methyl ester of ALA (MAL) is based on the photosensitization of the target tissue by ALA- or MAL-induced porphyrins and subsequent irradiation with red light, inducing cell death in a dose-dependent manner via generation of reactive oxygen species (ROS).

Up to now topical ALA-PDT has been successfully used for the management of pre-cancerous lesions, including actinic keratoses (AKs) and Bowen's disease (see Ch. 6), and superficial, nonmelanoma skin tumors, mainly basal cell carcinoma (BCC) and early stages of squamous cell carcinoma (SCC). The efficacy of both ALA- and MAL-PDT in the treatment of patients with AKs and superficial or nodular BCCs has been investigated in several phase II and III clinical trials. In Europe, Australia, South America, and New Zealand MAL (Metvix, Photocure AS, Norway; Galderma SA, France) is approved for the PDT of superficial and nodular BCCs and AKs in combination with red light. In the USA, MAL has been approved (July 2004) for the treatment of AK in combination with red light (marketed under the name Metvixia). ALA (Levulan Kerastick, DUSA, Wilmington, MA) has been approved since 2000 in the USA for PDT of AKs in combination with blue light.

Other potential indications for topical ALA-PDT are cutaneous T-cell lymphoma, metastatic breast carcinoma, and metastasis from malignant melanoma, but for these indications clinical results have been either disappointing or the evidence from the literature is weak. Therefore, in this chapter only the two established indications for topical PDT of skin tumors, BCC and early incipient SCC, will be discussed in detail.

SCC is a malignant, potentially metastasizing tumor arising from the keratinocytes of the epidermis. Cumulative excessive lifetime exposure to sunlight is the major cause of SCC. In situ forms of SCC are AKs or Bowen's disease. SCC begins when atypical keratinocytes break through the basement membrane and begin to invade the dermis. Surgery or radiotherapy are the most common approaches to treat invasive SCC. However, for early invasive SCC, topical ALA-PDT may also be effective and offers pleasing cosmetic results.

BCC is a malignant, but exceedingly rare metastasizing tumor of the skin that arises from basal cells in the epidermis. It is the most common malignant tumor of the skin in white races. BCCs are usually located in sun-exposed areas of the skin: the face, head and neck region, trunk, and upper extremities (Table 7.1). Treatment of BCC depends on tumor size, location, and clinical type (Fig. 7.1).

Nodular BCCs have well-defined borders and grow vertically. Owing to the greater thickness of the tumor, nodular BCCs should be preferentially treated by surgery. Pigmented BCCs do not allow an optimal penetration of light and are therefore not an indication for PDT. Morpheaform BCCs grow with diffuse borders and are often larger than expected. Therefore, the treatment of morpheaform BCC should be surgical, with a preference for Mohs micrographic surgery with pathologic control of excision margins (Fig. 7.2). Superficial BCCs usually occur on the trunk and are often multiple. Several modalities exist for their treatment: cryotherapy, curettage and cautery, cytotoxic agents, radiotherapy, and excisional surgery. Surgery may be complicated by obvious scars and the requirement for complex reconstruction, while cryotherapy and topical chemotherapy may require multiple treatments and may result in poor cosmetic results or recurrence of the tumor. Therefore, topical PDT offers a tissue-sparing modality with excellent cosmesis. Topical PDT with ALA or MAL in patients with superficial BCC achieves clearance rates of up to 100% following a single treatment.

The aim of curative PDT of skin tumors is the complete destruction of the tumor. Owing to the limited penetration of red light into tissue, the thickness of tumors should not exceed 2–3 mm when surface illumination is used. When treating nodular BCCs by single ALA-PDT, the cure rate is rather low (on average below 50%). In order to ameliorate poor outcome after PDT of thicker BCC lesions, ALA-PDT has been performed by Thissen et al 3 weeks after debulking of the tumor. The former tumor areas were excised 3 months later and histopathologically evaluated for residual tumor. Clinically and

Table 7.1 Localization of BCCs

Region	Percent
Head, neck	85
Nose	30
Face	21
Front	15
Ear	7
Trunk, extremities	15

Adapted from Kopf AW Journal of Dermatol 1979; 6:267–281

histologically, a complete response was observed in 92% of the treated lesions.

ALA-PDT can also be used for adjuvant therapy in combination with Mohs surgery, as reported recently by Kuijpers et al. In four patients who underwent Mohs micrographic surgery for extensive BCC, first the central infiltrating tumor part was excised. After re-epithelialization, ALA-PDT of the surrounding tumor rims (2–5 cm) bearing the remaining superficial tumor parts was performed. This led to a complete remission of the tumors with excellent clinical and cosmetic results (follow-up period 27 months).

Remission rates after ALA-PDT probably can be improved by also using other modified treatment modali-

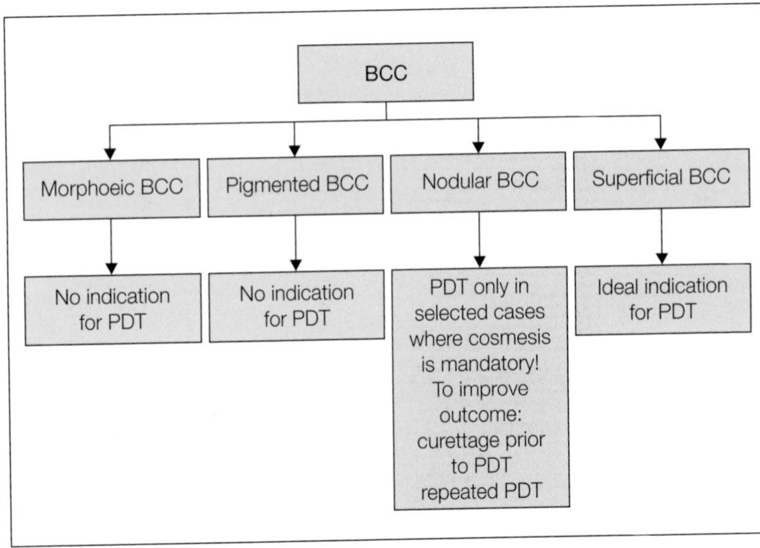

Fig. 7.1 BCC: indication for topical PDT

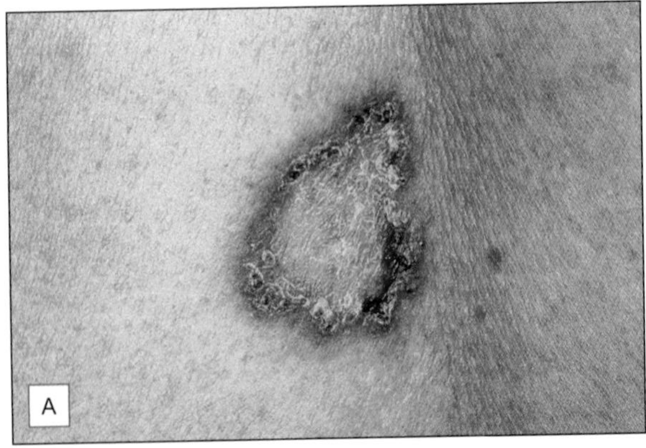

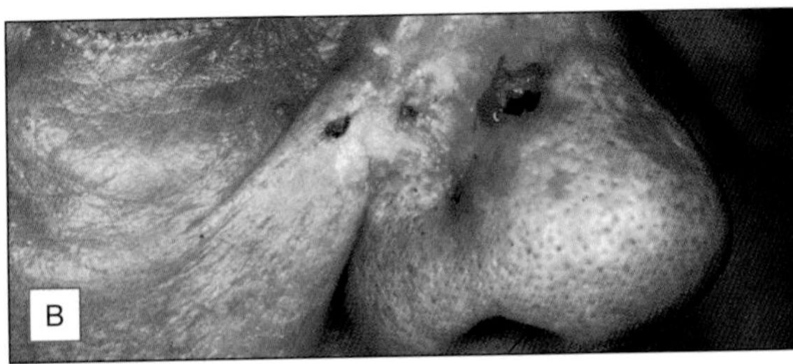

Fig. 7.2 (**A**) Pigmented and (**B**) morpheaform BCC. Both histologic subtypes of BCC are not suitable for topical ALA-PDT

ties, such as repeated treatments or addition of penetration enhancers like dimethyl sulfoxide (DMSO) or ethylenediamine tetra-acetic acid (EDTA).

The methods of PDT are continuously advancing. So far the proven advantages of PDT include comparable clinical outcomes to standard treatments, the simultaneous treatment of multiple tumors and incipient lesions, relatively short healing times, tumor control in immunocompromised patients (i.e. transplant recipients), good patient tolerance, and excellent cosmesis.

PATIENT SELECTION

Except for exclusion of patients with a known history of porphyria or allergic reactions to active ingredients of the applied sensitizers, no severe contraindications for ALA/MAL-PDT are known. ALA/MAL-PDT should be considered in particular for patients who have extensive, widespread or multiple low-risk superficial lesions, such as those in nevoid BCC syndrome. Also, immunosuppressed patients after organ transplantation, who often suffer from multiple lesions, are good candidates for PDT. Elderly patients who would require hospitalization for surgery or in whom radiation therapy would involve multiple daily treatment sessions benefit from PDT, since PDT is usually performed on an outpatient basis, is not invasive, and does not require local anesthesia (Box 7.1).

Box 7.1 Who is the ideal patient for ALA/MAL-PDT?

- Diagnosis of superficial BCC
- Multiple superficial BCCs
- Extensive, large or widespread superficial BCCs
- Nevoid BCC syndrome
- Site of BCC where disfigurement or poor healing from conventional therapies is a risk
- Contraindications for surgery, e.g. anticoagulants
- Immunosuppressed patients after organ transplantation, who suffer from multiple lesions

PDT can be repeated several times, and even in areas with prior exposure to ionizing irradiation PDT is possible.

EXPECTED BENEFITS

ALA-PDT for BCC has been studied extensively in a variety of surveys (Table 7.2). The weighted average of complete clearance rates, after follow-up periods varying between 3 and 36 months, was 87% in 12 studies treating 826 superficial BCCs and 53% in 208 nodular BCCs, as reviewed by Peng et al. Available compiled data by Zeitouni et al from other trials have shown an average of 87% for superficial BCCs, and 48% for nodular BCCs (Figs 7.3–7.5).

MAL-PDT for BCC achieves clearance rates of around 80% for nodular (debulking prior to PDT) and superficial BCC after two PDT sessions administered 7 days apart (Table 7.3).

In a prospective phase III trial comparing ALA-PDT with cryosurgery, Wang et al included 88 superficial and nodular BCCs. A 20% ALA/water-in-oil cream was applied for 6 h under an occlusive dressing, followed by irradiation with a laser at 635 nm (80 mW/cm^2, 60 J/cm^2). In the cryosurgery arm, lesions were treated with liquid nitrogen employing the open spray technique using two freeze–thaw cycles for 25–30 s each time. After 3 months, punch biopsies were performed and revealed a recurrence rate of 25% in the PDT group and 15% in the cryosurgery group. However, the clinical recurrence rates were only 5% for ALA-PDT and 13% for cryosurgery. Besides a better cosmetic outcome, the healing time was also shorter in the PDT-treated group.

Tumor thickness is a determinant of the response of BCC to ALA-PDT. A clearance rate of 100% was achieved by Morton with an ALA application time of 6 h for BCCs less than 2 mm in thickness.

Table 7.2 Summary of results of clinical studies using topical ALA-PDT for the treatment of BCC

Study	Indication/procedure	Number of lesions	Complete remission (%)	Follow-up (months)
Fink-Puches (1998)	Superficial BCC	95	50	36
Morton et al (1998)	Superficial BCC < 2 mm thickness, 6-h incubation	26	100	6–16
Thissen et al (2000)	Nodular BCC (debulking 3 weeks prior to PDT)	24	92	3 (histologic control)
Haller et al (2000)	Superficial BCC (double treatment within 7 days)	2	96	15–45
Wang et al (2001)	Superficial and nodular BCC	44	75 (histologically) 95 (clinically)	3 (histologic control)
Varma et al (2001)	Superficial BCC	61	82	12
Clark et al (2003)	Superficial BCC	87	97	12

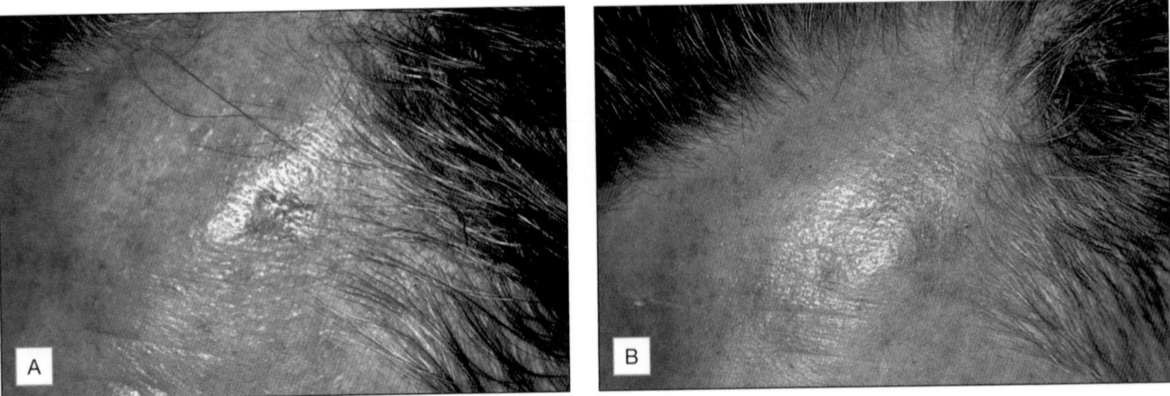

Fig. 7.3 (**A**) A 65-year-old man with superficial BCC on his left forehead prior to ALA-PDT. (**B**) 3 months after a single course of PDT with excellent clinical result—slight erythema only is present

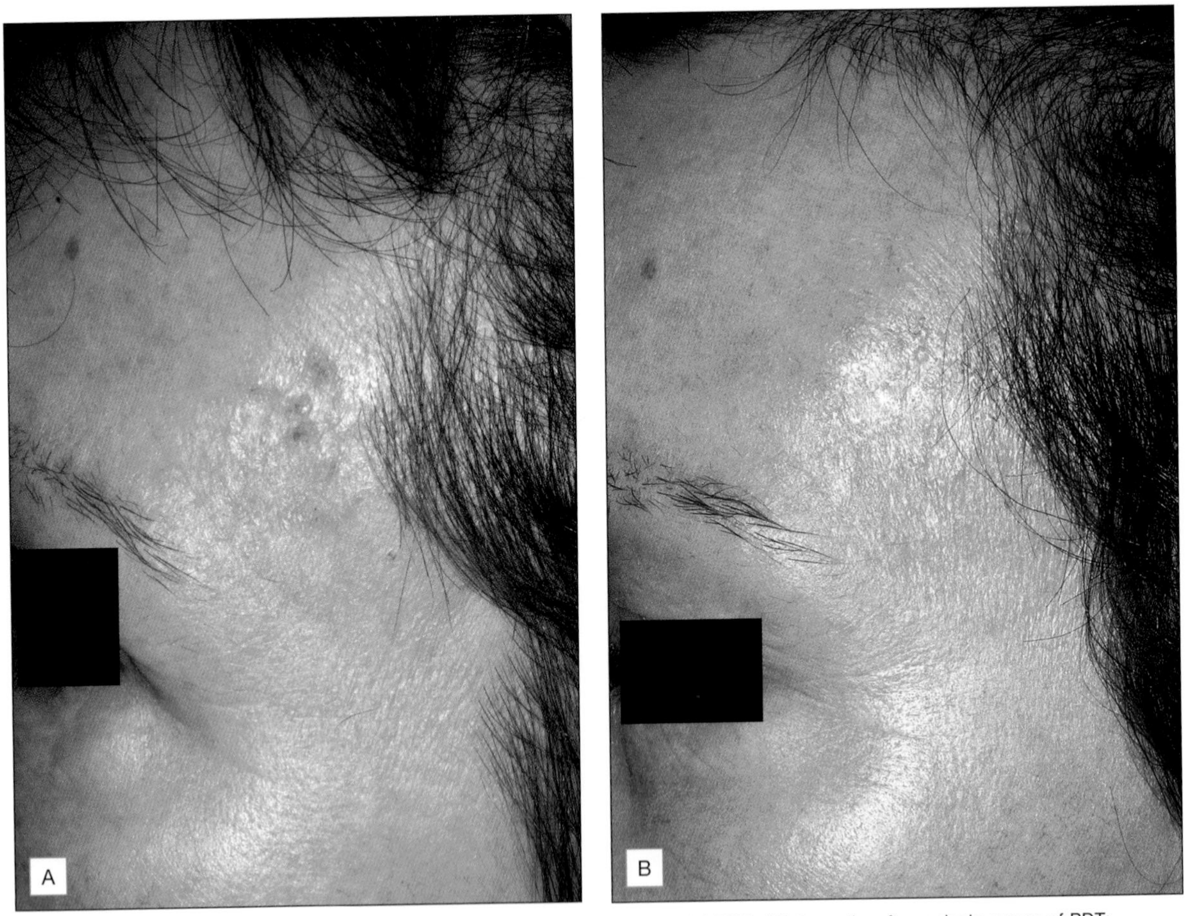

Fig. 7.4 (**A**) A 37-year-old woman with superficial BCC on her left temple prior to ALA-PDT. (**B**) 6 months after a single course of PDT: complete clearance and excellent cosmetic result

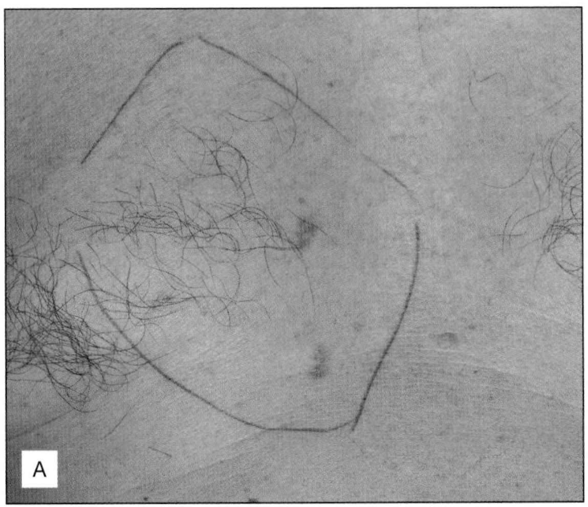

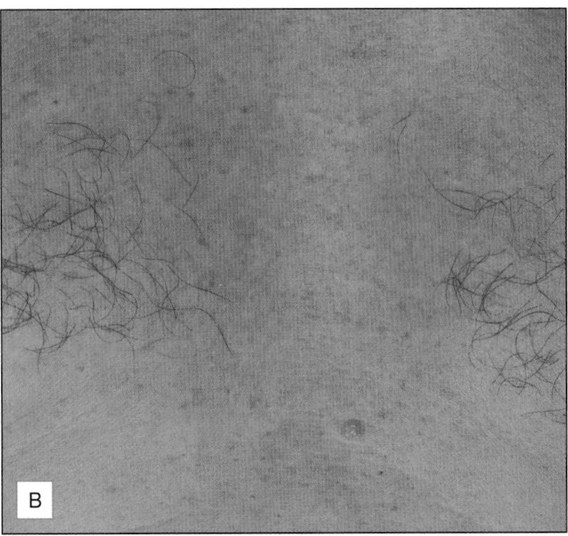

Fig. 7.5 (**A**) A 60-year old man with several superficial BCCs on his right breast prior to MAL-PDT. (**B**) 24 months after two courses of MAL-PDT: complete remission and excellent cosmetic result

Table 7.3 Summary of results of clinical studies using topical MAL-PDT for the treatment of BCC

Study	Indication/procedure	Number of lesions	Complete remission (%)	Follow-up (months)
Soler et al (2001)	Nodular and superficial BCC (debulking of nodular BCC, double treatment within 7 days)	350	79	35
Horn et al (2003)	Nodular and superficial BCC (double treatment within 7 days, nonresponders re-treated after 3 months)	123	82	24
Tope et al (2004)	Nodular BCC (double treatment within 7 days, nonresponders re-treated after 3 months)	56	79	6 (histologic control)
Basset-Seguin et al (2006)	Superficial BCC (single treatment, nonresponders re-treated after 3 months)	60	78	60
Eibenschutz et al (2006)	Large superficial and nodular BCCs (diameter up to 10 cm, re-treatment upon recurrence in 7 cases)	37	81	12
Rhodes et al (2006)	Nodular BCC (double treatment within 7 days, nonresponders re-treated after 3 months)	52	86	60
Vinciullo et al (2006)	"High risk" BCC (double treatment within 7 days, nonresponders re-treated after 3 months)	148	80	48

Although cure rates of up to 100% after PDT of superficial BCC have been shown in several studies, some studies have shown a decrease in the cure rate to 50–60% after long-term follow-up. We have observed recurrences of BCC even after 3 years following ALA-PDT in single patients. Therefore, a long-term follow-up of at least 12 months and preferably 5 years after PDT is mandatory for early detection of recurrent tumors. In the case of tumor recurrence, we would recommend re-treatment by surgery since this therapy allows histologic examination.

There are few studies on ALA-PDT of SCC. Most studies showed recurrence rates of greater than 50%.

Owing to the high recurrence rates and the metastatic potential of SCC, PDT should be reserved for patients with initial SCC in whom surgery is strongly contraindicated or for immunosuppressed patients requiring field reduction of numerous, early, incipient, superficial SCCs prior to more targeted surgical treatment of more invasive, larger SCCs that persist.

Besides clinical efficacy, cost-effectiveness is an important aspect of determining the overall benefit of PDT. Cost analysis indicates that with relatively low costs for permanent equipment, topical ALA/MAL-PDT is comparable in cost to other therapies when morbidity costs of standard treatments are included, and PDT is more economical in patients with multiple tumors who can be treated in a single PDT session.

OVERVIEW OF TREATMENT STRATEGY

• Treatment approach

Patients with superficial nonmelanoma skin tumors, mainly superficial BCC and in selected cases initial SCC, are eligible for ALA/MAL-PDT. The advantages and disadvantages of the different treatment modalities for superficial BCC are summarized in Table 7.4.

PATIENT INTERVIEWS

In order to identify the best therapeutic option for the patient, it is of utmost importance to take a very careful history of the patient. The patient should be asked the following questions:

1. Do you suffer from porphyria or do you know about a specific allergy against active ingredients of the ALA or MAL preparation? (*Reason: to exclude possible risk of induction of porphyria by topical administration of ALA or MAL.*)
2. Do you take anticoagulants or aspirin? (*Reason: to exclude possible bleeding in case of lesion preparation/curettage before PDT; anticoagulation itself is not a contraindication for PDT.*)
3. Do you take antioxidants, which might interfere with the photodynamic reaction? (*Reason: to minimize the risk of presence of high levels of antioxidants [vitamin C, E etc.], which perhaps quench the photodynamic reaction.*)
4. Do you take nonsteroidal anti-inflammatory drugs? (*Reason: to minimize the risk of presence of high levels of suppressors of the arachidonic pathway, which is vital for the inflammatory reaction that contributes to the direct toxic effect of the induction of ROS.*)
5. Do you take other photosensitizing drugs such as antimalarials, diuretics, antibiotics, etc? (*Reason: to minimize the risk of overintensity of the phototoxic effect.*)
6. Do you take HMG-CoA reductase inhibitors (statins) or cytostatic drugs such as hydroxyurea, azathioprine or others? (*Reason: to minimize the risk of prolonged healing/re-epithelialization after PDT.*)

PATIENTS

For patients with a clinical diagnosis of superficial BCC, there are several efficient alternative treatments for therapy of single lesions, including cryotherapy, curettage or surgery. For therapy of multiple superficial BCCs, PDT is a first-line modality (e.g. in basal cell nevus syndrome,

Table 7.4 Advantages and disadvantages of different treatment options for superficial BCC

Treatment	Advantages	Disadvantages
Topical ALA-PDT	Excellent cosmesis Noninvasive Safe Simultaneous treatment of multiple tumors Short healing time Cost effective	Pain during PDT Time consuming No histology
Curretage	Cheap and easy to perform Histology	Local anesthesia Scarring Recurrence rate
Cryotherapy	Cheap and fast to perform	Pain during treatment Blistering Delayed wound healing Scarring Hypopigmentation Skin atrophy No histology
Surgery (simple excision)	Safe Histology	Invasive Local anesthesia Scarring

immunosuppressed patients after organ transplantation). PDT may also be used in patients with a histologic or clinical diagnosis of nodular BCC or a histologic diagnosis of early or incipient SCC, if other established treatment modalities are contraindicated.

EQUIPMENT

PDT is a two-step procedure. For application of the drug, standard material-like bandages or occlusive dressings are necessary. For large, exophytic tumors or extensive hyperkeratosis, pre-PDT debulking with a ring curette or scalpel is required (see Figs 7.6–7.10).

For the second step, a specific light source is necessary.

LIGHT SOURCES

For irradiation of skin cancer, most often incoherent red light sources are used, and these are typically lamps (PDT 1200L, Waldmann Medizintechnik, Germany) or light-emitting diodes (LEDs) (Aktilite, Galderma or Omnilux, Photo Therapeutics Ltd., UK), which match the absorption maxima of the ALA- or MAL-induced porphyrins.

Small areas or single lesions can also be efficiently illuminated with different lasers (e.g. argon-ion pumped-dye lasers [PDLs] at 630 nm, gold vapor lasers at 628 nm, diode lasers) as long as they match the specific absorption maximum of the photosensitizer used. However, the costs of purchase and maintenance of laser systems is greater than for incoherent light sources.

For tissue destruction using ALA-PDT, red light (580–700 nm)—of 120–180 J/cm^2 (100–200 mW/cm^2)—may be chosen. For the more narrow emission spectra of the LED systems (bandwidth approximately 30 nm), the fluence values are significantly lower (37–50 J/cm^2). Therefore, for MAL-PDT using the Aktilite LED system, a light dose of 37 J/cm^2 is recommended both for AK and BCC. In any case, the light intensity should not exceed 200 mW/cm^2 to avoid hyperthermic effects. During

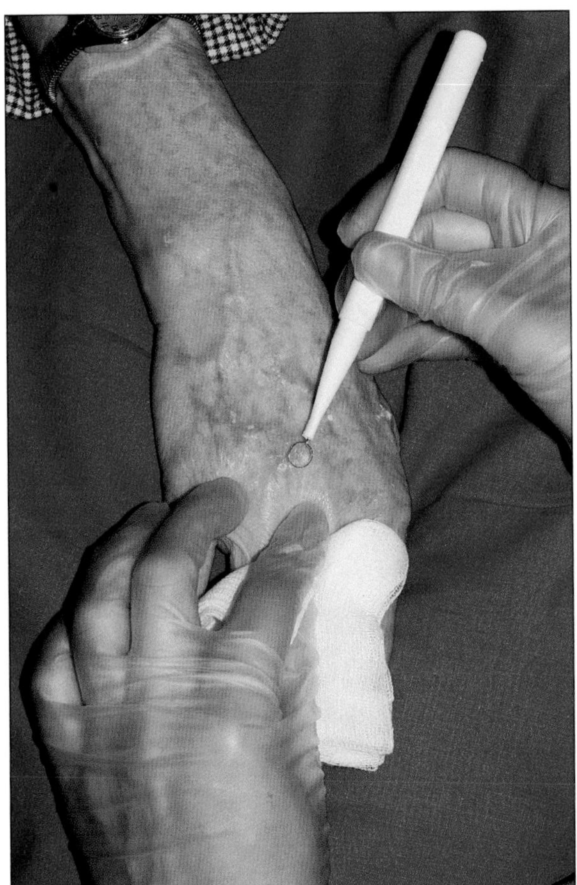

Fig. 7.6 A 74-year-old patient with initial SCC on the back of the hands. Curettage of the hyperkeratotic parts of the tumor with a Stiefel curette

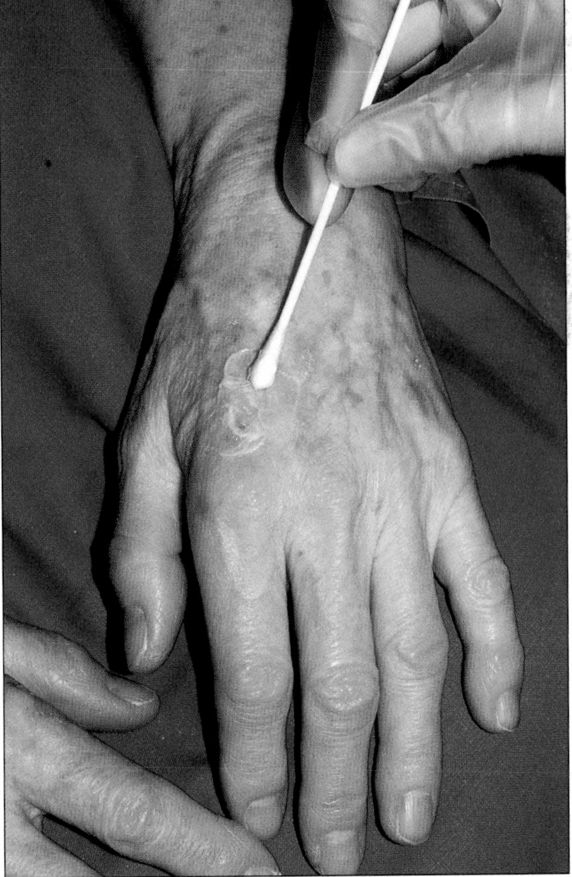

Fig. 7.7 Application of ALA cream (20% ALA in unguentum emulsificans). Either a swab or a wooden spatula can be used for application. Drug should be applied with 1-mm thickness and a minimum of a 0.5–1-cm overlap

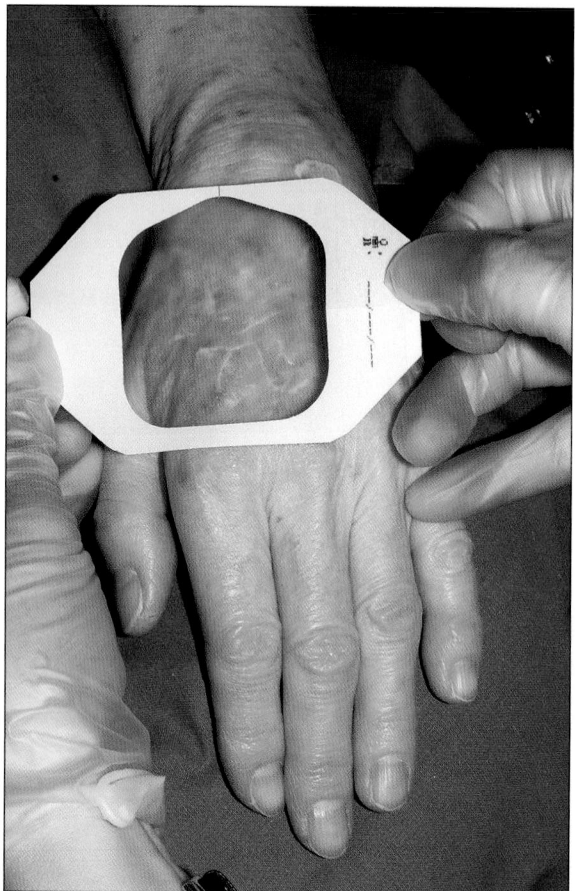

Fig. 7.8 Application of Tegaderm (3M, USA) for occlusion

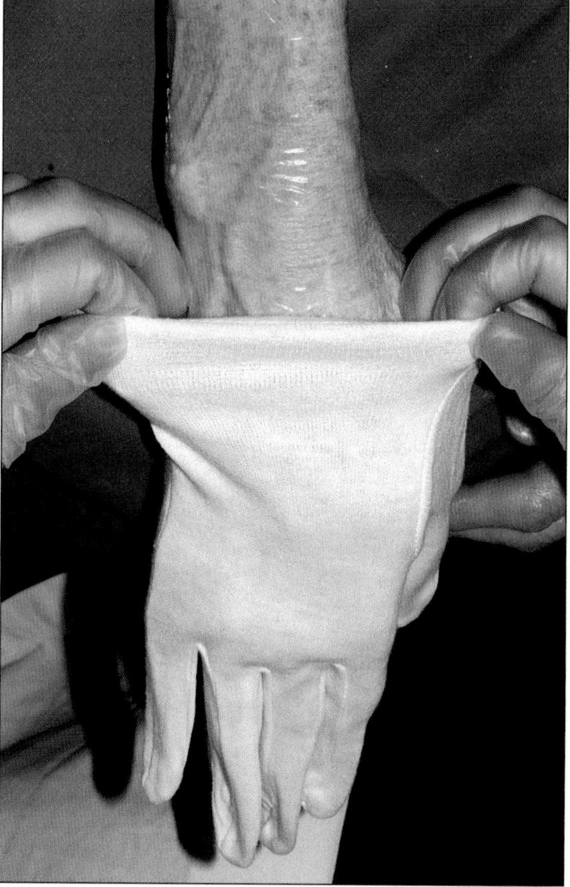

Fig. 7.9 Use of gloves for light protection. In case of lesions on the face, aluminum foil or simply a hat or cap can be used. Direct contact of aluminum foil with ALA-preparation should be avoided due to the acidity of this preparation

illumination, both the patient and clinic staff should wear protective goggles in order to avoid the risk of eye damage.

In a comparative trial it was shown that light at shorter wavelengths is less effective in the treatment of Bowen's disease at a theoretically equivalent dose; therefore, only red light is recommended for PDT of skin tumors in order to maximize tissue penetration.

Meanwhile, intense pulsed light systems (IPL) have been used also for the treatment of skin cancer with PDT. Although these systems offer a very short illumination time and significantly lower pain levels compared to the continuous wave (CW) light sources, their use for the treatment of BCC, SCC or Bowen's disease should be considered carefully. There might be the risk of underexposure of light to certain parts of the tumor due to the small size of the illumination field, which then requires an overlap of the light pulses.

PHOTOSENSITIZER

MAL is more lipophilic than ALA and might therefore result in an increased tumor penetration after topical application. However, Kuijpers et al found no difference in therapeutic outcome (histologically proven) in a short-term efficacy study with ALA- versus MAL-PDT in the treatment of nodular BCCs (follow-up period 2 months).

For the treatment of skin tumors, ALA, usually as hydrochloride (Crawford Pharmaceuticals, UK; Photonamic GmbH, Germany) is applied in custom-made formulations, either oil-in-water creams or gels, at a concentration of 20%. However, no comparative data on different formulations exist. ALA preparations are mostly applied to the lesions under occlusion and, in addition, a light protecting dressing or clothing for 4–6 h prior to irradiation.

For the MAL ointment (Metvix, Photocure AS, Norway; Galderma SA, France), a shorter incubation time of 3 h is sufficient due to its preferential uptake and higher selectivity. The entire area is then covered with an occlusive foil to allow for better penetration.

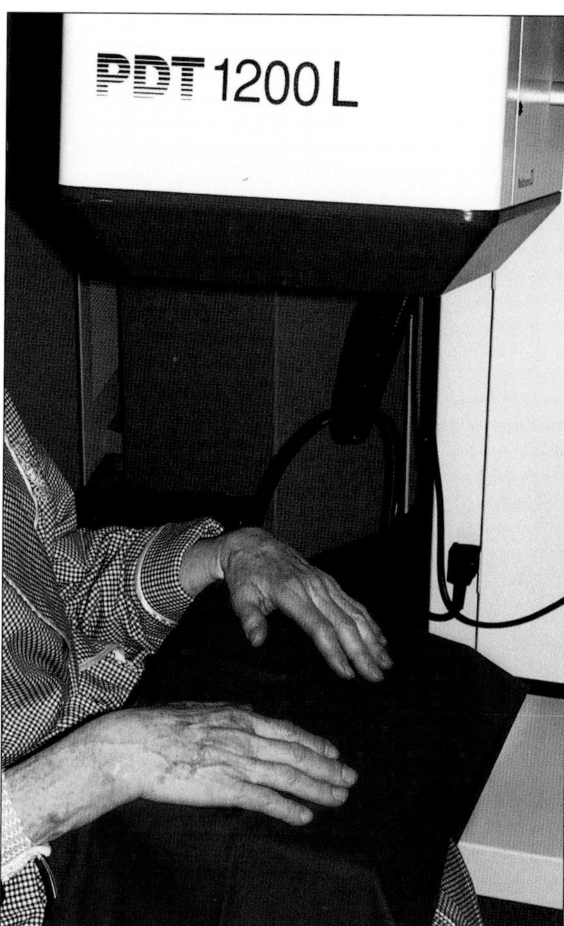

Fig. 7.10 Illumination with incoherent light source after an incubation period of 6 h (Waldmann PDT 1200 L, Waldmann Medizintechnik, Villingen-Schwenningen, Germany)

Enhancement of ALA-PDT has been studied using the penetration enhancer DMSO and the iron chelators desferrioxamine and EDTA, but there are no randomized comparison data.

• Treatment algorithm

1. Check patient eligibility for MAL/ALA-PDT:
   - Check indication (if necessary perform a biopsy to prove the diagnosis)
   - Check exclusion criteria: pregnancy, allergy to components of the MAL/ALA preparation, porphyria, etc
   - Obtain written informed consent
   - Obtain exact documentation of the localization and size of the lesion (photodocumentation prior to therapy might be suitable).
2. Treatment:
   - Select the area to be treated
   - Check whether crusts or prominent tumor parts are present which might be removed prior to the PDT procedure (Fig. 7.6)
   - Apply the 20% ALA formulation or the MAL preparation (1-mm thick) to the lesion with little overlap (about 0.5–1 cm) to the surrounding tissue (Fig. 7.7)
   - Cover the entire area with an occlusive foil to allow better penetration (Fig. 7.8)
   - Then cover the incubated area also with a light protecting dressing or clothing to avoid photobleaching of the induced porphyrins (Fig. 7.9)
   - Advise the patient to come back in 3 h (when MAL is applied) or 4–6 h (when ALA is applied)
   - Remove the dressing and emulsion after 3 h (for MAL) or 4–6 h (for ALA) of incubation
   - Place the lamp/laser the right distance from the lesion (Fig. 7.10)
   - Irradiate with the irradiation parameters advised for the specific illumination system
   - After irradiation cover the lesion to avoid exposure to sunlight
   - Tell the patient that there will be crusting of the lesion 2–3 days following PDT, which will resolve within the next 2 weeks
   - Tell the patient to come back if infection of the treated area or any other problem occurs
   - No specific post-PDT treatment is required besides avoidance of the sun, sun protection with sunscreens for the next 4–6 weeks
   - Careful follow-up is mandatory for early detection of recurrence, and recommended intervals are: 4 weeks after PDT, and 3, 6, 12, 18, 24, and 36 months after PDT
   - If thicker tumors (>3 mm) are treated with ALA-PDT, a second treatment session (3–5 weeks apart) is recommended to improve the therapeutic outcome. For MAL-PDT, a second treatment after 7 days is routinely recommended for all tumors treated.

With red light, superficial lesions can be treated in a single session as described earlier. However, thicker lesions can be treated repeatedly with the same parameters starting 3–5 weeks after the first PDT session. Efficacy of PDT in thicker lesions can also be improved by tissue preparation (debulking) prior to PDT. For tissue preparation, a slight curettage without major bleeding is sufficient.

Irradiation should be performed preferentially with red light due to the likelihood of deeper tissue penetration. Irradiation with blue or green light for skin cancer is contraindicated.

The advantages of PDT as compared to surgery or cryotherapy are the good cosmetic results and good tolerability despite a certain discomfort, particularly when larger areas are treated. Further, large areas can be treated in one session. In an overwhelming majority of patients treated for oncologic indications, PDT is very well accepted.

TROUBLESHOOTING, SIDE EFFECTS, AND COMPLICATIONS

A list of possible complications of ALA/MAL-PDT is provided in Table 7.5.

The well-known stinging or burning sensation during topical PDT is usually well tolerated when small areas are treated. However, in case of larger areas (mostly in severely sun-damaged skin) significant discomfort can make analgesia with metamizole or piritramide, or even general or local anesthesia, necessary. Pain perception can also be alleviated by a fan, cold air stream or by pouring water onto the treated area during the illumination procedure. Application of a tetracaine gel 1-h pre-irradiation did not significantly reduce pain during and after PDT in a randomized, double-blind, placebo-controlled study by Holmes et al. Application of a eutectic mixture of prilocaine/lidocaine (EMLA) should be avoided due to the high pH of this preparation, which might interfere with the acidity of the ALA preparation, leading to a chemical inactivation of the photosensitizer. In addition, topically applied anesthetics also induce local vasoconstriction, which interferes with the generation of sufficient amounts of ROS. Stinging pain and a burning sensation are usually restricted to the time span of illumination and a few hours thereafter.

After light exposure, for several days, localized erythema and edema in the treated area is usually seen, and is followed by a dry necrosis sharply restricted to the tumor. After 10–21 days, formed crusts come off and complete re-epithelialization is observed. During this phase, most patients report only slight discomfort.

The cosmetic outcome of the completely responding lesions is good or very good in most patients. In about 2%, minor scarring occurs, and also uncommon (2%) are pigmentary changes. Some patients experience a temporary pigmentary change with a residual erythematous hue. Irreversible alopecia has not yet been observed in the vast majority of the treated patients; however, due to the concomitant sensitization of the pilosebaceous units, this potential effect should be taken into account.

When treating invasive tumors, e.g. invasive SCC, the lack of a histologic control and the limited depth of tissue penetration of a single topical PDT treatment must be borne in mind. Therefore, usually only superficial lesions should be treated by PDT and regular follow-up is needed to recognize recurrence of the tumor.

Table 7.5 Side effects of ALA-PDT

Frequency	Possible side effects of ALA-PDT
Usually	Stinging or burning sensation during irradiation Localized erythema and edema after irradiation Crusting and dry necrosis of tumor
Occasionally	Stinging or burning for some hours after irradiation
Rarely	Minor scarring Pigmentary changes (usually resolve) Alopecia in the treatment area

TREATMENT TIPS FOR EXPERIENCED PRACTITIONERS

To improve treatment results, several studies have tried various modifications of the treatment protocol (Tables 7.6, 7.7). Several workers proposed double or even multiple ALA-PDT treatments to improve therapy outcome. In contrast to ALA-PDT, topical MAL with PDT is routinely performed twice within 7 days.

For lesions less than 1 cm in diameter, Fritsch et al reported 60%, 80%, and 100% recurrence-free complete response rates with, respectively one, two, and three treatments (follow-up 12–24 months). In this study the treatments were given at 1-month intervals until complete response was achieved. Similarly, Calzavara-Pinton and co-workers repeated ALA-PDT every alternate day (up to a maximum of three treatments) until no tumor was

Table 7.6 Protocol for topical ALA-PDT of nonmelanoma skin cancer

Photosensitizer	20% ALA in water in oil emulsion
Lesion preparation	Debulking of exophytic tumor parts or hyperkeratotic crusts using a curette or scalpel
Application	Topical application with little overlap (about 1 cm) to the surrounding tissue, occlusive and light-impermeable dressing
Incubation time	4–6 h
Light source	Red light from an incoherent lamp or laser emitting 635 nm
Irradiation parameters	Light intensity 100–180 mW/cm^2 Light dose 120–180 J/cm^2
Frequency of treatment	Usually single treatment, for larger or thicker tumors repeated treatments (not established)

Table 7.7 Protocol for topical MAL (Metvix)-PDT of BCC	
Photosensitizer	MAL 160 mg/g topical cream (Metvix)
Lesion preparation	Debulking of exophytic tumor parts or hyperkeratotic crusts using a curette or scalpel
Application	Topical application (1-mm thick, with 0.5–1 cm overlap to the surrounding tissue), adhesive occlusive dressing
Incubation time	3 h
Light source	Red light from an incoherent lamp or LED (light-emitting diode)
Irradiation parameters	For lamp: light intensity < 200 mW/cm^2; light dose 120–180 J/cm^2 For LED: light intensity approx. 50–100 mW/cm^2; light dose 37 J/cm^2
Frequency of treatment	Routinely two sessions 1 week apart, repeated if required at 3-month follow-up

apparent, and achieved a 100% complete response rate at 30 days, with a recurrence rate of 13% over a follow-up period of 24–36 months. Haller et al chose a 7-day interval between initial and second treatment to provide time for maximum photodynamic damage to develop and for some healing to occur between treatments. With a routine double treatment they achieved a complete response rate of 96% after a median follow-up of 27 months.

However, the optimal timing of repeated treatments remains unknown. Whether it is preferable to observe patients regularly and only re-treat when necessary, or to give a standardized double treatment to all patients, is still an open question. Using a routine double treatment would result in about 50% of patients receiving a second PDT that would not have otherwise been required.

FURTHER READING

Basset-Seguin N, Ibbotson S, Emtestam L et al 2006 MAL-PDT vs. cryotherapy for treatment of primary superficial basal cell carcinoma: results of a five years prospective randomized trial. Journal of Investigative Dermatology 126 (Suppl 2):S34

Braathen LR, Szeimies RM, Basset-Seguin N et al 2007 Guidelines on the use of photodynamic therapy (PDT) for non-melanoma skin cancer: an international consensus. International Society for Photodynamic Therapy in Dermatology. Journal of the American Academy of Dermatology 56:125–143

Calzavara-Pinton PG 1995 Repetitive photodynamic therapy with topical delta-aminolevulinic acid as an appropriate approach to the routine treatment of superficial non-melanoma skin tumors. Journal of Photochemistry and Photobiology 29:53–57

Clark C, Bryden A, Dawe R et al 2003 Topical 5-aminolaevulinic acid photodynamic therapy for cutaneous lesions: outcome and comparison of light sources. Photodermatology, Photoimmunology & Photomedicine 19:134–141

Eibenschutz L, Marenda S, Mariani G et al 2006 MAL-PDT in the treatment of large cell basal cell carcinomas. Journal of Investigative Dermatology 126 (Suppl 2):s16

Fink-Puches R, Soyer HP, Hofer A, Kerl H, Wolf P 1998 Long-term follow-up and histological changes of superficial nonmelanoma skin cancers treated with topical delta-aminolevulinic acid photodynamic therapy. Archives of Dermatology 134:821–826

Foley P 2003 Clinical efficacy of methyl aminolevulinate (Metvix) photodynamic therapy. Journal of Dermatologic Treatment 14 (Suppl 3):15–22

Guillen C, Sanmartin O, Escudero A et al 2000 Photodynamic therapy for in situ squamous cell carcinoma on chronic radiation dermatitis after photosensitization with 5-aminolevulinic acid. Journal of the European Academy of Dermatology 14:298–300

Haller JC, Cairnduff F, Slack G et al 2000 Routine double treatments of superficial basal cell carcinomas using aminolaevulinic acid-based photodynamic therapy. British Journal of Dermatology 143:1270–1274

Holmes MV, Dawe RS, Ferguson J et al 2004 A randomized, double-blind, placebo-controlled study of the efficacy of tetracaine gel (Ametop) for pain relief during topical photodynamic therapy. British Journal of Dermatology 150:337–340

Horn M, Wolf P, Wulf HC et al 2003 Topical methyl aminolevulinate photodynamic therapy in patients with basal cell carcinoma prone to complications and poor cosmetic outcome with conventional treatment. British Journal of Dermatology 149:1242–1249

Karrer S, Szeimies RM, Hohenleutner U et al 2001 Role of lasers and photodynamic therapy in the treatment of cutaneous malignancy. American Journal of Clinical Dermatology 2:229–237

Kuijpers DIM, Smeets NWJ, Krekels GAM et al 2004 Photodynamic therapy as adjuvant treatment of extensive basal cell carcinoma treated with Mohs micrographic surgery. Dermatologic Surgery 30:794–798

Kuijpers DI, Thissen MR, Thissen CA, Neumann MH 2006 Similar effectiveness of methyl aminolevulinate and 5-aminolevulinate in topical photodynamic therapy for nodular basal cell carcinoma. Journal of Drugs in Dermatology 5:642–645

Morton CA, Brown SB, Collins S et al 2002 Guidelines for topical photodynamic therapy: report of a workshop of the British Photodermatology Group. British Journal of Dermatology 146:552–567

Morton CA, MacKie RM, Whitehurst C et al 1998 Photodynamic therapy for basal cell carcinoma: effect of tumor thickness and duration of photosensitizer application on response. Archives of Dermatology 134:248–249

Morton CA, Whitehurst C, McColl JH et al 2001 Photodynamic therapy for large or multiple patches of Bowen disease and basal cell carcinoma. Archives of Dermatology 137:319–324

Pagliaro J, Elliott T, Bulsara M et al 2004 Cold air analgesia in photodynamic therapy of basal cell carcinomas and Bowen's disease: an effective addition to treatment: a pilot study. Dermatologic Surgery 30:63–66

Peng Q, Warloe T, Berg K et al 1997 5-ALA based photodynamic therapy. Cancer 79:2282–2308

Rhodes LE, de Rie M, Enström Y et al 2006 A randomized European comparison of MAL-PDT and excision surgery in nodular basal cell carcinoma: results from a 60 month follow-up study. Journal of Investigative Dermatology 126 (Suppl 2):s34

Rowe DE 1995 Comparison of treatment modalities for basal cell carcinoma. Clinical Dermatology 13:617–620

Siddiqui MAA, Perry CM, Scott LJ 2004 Topical methyl aminolevulinate. American Journal of Clinical Dermatology 5:127–137

Soler AM, Warloe T, Berner A, Giercksky KE 2001 A follow-up study of recurrence and cosmesis in completely responding superficial and nodular basal cell carcinomas treated with methyl 5-aminolaevulinate-based photodynamic therapy alone and with prior curettage. British Journal of Dermatology 145:467–471

Soler AM, Warloe T, Tausjo J et al 1999 Photodynamic therapy by topical aminolevulinic acid, dimethylsulphoxide and curettage in nodular basal cell carcinoma: a one-year follow-up study. Acta Dermato-Venerologica 79:204–206

Szeimies RM, Morton CA, Sidoroff A, Braathen LR 2005 Photodynamic therapy for non-melanoma skin cancer. Acta Dermato-Venerologica 85:483–490

Thissen MRTM, Schroeter CA, Neumann HAM 2000 Photodynamic therapy with delta-aminolaevulinic acid for nodular basal cell carcinomas using a prior debulking technique. British Journal of Dermatology 142:338–339

Tope WD, Menter A, El-Azhary RA et al 2004 Comparison of topical methyl aminolevulinate photodynamic therapy versus placebo photodynamic therapy in nodular BCC. Journal of the European Academy of Dermatology and Venereology 18 (Suppl 2):413–414

Varma S, Wilson H, Kurwa HA et al 2001 Bowen's disease, solar keratoses and superficial basal cell carcinomas treated by photodynamic therapy using a large-field incoherent light source. British Journal of Dermatology 144:567–574

Vinciullo C, Elliott T, Francis D 2006 MAL-PDT in "difficult-to-treat" basal cell carcinoma, an Australian study: 48 month follow-up data. Journal of Investigative Dermatology 126 (Suppl 2):s34

Wang I, Bendsoe N, Klinteberg CAF et al 2001 Photodynamic therapy vs. cryosurgery of basal cell carcinomas: results of a phase III clinical trial. British Journal of Dermatology 144:832–840

Zeitouni NC, Oseroff AR, Shieh S 2003 Photodynamic therapy for nonmelanoma skin cancers. Molecular Immunology 39:1133–1136

8 Treatment of Basal Cell Nevus Syndrome

Dany J. Touma

INTRODUCTION

Basal cell nevus syndrome (BCNS), also known as nevoid basal cell carcinoma syndrome or Gorlin syndrome, is a systemic autosomal dominant disease, mapped to chromosome 9q23.1–q31. The basic genetic defect is a mutation of a tumor suppressor gene, which is analogous to the *Drosophila* fruit fly's PATCHED gene, with variable expression and under-reporting of this disease. BCNS most commonly affects Caucasians, although all skin types are affected. There is no sex predilection.

While individuals affected with BCNS are phenotypically vastly heterogenous, they are generally characterized by the occurrence of multiple basal cell carcinomas (BCCs) at an early age, pathognomonic palmo-plantar pitting, epidermal cysts of the skin, painful and aggressive odontogenic cysts occurring early in life, calcification of the falx cerebri, and skeletal abnormalities such as frontal bossing, broad nasal bridge, and spinal abnormalities. Fibromas of the ovaries and heart, medulloblastomas, and meningiomas are also seen. The associated features of BCNS are often devastating; however, most patients with BCNS suffer mostly from the overwhelming occurrence of BCC lesions. These patients are extremely sensitive to sun exposure, and radiation therapy tends to trigger overgrowth of tumors in the treatment field. Tumors typically develop at a young age, generally beginning at puberty, but rarely during childhood. Patients with BCNS may initially present with tens if not hundreds of these tumors (Fig. 8.1), and those under surveillance continuously develop new and recurrent growths. This debilitating condition, while rarely fatal, results in numerous regular treatments over the years, scarring, reduced quality of life, and excessive medical cost.

TRADITIONAL MANAGEMENT

Patients with BCNS are typically managed with a multidisciplinary approach. Most dermatologists examine these patients every 3 months, and treat newly appearing lesions as they develop. Tumors of the face may be best treated with Mohs micrographic surgery, not only to achieve optimal margin control and minimize recurrences, but also to obtain maximal tissue preservation and to limit long-term disfigurement which might occur after innumerable tumors are surgically removed. Patients are also treated with simple or punch excision, destructive modalities such as cryotherapy, and electrodessication and curettage, particularly for lesions on the trunk. Often, however, and as patients become tired of repeated treatments, lesions are grouped and treated in larger sessions, or patients may delay treatment altogether, which may result in the emergence of larger, more-difficult-to-treat lesions. In addition, some of the tumors in BCNS patients, particularly those that are recurrent or those that are in the T-zone of the face, are inherently more difficult to diagnose and treat.

Patients with BCNS are advised to adhere to lifelong strict sun protection, and in order to perhaps reduce the occurrence of new tumors and treat subclinical lesions, a few topical chemotherapeutic and chemopreventive agents are sometimes used. A combination of tretinoin 0.1% and 5-fluorouracil 5% (5-FU) has been found to be helpful in the prophylaxis and treatment of superficial BCCs in BCNS, and is often recommended to patients, with large surface application of this combination proven to be safe. In practice, many patients and physicians tend to minimize the use of 5-FU because it is highly irritating and poorly tolerated. Imiquimod, an immune response modifier, has been used for the management of multiple BCCs in BCNS. In one study, four patients were treated with three to five applications/week for 8–14 weeks. Thirteen of 17 tumors resolved. In all studies, however, prolonged mild-to-severe erythema and superficial erosions were observed. Isotretinoin at low doses of 0.4 mg/kg/day has a suppressive role on BCCs in BCNS; however, tumors reappear upon cessation of treatment. The CO_2 laser is also used to treat multiple BCCs in the context of BCNS, but is associated with significant morbidity for about 2 weeks, and the possibility of scarring if the skin is too deeply vaporized.

Patients with BCNS are looking for simpler treatment of BCCs that minimizes the occurrence of new growths, decreases treatment morbidity, and improves cosmesis, quality of life, and cost. Photodynamic therapy (PDT) is a controlled method of skin cancer treatment and chemoprevention that has a proven record of efficacy and safety, fast healing times, and good-to-excellent cosmesis, and is well suited for patients with BCNS.

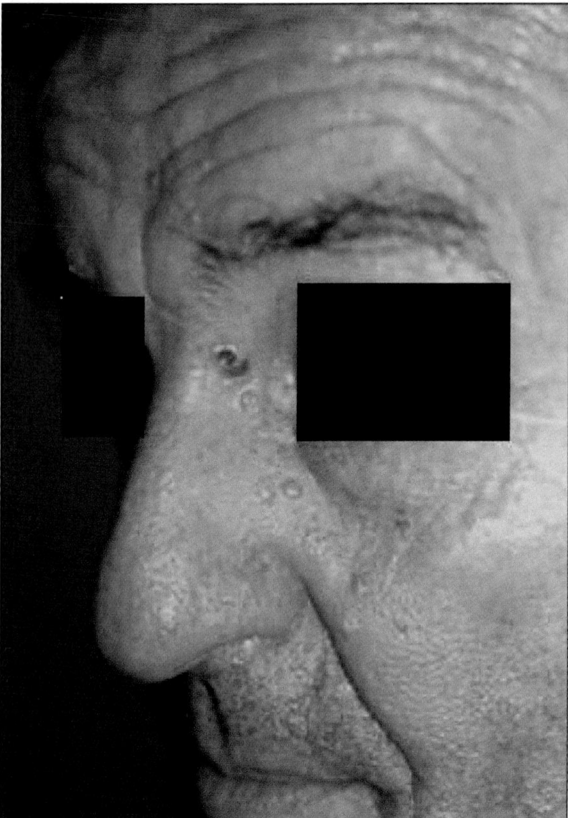

Fig. 8.1 Patient with BCNS. Note several tumors in the periorbital area

PHOTODYNAMIC THERAPY

Several systemic photosensitizers, including Photofrin, Photochlor, benzoporphyrin derivative (PBD), tin etiopurpurin (SnET2), mThPc, lutetium texafrin, Npe6, and human porphyrin derivative (HPD), activated by various light sources delivering a wavelength in the 630–743-nm range, have been used successfully to treat BCCs, whether in the context of BCNS or not. Using Photofrin, the most commonly used systemic photosensitizer, at a dose of 1.0 mg/kg followed 48–72 h later by a 630-nm red light dose of 150–275 J/cm^2 at 150 mW/cm^2, Oseroff et al achieved a 92.2% clearance rate at 6 months of BCCs, including tumors in BCNS patients. In this study, up to 51 tumors were treated over 2 days after a single Photofrin injection. Recurrence rates at 5 years were 28% and 15% for sporadic and BCNS tumors, respectively. Intravenous SnET2 was used successfully with light irradiation to clear all 13 treated lesions in a BCNS patient after a single treatment, with a follow-up of 6 months. Verteporfin, a much shorter-acting systemic photosensitizer, was used at a dose of 14 mg/m^2 with 688-nm red light emitting diode (LED) activation at various fluences 1–3 h after photosensitizer administration to treat 54 patients with 421 nonmelanoma skin cancers, including superficial and nodular BCCs and Bowen's disease. After a single treatment at 180 J/cm^2, clinical and histologic clearance rates were 95% at 24 months. Pain during treatment was a significant side effect, and 65% of treatment sites were judged to have good-to-excellent cosmesis at 24 months.

The limitations of systemic PDT include the complexity of drug administration, limited local control of treatment, and delayed generalized photosensitivity. These factors have limited the use of and interest in systemic PDT for the treatment of BCCs, although there is no question that many patients with diffuse thick tumors, such as those with BCNS, may continue to benefit from this approach, particularly with the newer shorter-acting photosensitizers.

Topical PDT using 20% 5-aminolevulinic acid (ALA) solution and the methyl ester of ALA (MAL) has been the main focus of recent research. Topical PDT is easy to use, accessible to the vast majority of dermatologists, relatively inexpensive, and lacks the delayed photosensitivity of systemic PDT. Numerous studies have shown the efficacy, safety, and excellent cosmetic outcome of using topical PDT for superficial-type and nodular BCCs, despite the fact that there is wide variation in their methodology, use of photosensitizer, and type of light activation (see Ch. 7). Complete responses (CR) for superficial BCCs range between 80% and 95%, and those for nodular and noduloulcerative BCCs reach 83–92%, with tumors less than 2-mm thick responding best. Morpheaform BCCs are usually unresponsive due to their deep fibrotic nature, but this type is not particularly common in BCNS patients. While no human studies have formally evaluated the chemopreventive role of PDT for patients at risk for multiple BCCs, clinical experience is strongly suggestive of that, with many anecdotal reports of reduced incidence of new BCCs in patients treated with broad application PDT. In mice, studies have demonstrated a role for topical PDT in preventing new-onset BCCs after repetitive UV irradiation.

At the technical level, studies of topical PDT in the treatment of BCCs have demonstrated that ALA is equivalent to MAL, with 6 h being an ideal incubation time. As for light sources, the 630-nm light sources are deeper penetrating and therefore more efficacious for BCCs, except for pigmented BCCs, which respond better to 390-nm light. Single treatments are rarely sufficient, while repeat treatments at 1–8-week intervals increases response. In fact, double treatment is now recommended for all tumors. Pre-treating the tumor with dimethylsulfoxide (DMSO), adding ethylenediamine tetra-acetic acid (EDTA) or the iron chelator desferrioxamine to the ALA vehicle, and pre-treatment curettage significantly enhance the CR of superficial and nodular BCCs, as does light dose fractionation and irradiating at low fluence rates. Results from these studies can be extrapolated to patients with BCNS, since these patients have a great increase in incidence of BCCs, but their tumors generally have a predictable response to the different available modalities for skin cancer, and topical PDT is no exception.

Few studies have examined the role of topical PDT in BCNS patients. Caty et al, using twice-weekly UV-irradiated PTCH transgenic mice, demonstrated that weekly topical MAL-PDT was highly effective at preventing the occurrence of new BCCs in 15 mice (no BCCs), compared to 20 non-treated UV-irradiated mice (19 BCCs). Itkin and Gilchrest reported the use of 20% ALA incubated for up to 5 h, and irradiated with 417-nm blue light at 10 J/cm^2, to treat two BCNS patients. Two sets of double treatments separated by 1 week were done at 2–4-month intervals. Complete CR at 8 months from the initial treatment was observed in 8 of 9 facial superficial BCCs (89%), 18 of 27 lower extremity superficial BCCs (67%), and 5 of 16 nodular facial BCCs (31%). Partial response was seen in the residual tumors (Figs 8.2, 8.3). A decreased incidence of new tumors during the observation period was also reported. As expected from earlier studies, previous facial scarring and skin texture were improved. Similar results were reported using 1-h incubation with ALA and four treatments at 2–3-month intervals in another patient with BCNS. In a report by Oseroff and his group, three children with BCNS involving up to 25% of their body surface were treated with ALA, followed by activation with a pulsed-dye laser (PDL) and noncoherent light in one to three treatments, using up to 36 fields per session. They reported 85–98% tumor clearance, with excellent cosmetic outcome, and a follow-up up to 6 years.

Recently, intralesional ALA-PDT was introduced, which obviates the difficulties of controlling ALA penetration into tumors. Chapas et al recently evaluated intralesional ALA-PDT for nomelanoma skin cancer, including BCCs in BCNS patients. In this study, lesions were first anesthesized with xylocaine and epinephrine (adrenalin), and then injected with 20% ALA until blanching was seen, and covered with topical ALA. Incubation was for 1 h, followed by blue light at 10 J/cm^2, or PDL at 7.5 J/cm^2. Repeat treatments were necessary, with all tumors achieving complete or partial response. Protocols of intralesional PDT vary, much like those with PDT in general, and large studies are lacking; however, early results of this exciting new development are very promising (Figs 8.4A and B).

Because patients with BCNS have a lifelong risk of developing BCCs, concerns have been raised about the safety of repeated treatments with PDT. To that end, Haylett et al evaluated the possible clonogenic effect and DNA damage of ALA-PDT on BCNS fibroblasts and compared these to normal fibroblasts. There was no difference in terms of clonogenic survival. Minor DNA damage was measured in the BCNS fibroblasts, particularly at high doses, but was fully repaired within 24 h. While this and other studies have not evaluated the long-term effect of longitudinal and repeated PDT sessions, which might be required in BCNS patients, studies like this one are reassuring. In addition, the long-term follow-up of patients with erythropoietic protoporphyria, who have a continuous low-grade PDT reaction from daily exposure to sun and ambient light, does not demonstrate any increased incidence of skin cancer (and therefore no clinically significant DNA damage) in this group. Other studies have demonstrated the cost-effectiveness of repeated PDT, particularly when compared to simple excisions.

Finally, another useful application of PDT in BCNS patients is in fluorescence diagnosis and assisting in the treatment of tumors that are recurrent or clinically difficult to delineate.

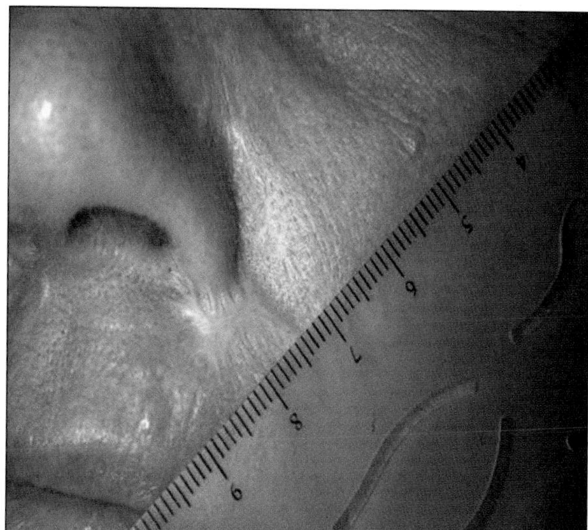

Fig. 8.2 Nodular BCC in a BCNS patient

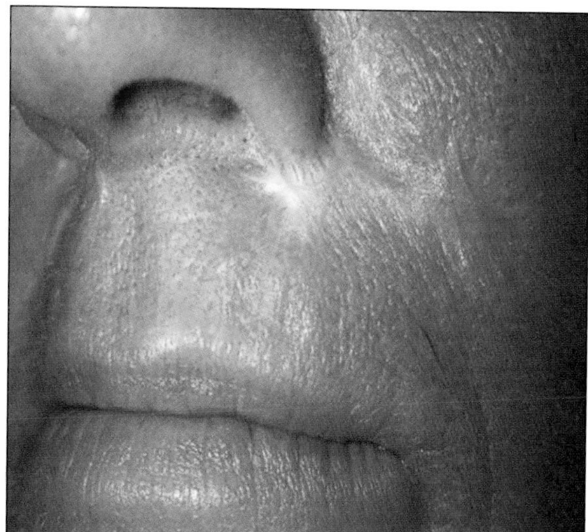

Fig. 8.3 Resolution after topical PDT using ALA 20% and blue light (Courtesy of Barbara Gilchrest, MD)

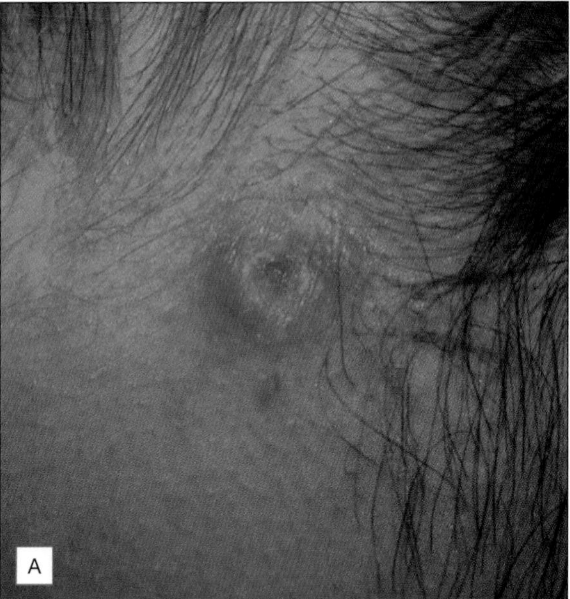

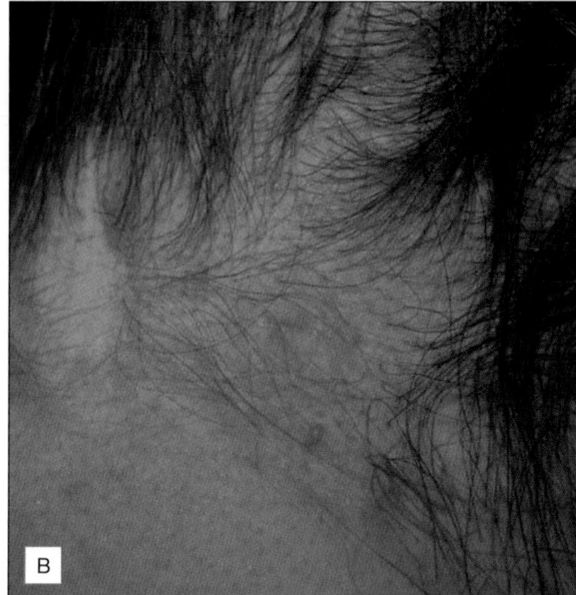

Fig. 8.4 (A) Nodular BCC in a BCNS patient **(B)** Resolution after a single PDT session using intralesional 20% ALA and blue light (Courtesy of Barbara Gilchrest, MD)

CONCLUSION

PDT is a valuable modality in the treatment of BCCs in BCNS. It is cost-effective, easy to use, and accessible in its topical form, and while cure rates of individual lesions are not necessarily superior to other established modalities, and treatment protocols are not standardized, the ability to treat multiple and subclinical lesions using broad surface treatments, the excellent cosmetic outcome, and the high patient acceptance make this modality very well suited for patients with BCNS.

FURTHER READING

Abels C 2001 Fluorescence diagnosis. In: Calzavara Pinton G, Szeimies RM, Ortel B (eds) Photodynamic Therapy and Fluorescence Diagnosis in Dermatology. Elsevier: Amsterdam, 165–176

Bellnier DA, Greco WR, Loewen GM et al 2006 Clinical pharmacokinetics of the PDT photosensitizers porfimer sodium (Photofrin), 2-[1-hexyloxyethyl]-2-devinyl pyropheophorbide-a (Photochlor) and 5-ALA-induced protoporphyrin IX. Lasers in Surgery and Medicine 38:439–444

Caekelbergh K, Annemans L, Lambert J et al 2006 Economic evaluation of methyl aminolaevulinate-based photodynamic therapy in the management of actinic keratoses and basal cell carcinoma. British Journal of Dermatology 155:784–790

Cappugi P, Mavilia L, Campolmi P, et al New proposal for the treatment of nodular basal cell carcinoma with intralesional 5-aminolevulinic acid. Journal of Chemotherapy 16:491–493

Caty V, Liu Y, Viau G et al 2006 Multiple large surface photodynamic therapy sessions with topical methylaminolaevulinate in PTCH heterozygous mice. British Journal of Dermatology 154:740–742

Chapas AM, Gilchrest BA 2006 Broad area photodynamic therapy for treatment of multiple basal cell carcinomas in a patient with nevoid basal cell carcinoma syndrome. Journal of Drugs in Dermatology 5 (2 Suppl):3–5

Chapas A, Zeltser R, Geronemus R et al 2006 Intralesional photodynamic therapy of nonmelanoma skin cancer. Lasers in Surgery and Medicine 18 (Suppl):27

Compton JG, Goldstein AM, Turner M, Bale AE 1994 Fine mapping of the nevoid basal cell carcinoma syndrome (NBCC) to chromosome 9q in three families. Journal of Investigative Dermatology 103:178–181

Ericson MB, Sandberg C, Stenquist B et al 2004 Photodynamic therapy of actinic keratosis at varying fluence rates: assessment of photobleaching, pain and primary clinical outcome. British Journal of Dermatology 151:1204–1212

Evans DGR, Ladusans E, Rimmer S et al 1993 Complications of the nevoid basal cell carcinoma syndrome: results of a population based study. Journal of Medical Genetics 30:460–464

Fardon PA, Del Mastro RG, Evans DGR et al 1992 Location of gene for Gorlin syndrome. Lancet 339:581–582

Fijan S, Honigsmann H, Ortel B 1995 Photodynamic therapy of epithelial skin tumors using delta-aminolevulinic acid and desferrioxamine. British Journal of Dermatology 133:282–288

Goldberg LH, Hsu SH, Alcalay J 1989 Effectiveness of isotretinoin in preventing the appearance of basal cell carcinomas in basal cell nevus syndrome. Journal of the American Academy of Dermatology 21:144–145

Golitz LE, Norritts DA, Leukens CA et al 1980 Multiple basal cell carcinomas of the palms and soles after radiation therapy. Archives of Dermatology 116:1159–1163

Gorlin R 1995 Nevoid basal cell carcinoma syndrome. Dermatology Clinics 13:1:113–125

Hahn H, Wicking C, Zaphiropoulos PG et al 1996 Mutations in the human analogue of *Drosophila patched* in the nevoid basal cell carcinoma syndrome. Cell 85:841–851

Haller JC, Cairnduff F, Slack G et al 2000 Routine double treatments of superficial basal cell carcinomas using aminolaevulinic acid-based photodynamic therapy. British Journal of Dermatology 143:1270–1275

Haylett AK, Ward TH, Moore JV 2003 DNA damage and repair in Gorlin syndrome and normal fibroblasts after aminolevulinic acid photodynamic therapy: a comet assay study. Photochemistry and Photobiology 78:337–341

Ibbotson SH, Moseley H, Brancaleon L et al 2004 Photodynamic therapy in dermatology: Dundee clinical and research experience. Photodiagnosis and Photodynamic Therapy 1:211–223

Itkin A, Gilchrest B 2004 5-Aminolevulinic acid and blue light photodynamic therapy for treatment of multiple basal cell carcinomas in two patients with nevoid basal cell carcinoma syndrome. Dermatologic Surgery 30:1054–1061

Kagy MK, Amonette R 2000 The use of imiquimod 5% cream for the treatment of superficial basal cell carcinomas in a basal cell nevus syndrome patient. Dermatologic Surgery 26:577–578

Krunic AL, Viehman GE, Madani S et al 1998 Microscopically controlled surgical excision combined with ultrapulse CO_2 vaporization in the management of a patient with the nevoid basal cell carcinoma syndrome. Journal of Dermatology 25:10–12

Kuijpers DI, Thissen MR, Thissen CA et al 2006 Similar effectiveness of methyl aminolevulinate and 5-aminolevulinate in topical photodynamic therapy for nodular basal cell carcinoma. Journal of Drugs in Dermatology 5:642–625

Lui H, Hobbs L, Tope WD et al 2004 Photodynamic therapy of multiple nonmelanoma skin cancers with verteporfin and red light-emitting diodes: two-year results evaluating tumor response and cosmetic outcomes. Archives of Dermatology 140:26–32

Liu Y, Viau G, Bissonnette R 2004 Multiple large-surface photodynamic therapy sessions with topical or systemic aminolevulinic acid and blue light in UV-exposed hairless mice. Journal of Cutananeous Medicine and Surgery 8:131–139

Micali G, Lacarrubba F, Nasca MR et al 2003 The use of Imiquimod 5% cream for the treatment of basal cell carcinoma as observed in Gorlin's syndrome. Clinical and Experimental Dermatology 28 (Suppl):19–23

Morton CA, MacKie RM, Whitehurst C et al 1998 Photodynamic therapy for basal cell carcinoma: effect of tumor thickness and duration of photosensitizer application on response. Archives of Dermatology 134:248–249

Nielsen KP, Juzeniene A, Juzenas P et al 2005 Choice of optimal wavelength for PDT: the significance of oxygen depletion. Photochemistry and Photobiology 81:1190–1194

Oseroff AR, Dozier SE 1998 Lasers and photodynamic therapy. In: Miller SJ, Maloney ME, (eds) Cutaneous Oncology. Oxford: Blackwell Science, 534–541

Oseroff AR, Shieh S, Frawley NP et al 2005 Treatment of diffuse basal cell carcinomas and basaloid follicular hamartomas in nevoid basal cell carcinoma syndrome by wide area 5-aminolevulinic acid photodynamic therapy. Archives of Dermatology 141:60–67

Oseroff AR, Blumenson LR, Wilson BD et al 2006 A dose ranging study of photodynamic therapy with porfimer sodium (Photofrin) for treatment of basal cell carcinoma. Lasers in Surgery and Medicine 38:417–426

Peng Q, Warloe T, Berg K et al 1997 5-ALA based photodynamic therapy. Cancer 79:2822–2308

Rhodes LE, de Rie M, Enstrom Y et al 2004 Photodynamic therapy using topical methyl aminolevulinate vs surgery for nodular basal cell carcinoma: results of a multicenter randomized prospective trial. Archives of Dermatology 140:17–23

Rifkin R, Reed B, Hetzel F et al 1997 Photodynamic therapy using SnET2 for basal cell nevus syndrome: a case report. Clinical Therapeutics 19:639–641

Shanley S, Ratcliffe J, Hockey A et al 1994 Nevoid basal cell carcinoma syndrome: review of 118 affected individuals. American Journal of Medical Genetics 50:282–290

Soler AM, Angell-Petersen E, Warloe T et al 2000 Photodynamic therapy of superficial basal cell carcinoma with 5-aminolevulinic acid with dimethylsulfoxide and ethylendiaminetetraacetic acid: a comparison of two light sources. Photochemistry and Photobiology 71:724–729

Soler AM, Warloe T, Berner A, Giercksky KE 2001 A follow-up study of recurrence and cosmesis in completely responding superficial and nodular basal cell carcinomas treated with methyl 5-aminolevulinate-based photodynamic therapy alone and with prior curettage. British Journal of Dermatology 145:467–471

Star WM, van't Veen AJ, Robinson DJ et al 2006 Topical 5-aminolevulinic acid mediated photodynamic therapy of superficial basal cell carcinoma using two light fractions with a two-hour interval: long-term follow-up. Acta Dermato-Venerologica 86:412–417

Stockfleth E, Ulrich C, Hauschild A et al 2002 Successful treatment of basal cell carcinomas in a nevoid basal cell carcinoma syndrome with topical 5% imiquimod. European Journal of Dermatology 12:569–572

Strange PR, Lang PG Jr 1988 Long term management of basal cell nevus syndrome with topical tretinoin and 5-fluorouracil. Journal of the American Academy of Dermatology 27:842–845

Stummer W, Reulen HJ, Novotny A, Stepp H, Tonn JC 2003 Fluorescence-guided resections of malignant gliomas – an overview. Acta Neurochirurgica 88 (Suppl):9–12

Thissen MRTM, Schroeter CA, Neumann HAM 2000 Photodynamic therapy with delta-aminolaevulinic acid for nodular basal cell carcinomas using a prior debulking technique. British Journal of Dermatology 142:338–339

Touma D, Yaar M, Whitehead S, Konnikov N, Gilchrest B 2004 Evaluation of short incubation photodynamic therapy for actinic keratosis and photodamage. Archives of Dermatology 140:33–40

Varma S, Wislon H, Kurwa HA et al 2001 Bowen's disease, solar keratoses and superficial basal cell carcinomas treated by photodynamic therapy using a large field incoherent light source. British Journal of Dermatology 144:567–574

9 Treatment of Human Papilloma Virus

Ida-Marie Stender

INTRODUCTION

Based on the promising results from randomized as well as nonrandomized clinical trials, this chapter will describe treatment of recalcitrant hand and foot warts with 5-aminolevulinic acid (ALA) photodynamic therapy (PDT). ALA-PDT treatment of condyloma and human papilloma virus (HPV)-related conditions, such as intraepithelial neoplasia, will be discussed; however, the methodology will not be described in detail, since treatment modalities are not yet standardized.

HUMAN PAPILLOMA VIRUS IN HAND AND FOOT WARTS

• Etiology

HPV is a double-stranded DNA virus of the papova virus family. More than 70 genotypes of HPV have been identified. Hand and foot warts are mainly caused by HPV 1, 2, and 4, and genital warts by HPV 6, 11, 16, and 18.

Warts are transmitted by direct or indirect cutaneous infection with the HPV.

• Prevalence

The exact prevalence of warts is not known. About 22% of schoolchildren have warts.

• Clinical appearance and diagnosis

HPV infection can present on skin as foot and hand warts, flat warts, and genital warts. Warts can be classified by clinical appearance, location, histology, and type of virus.

The clinical judgment of an experienced dermatologist is usually sufficient for the correct diagnosis of a wart.

• Histology

Hand and foot warts are characterized by hyperplasia of all layers of the epidermis. Acanthosis, papillomatosis, hyperkeratosis with parakeratosis, and thrombosed capillaries in dermal papillae are seen. Elongated ridges curve towards the center of the wart. Vacuolated cells, called koilocytotic cells, are located in the mid to upper dermis.

• Therapeutic challenges

Reasons for wart removal include functional, cosmetic, and psychosocial concerns. Although there is no fully reliable cure for warts, there is an intense wish from patients to be treated because of the unsightly appearance, pain, and concern that the warts might spread.

• Patient selection

Patients with warts remaining after standard treatments administered by a dermatologist for more than at least 3 months may be offered ALA-PDT.

Pain during and after ALA-PDT should be considered a relative contraindication for treatment, particularly in children. Pregnant and nursing women should not be offered ALA-PDT because of lack of treatment experience and safety data in this subgroup. Patients with porphyria or other photo-induced or exacerbated diseases, as well as patients allergic to the content of the ALA cream, also should not be offered ALA-PDT.

• Expected benefits

A series of six ALA-PDT treatments during a 9-week period has proven effective for the treatment of recalcitrant warts.

Efficacy of the treatment can be measured as the relative change in wart area as well as the treatment-related change in wart count. Reappearance of skin ridges indicates that the wart is no longer present. If paring reveals no capillaries, wart resolution is further confirmed. ALA-PDT is superior to placebo-PDT when both wart area and number of resolving warts are considered. In one double-blinded study, a total of 232 foot and hand warts in 45 patients were randomized to receive either ALA-PDT or placebo-PDT. Prior to irradiation with a broadband light source, 20% ALA cream or placebo cream was applied for 4 h, and the treatment was repeated weekly for 3 weeks. Patients were followed up 1 month later, and if warts persisted, they were re-treated for a further three weekly treatments and assessed at weeks 14 and 18. Study results indicated a significant decrease in wart area in the active treatment group at weeks 14 and 18, with a median difference of 46% and 29%, respectively ($P = 0.006$, $P = 0.008$). Complete clearance of warts by week 18 was seen in 56% of patients in the active treatment group, compared with 42% in the placebo-treated group ($P < 0.05$). Both the number of resolving warts and the difference in relative wart area at weeks 14 and 18 were significant ($P < 0.05$) in favor of ALA-PDT (Tables 9.1, 9.2).

It is inconvenient for patients to come to the clinic for application of ALA-containing cream and return 4 h later for irradiation. Patients, however, can easily be taught how to pare the warts and apply the ALA cream themselves. No serious local or systemic adverse events were reported in patients given six ALA-PDT treatments over 9 weeks. Scarring, other skin abnormalities, and functional disturbance were not noted. Additionally, transient pain is frequently seen. ALA-PDT produces no plume and no bleeding, and therefore it reduces risk of transfer of HPV particles.

• Cost/benefit

Taking Denmark as an example in 2006, 2 g of a commercialized cream containing methylester ALA (MAL) will cost around €300 (c. US$300). Such a quantity may be sufficient for repeated treatments of two to three medium-sized warts. Commercially available noncoherent light lamps suitable for PDT range in price from €6000 to €19 000.

For patients with recalcitrant warts, the spending of €300 for a 58% likelihood of cure within a few weeks is for many an attractive trade-off. In most countries, public health systems or various health insurance schemes are setting guidelines for which therapies can be used. Most such schemes, however, do not take into account the total cost of wart treatment. In addition to direct medical costs, indirect but significant costs such as lost work time, travel time to and from clinics for patients and accompanying relatives, and the spreading of the virus to others may not be considered by policymakers. In the narrow traditional cost–benefit perspective, the additional cost of ALA is typically only compared to the likely cost of additional patient- and physician-administered therapies (salicylic acid-containing ointments, cryotherapy, curettage, cantharidine, etc.) that may be required. Since the exact number of required visits for wart treatment may be unknown, such trade-off analyses tend to be biased towards whichever treatment modality is cheapest per treatment. As PDT is an emerging therapy, its availability is expected to increase over time as its cumulative efficacy becomes apparent and the unit cost of treatment is reduced by improved technology and volume-related savings.

For the dermatologist, the curing of a patient in fewer visits entails a superior use of resources. However, if the dermatologist is not paid for offering PDT either by the patient or by the health system, there is no incentive to invest in PDT lamps(s), train personnel or acquire and administer the more expensive ALA medication. Wart removal has traditionally not been among the most prestigious dermatologic skills, but for patients affected with this troublesome, often intractable problem, an expeditious cure is highly valued.

CONDYLOMA AND INTRAEPITHELIAL NEOPLASIA

Condyloma acuminata is a common sexually transmitted disease for which no treatment is completely satisfactory. HPV infection with certain oncogenic viral types can lead to the development of intraepithelial neoplasia (IN) of the cervix (CIN), vagina, vulva (VIN), and anus. Diagnosis is based upon biopsy.

Conventional treatment for condyloma involves topical medications, cryotherapy, and laser, whereas the treatment of IN often involves surgical excision with wide margins and laser ablation. ALA-PDT is a potentially effective treatment for condylomata acuminata, with an overall cure rate of 72.9% (ALA 20% cream, irradiation with optical system made at Forth-IESL, 400–800 nm, 70–100 J/cm^2, 70 mW/cm^2). In one protocol, ALA gel (10%) was applied to vulvar and vaginal lesions followed by occlusion with a dressing for a mean interval of 154 min and ultimate illumination with a 635-nm dye laser. Evalu-

Table 9.1 Number (%) of persisting and vanishing warts in ALA-PDT and placebo-PDT groups

Week	ALA-PDT		Placebo-PDT		P
	Number persisting (%)	Number vanishing (%)	Number persisting (%)	Number vanishing (%)	
0	117 (100)	0	115 (100)	0	—
7	98 (85)	18 (16)	96 (84)	19 (17)	0.835
14	49 (50)	49 (50)	64 (65)	34 (35)	0.030
18	50 (44)	64 (56)	65 (58)	47 (42)	0.033

Data from Stender IM, Na R, Fogh H, Gluud C, Wulff HC 2000 Photodynamic therapy with 5-aminolevulinic acid or placebo for recalcitrant foot and hand warts: randomized double-blind trial. Lancet 355:963–966

Table 9.2 Relative change in wart area and area of persisting warts compared with area at entry (%) at weeks 7, 14, and 18

Week number	ALA-PDT	Placebo-PDT	Difference (CI)	P
7				
Area of warts compared with area at entrance Median Quartiles Range	−33 (−74.0) (−100 to 483)	−12 (−60.0) (−100 to 100)		0.07
Area of persisting warts compared with area at entrance Mean change (SE)	−16.4 (6.1)	−11.2 (6.1)	−5.2 (19.4, 9.0)	Not significant
14				
Area of persisting warts compared with area at entrance Median Quartiles Range	−98 (−100, −55) (−100, −56)	−52 (−100.0) (−100, −25)		0.0006
Area of warts compared with area at entrance Mean change (SE)	−45.3 (5.5)	−16.7 (4.8)	−28.6 (−15.9, 41.4)	0.00001
18				
Area of warts compared with area at entrance Median Quartiles Range	−100 (−100, −57) (−100 to 56)	−71 (−100.0) (−100 to 60)		0.008
Area of persisting warts compared with area at entrance Mean change (SE)	−38.2 (6.3)	−20.1 (5.3)	−18.1(−3.6, −32.6)	0.015

Data from Stender IM, Na R, Fogh H, Gluud C, Wulff HC 2000 Photodynamic therapy with 5-aminolevulinic acid or placebo for recalcitrant foot and hand warts: randomized double-blind trial. Lancet 355:963–966

ation after 2 months revealed clearance of lesions in 66–73% of the condyloma patients and 37–57% of patients with IN. In vivo study of fluorescence kinetics and PDT in condylomata indicated that optimal time for irradiation varied among patients from 6 to 11 h. Urethral condyloma given topical ALA followed by intraurethral PDT showed a complete cure rate of 95% and the recurrence rate was 5% after 6–24 months of follow-up. Topical ALA-PDT is a potential effective treatment of CIN with comparable results to cold-knife conization. PDT using intravenously injected metatetrahydroxyphenylchlorin (Foscan) followed by irradiation 96 h later with 632-nm light from a diode laser showed promising effect with low recurrences after 2 years of observation. CIN treated with intravenously injected Photofrin (polyhematoporphyrin ether/ester) and 48–60 h later exposed to Excimer dye laser or YAG-OPO laser showed a complete response rate of 90% at 3-months follow-up. Seventy-two percent of HPV-positive patients were HPV-negative 12 months following PDT. ALA-PDT appears to be a promising future treatment for condyloma accuminata as well as for intraepithelial neoplasia.

MECHANISM BEHIND ANTIVIRAL EFFECT OF PDT

PDT acts in HPV infection mainly by the destruction of infected keratinocytes and inactivation of viral particles of nonenveloped viruses. Photosentizing molecules may bind to the viral surface glycoproteins, resulting in an inhibition of the early phases of viral infection.

OVERVIEW OF TREATMENT STRATEGY FOR HAND AND FOOT WARTS (Fig. 9.1)

TREATMENT APPROACH

A 20% ALA-containing cream prepared in the local hospital pharmacy was used in a double-blinded treatment study of warts.

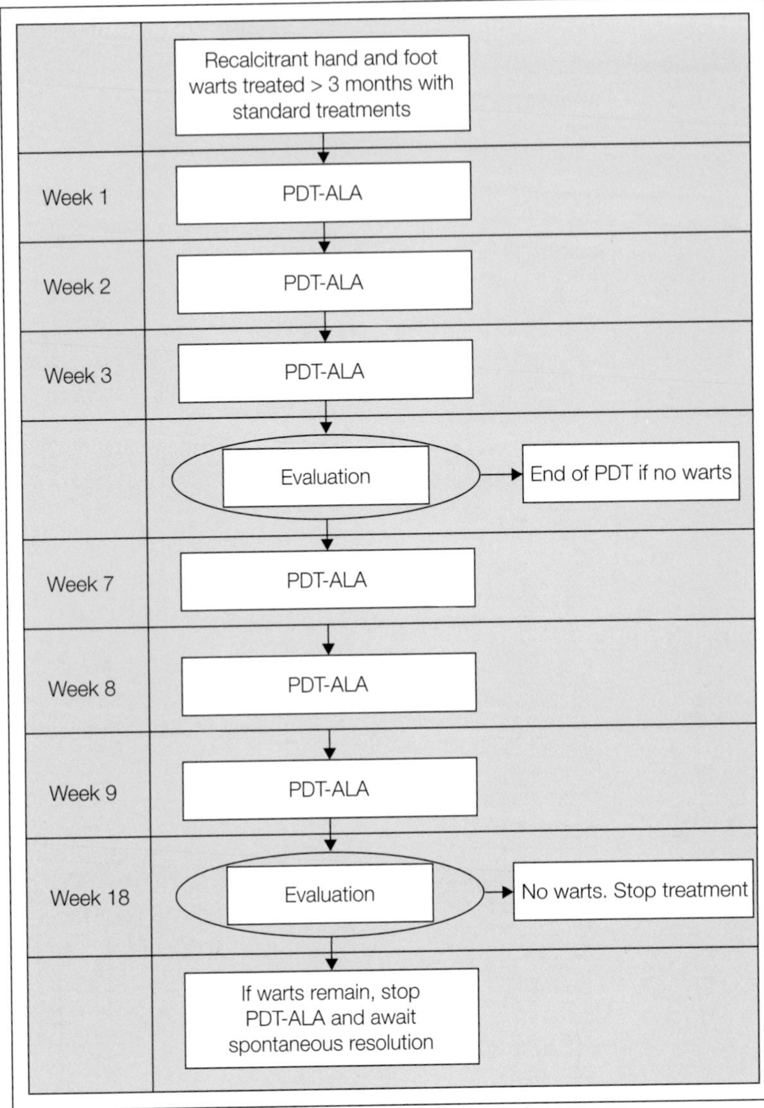

Fig. 9.1 PDT flowchart for treatment of hand and foot warts

An appropriate light source for ALA-PDT emits light in a wavelength range including the absorption peaks of protoporphyrin IX (PpIX). Lasers as well as nonlaser light sources can be used. The optimal wavelength of light, whether it is applied as a low dose for a relatively long exposure time or as a high dose for short exposure time, is still not well defined. Total energy doses for PDT light sources have also not been standardized and may vary from 60 to 250 J/cm^2 for laser lights and from 30 to 540 J/cm^2 for nonlasers. In our study, warts were exposed to a fluence of 50 mW/cm^2 for 23 min, which corresponded to a total dose of 70 J/cm^2.

For ALA-PDT treatment of warts, a commonly used and effective light source is the commercially available Waldmann PDT 1200 lamp (Waldmann-Medizin-technik, Villingen-Schwenningen, Germany), which emits in the range 590–700 nm, including the PpIX absorption peaks at 630 nm and 690 nm. Another useful light device is the Actilite (Galderma), which is portable, easy to use, and has an built-in cooling fan.

PATIENTS

Indications for treatment of warts are pain, interference with functioning or cosmetic embarrassment. Patients with recalcitrant hand and foot warts who have previously been offered various unsuccessful treatments should be offered ALA-PDT.

EQUIPMENT

- 20% ALA (Sigma Co, St Louis, MO) prepared in a cream base, Metvix, or similar formulation
- Lamp (e.g. Waldmann, Actilite, or other convenient lamps)
- Scalpel
- Bandages
- Spray bottle for water-cooling

• Treatment algorithm

During the 18-week period of ALA-PDT treatment, patients are expected to pare their warts with a scalpel and apply keratolytics twice a week. Paring of warts and application of ALA cream can be performed by patient or nurse (Fig. 9.2):

1. The warts are pared with a scalpel to remove the horny layer prior to ALA cream application (Fig. 9.3). In case of bleeding, treatment should be deferred until bleeding has stopped.
2. Apply a visible layer of ALA cream on the warts and to a 0.5–1-cm margin beyond the warts (Figs 9.4, 9.5).
3. Cover the warts with an occlusive dressing (e.g. Tegaderm R, 3M) (Fig. 9.6).
4. Cover the dressing with extra fixation. Apply the bandage to the lateral side of the feet to avoid loosening when the patient walks (Fig. 9.7).

Patients can apply the cream in the morning and come to the clinic for irradiation 3–4 h later. Some patients prefer to apply the cream at 5:00 am and come for irradiation on their way to work.

Irradiation is performed by a nurse as follows:

1. Remove the bandages and ointment (Fig. 9.8).
2. Patient and nurse should use protective glasses during the irradiation period since the red light can irritate the eyes.
3. Place the lamp in the correct position and start illumination. Using the Actilite (Galderma), appropriate parameters are a distance of 8–11 cm from the wart (Fig. 9.9) with irradiation (570–670 nm, 75 J/cm^2) for 7 min (Fig. 9.10). Using the PDT Waldmann 1200, the parameters are 590–700 nm, 50 mW/cm^2 for 23 min (70 J/cm^2). Make the patient as comfortable as possible (Fig. 9.11). In case of pain, apply water with a spray bottle (Fig. 9.12). If pain relief is not sufficient, increase the distance from the light to the irradiated area or take breaks during the irradiation procedure.
4. Turn the light off when the proper dose has been given.
5. Treated lesions should be protected against direct sun and direct light during the following 48 h.

Special post-treatment care, except avoiding light exposure, is not necessary. As per previous studies, the earlier described PDT procedure should be repeated three times with 1-week intervals between treatments; then, 1 month of observation should, in case of persisting warts, be followed by three more PDT treatments. After the last treatment, patients should continue to pare their warts twice a week followed by local application of a keratolytic.

TROUBLESHOOTING, SIDE EFFECTS, AND COMPLICATIONS

Final evaluation of the effect too soon after the last PDT treatment may lead to disappointing results. Do not evaluate response before 2 months after the last PDT treatment.

Multiple PDT treatments are needed. One treatment is not effective.

Preparation of the warts before treatment as well as home treatment by the patient is necessary.

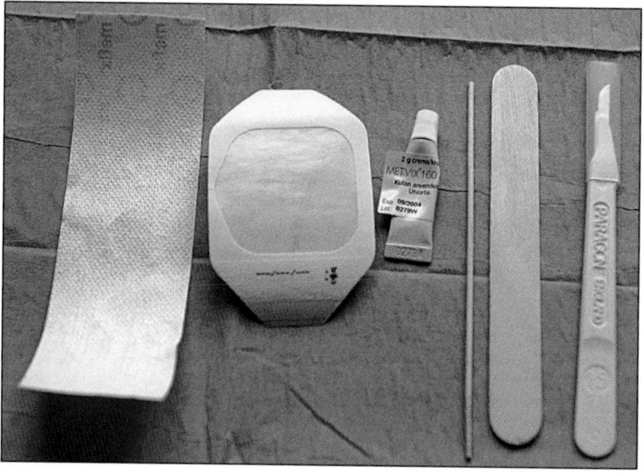

Fig. 9.2 Bandage, foil, ALA cream, application tools, and scalpel

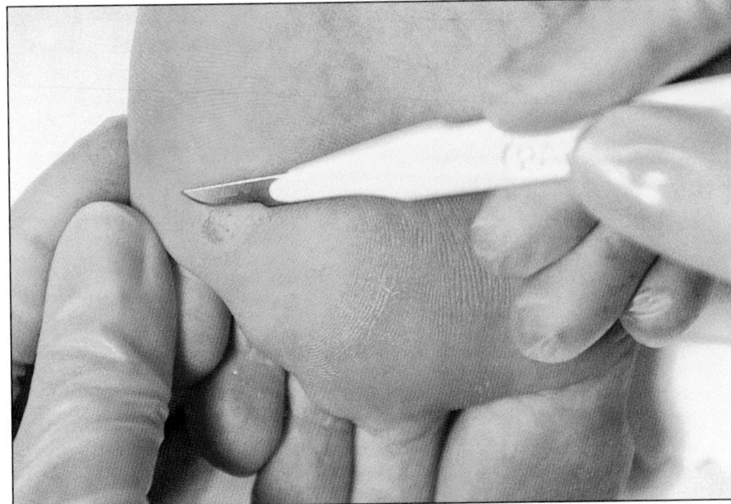

Fig. 9.3 Paring of wart with scalpel

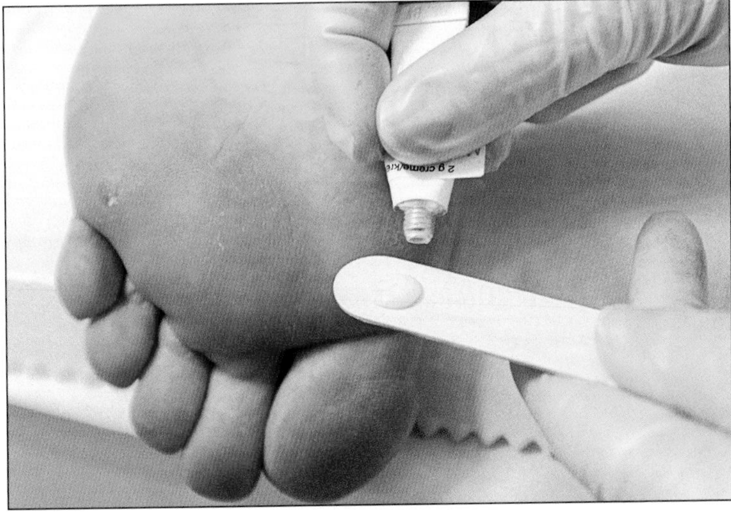

Fig. 9.4 Use a spatula for reasons of hygiene

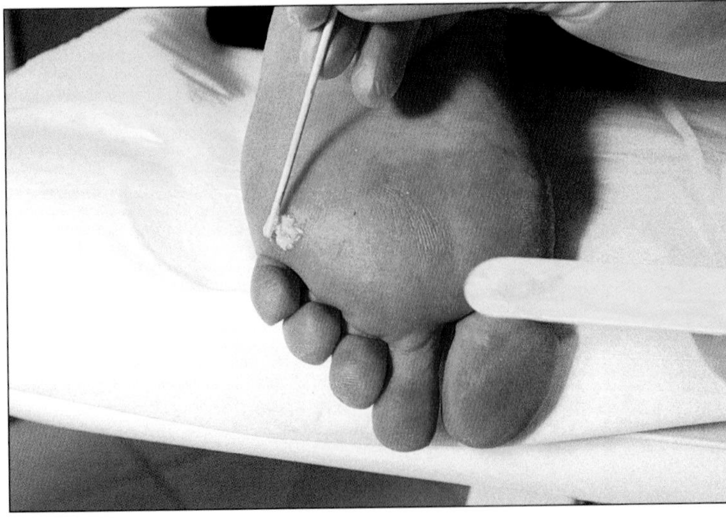

Fig. 9.5 Apply a visible layer of cream to the lesion

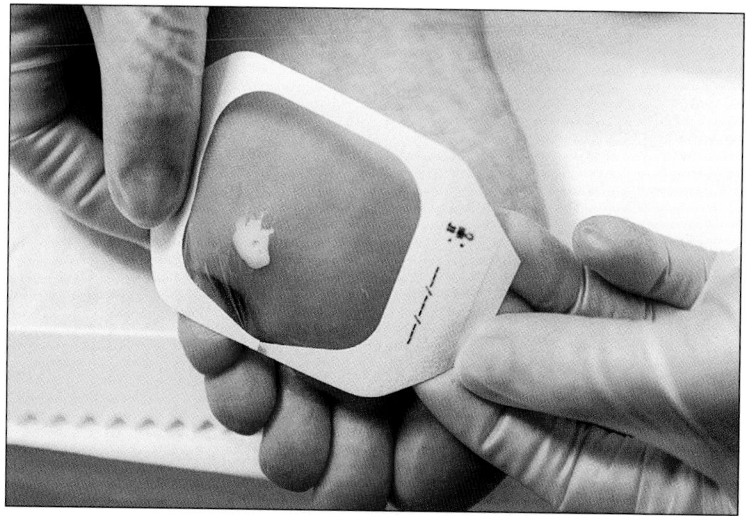

Fig. 9.6 Wart being covered by foil

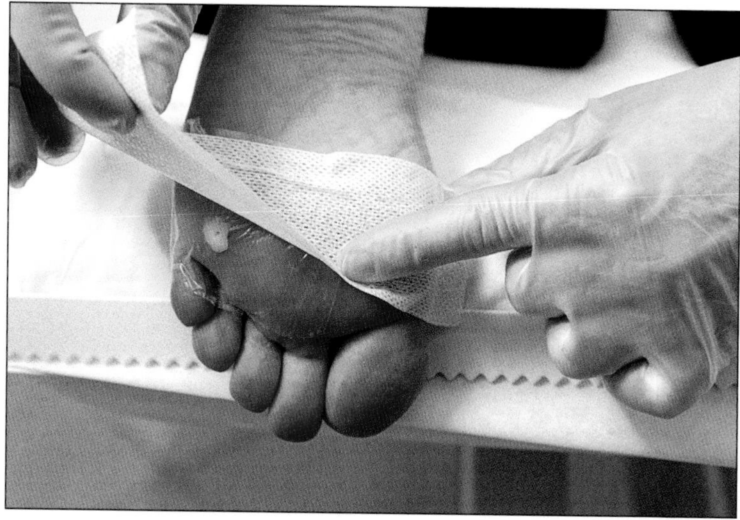

Fig. 9.7 Extra fixation bandage

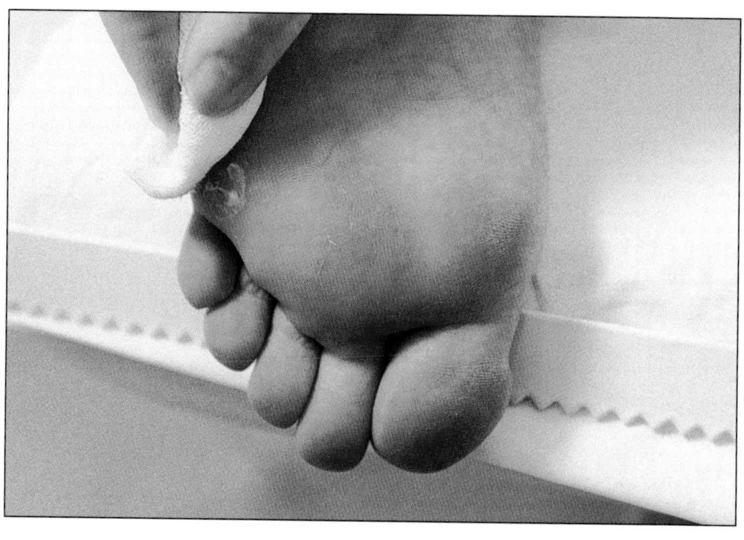

Fig. 9.8 Removal of bandage

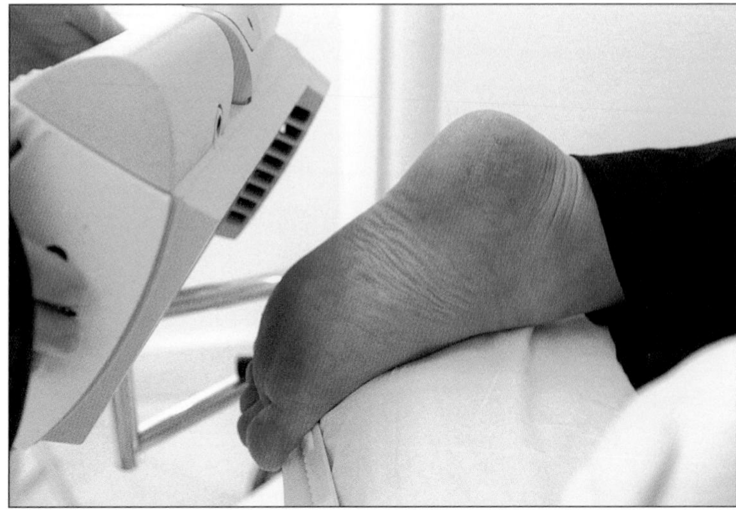

Fig. 9.9 Place lamp in right position depending on lamp

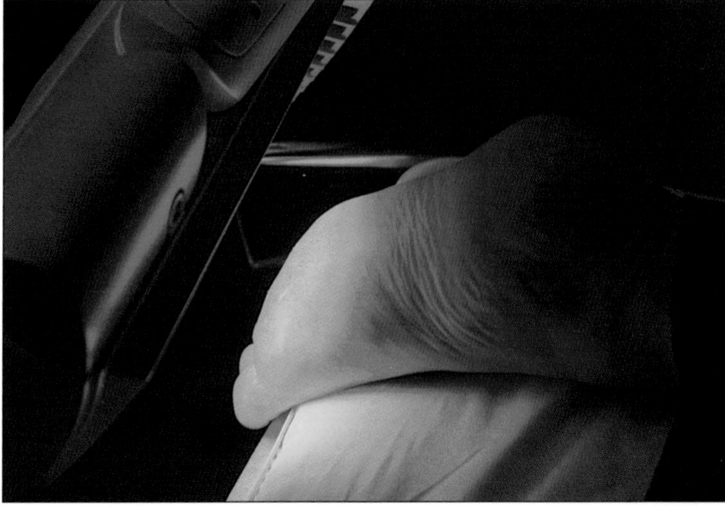

Fig. 9.10 Irradiation for 7 min (depending on lamp) (Photocure lamp: 7 min, 570–670 nm, 75 J/cm^2)

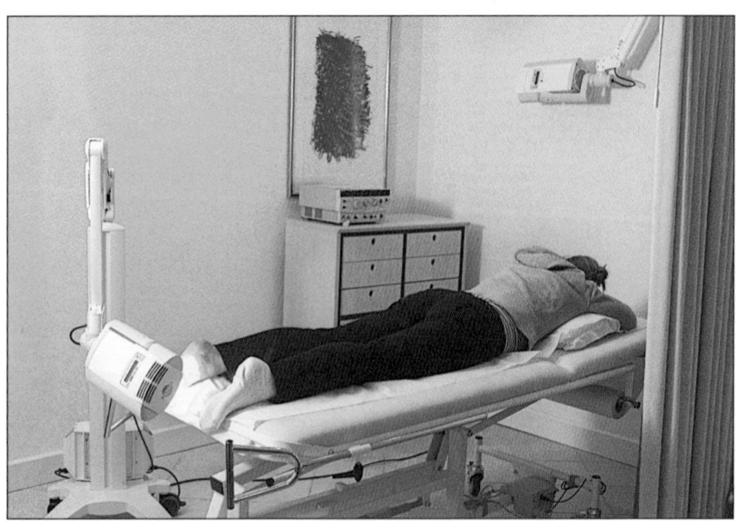

Fig. 9.11 Position the patient comfortably for the irradiation period

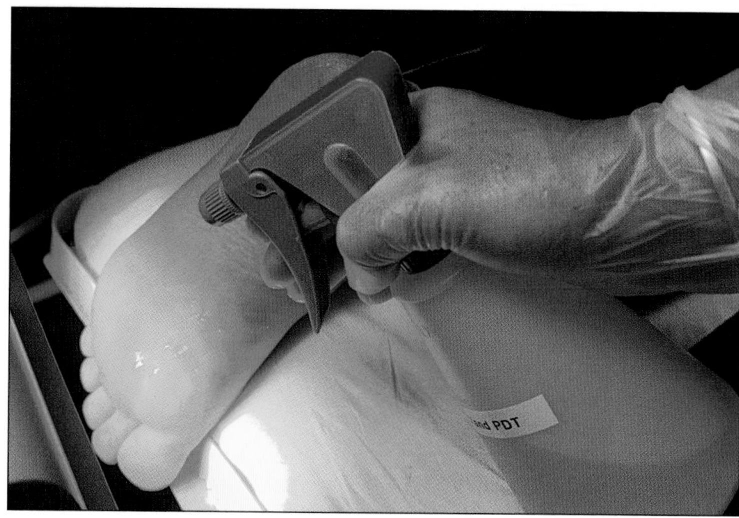

Fig. 9.12 Spray water to soothe pain

Pain is one of the major side effects of ALA-PDT and shows wide inter-patient variation. Some patients do benefit from systemic analgesia before and after PDT treatment. If burning and stinging occur during and after PDT treatment, application of cold water may help to relieve the pain. Usually pain resolves within 48 h after irradiation of the warts.

During irradiation the pain may be unacceptable in about 10% of the lesions treated. If this occurs, light intensity may be reduced by increasing the distance from the lamp to the warts. In case this maneuver is not sufficient, briefer light therapy may be delivered.

Severe complications after PDT treatment are extremely rare.

Only patients who have tried various conventional and nonconventional wart treatments are treated with ALA-PDT. It is a valid management option to leave warts untreated.

FURTHER READING

Bodner K, Bodner-Adler B, Wierrani F et al 2003 Cold-knife conization versus photodynamic therapy with topical 5-aminolevulinic acid (5-ALA) in cervical intraepithelial neoplasia (CIN) II with associated human papillomavirus infection: a comparison of preliminary results. Anticancer Research 23:1785–1788

Campbell SM, Gould DJ, Salter L et al 2004 Photodynamic therapy using meta-tetrahydroxyphenylchlorin (Fosca) for the treatment of vulval intraepithelial neoplasia. British Journal of Dermatology 151:1076–1080

El-Said A-H, Martin-Hirsch P, Duggan-Keen M et al 2001 Immunological and viral factors associated with the response of vulval intraepithelial neoplasia to photodynamic therapy. Cancer Research 61:192–196

Fabbrocini G, Di Constanzo MP, Riccardo AM et al 2001 Photodynamic therapy with topical δ-aminolaevulinic acid for the treatment of plantar warts. Journal of Photochemistry and Photobiology B: Biology 61:30–34

Fehr MK, Hornung R, Degen A et al 2002 Photodynamic therapy of vulvar and vaginal condyloma and intrapithelial neoplasia using topically applied 5-aminolevulinic acid. Lasers in Surgery and Medicine 30:273–279

Ibbotson SH 2002 Topical 5-aminolaevulinic acid photodynamic therapy for the treatment of skin conditions other than non-melanoma skin cancer. British Journal of Dermatology 146: 178–188

Stefanaki IM, Georgiou S, Themelis GC et al 2003 In vivo fluorescence kinetics and photodynamic therapy in condylomata acuminata. British Journal of Dermatology 149: 972–976

Stender IM, Na R, Fogh H et al 2000 Photodynamic therapy with 5-aminolaevulinic acid or placebo for recalcitrant foot and hand warts: randomised double-blind trial. Lancet 355: 963–966

Wang XL, Wang HW,Wang HS et al 2004 Topical 5 aminolevulinic acid-photodynamic therapy for the treatment of urethral condylomata acuminata. British Journal of Dermatology 151:880–885

Yamaguchi S, Tsuda H, Takemore M et al 2005 Photodynamic therapy for cervical intraepithelial neoplasia. Oncology 69: 110–116

10 Treatment of Cutaneous T-Cell Lymphoma, Psoriasis, and Port Wine Stain Birthmarks

Tanya Kormeili, Kristen M. Kelly

INTRODUCTION

Photodynamic therapy (PDT) utilizes a photosensitizer and light to generate reactive oxygen species (ROS) which cause tissue damage. PDT involves a photochemical method of injury which is different from the heat-induced effects typically observed during many light–tissue interactions.

PDT has been utilized to treat a wide range of benign, premalignant, and malignant dermatologic disorders. Common uses such as treatment of actinic keratoses and skin cancers are discussed in other chapters. PDT has also been evaluated for treatment of other cutaneous disorders, including cutaneous T-cell lymphoma (CTCL), psoriasis, and port wine stain (PWS) birthmarks (Fig. 10.1).

PDT photosensitizers can be applied topically or delivered systemically (oral or intravenous). Because of ease of use and fewer potential side effects, dermatologic PDT most commonly utilizes topical photosensitizers. In the USA, the only FDA-approved topical photosensitizer is 5-aminolevulinic acid (ALA) (see Fig. 1.1A). During clinical use, nonfluorescent, nonphotodynamically active ALA is applied to the skin where it is transformed into highly fluorescent and photodynamically active protoporphyrin IX (PpIX) via the heme cycle (see Box 1.2). However, in some cases, systemic photosensitizer delivery may offer significant benefits, e.g. in treatment of PWS where such administration offers an opportunity for vascular compartmentalization and selective vascular destruction.

CUTANEOUS T-CELL LYMPHOMA

CTCL is a malignant neoplasm of T lymphocytes, specifically T-helper cells. CTCL presents clinically as patches, plaques, tumors or erythroderma and requires histologic correlation for definitive diagnosis (Fig. 10.2). Prognosis varies with the degree of systemic and cutaneous involvement, and severe disease requires aggressive systemic treatment. However, patients with disease limited to the skin may be candidates for ALA-PDT.

Many treatment options are available for CTCL, including topical corticosteroids, topical nitrogen mustard, retinoids, psoralen in combination with UV irradiation (PUVA), radiation therapy, excision, and CO_2 laser surgery. Each of these therapies has limitations related to adverse effects or efficacy, and as such, alternatives are often sought. Topical ALA-PDT is one option, which may be useful for treatment of localized CTCL. Selective ALA uptake into lesions occurs after application, with subsequent inhibition of malignant transformed T cells. Malignant blood cells may also have an increased ability to convert ALA into PpIX as compared to normal blood cells.

• Patient selection

Topical ALA-PDT may be appropriate for CTCL patients with difficult-to-treat lesions because of localized resistance, location or other health considerations.

• Expected benefits

Complete clinical remission of localized CTCL has been achieved with ALA-PDT, although not for all lesions (Table 10.1). Prolonged remission may occur and has been reported with follow-up as long as 3 years. However, it is also important to note that on occasion, clinical resolution is observed, but biopsy reveals persistent malignant lymphocytic infiltration. This may be most common when lesions appear to clear after one treatment. As such, careful monitoring post-treatment is required.

• Treatment techniques

No standardized protocol exists for treatment of CTCL with PDT. Table 10.1 lists some of the studies which have evaluated different treatment strategies. Twenty percent ALA has been used most commonly. Application time has varied in investigations, but a period of 4–6 h appears to be adequate, especially when the area is occluded (generally with a light-shielding dressing).

Oseroff et al evaluated the effect of light dose and intensity on clinical effectiveness. They found that response increased with fluence (starting at 10 J/cm^2), reaching a plateau at 75–100 J/cm^2. Intensity also affected treatment response, with 150 mW/cm^2 being more effective than lower fluence rates.

Edstrom et al studied the effects of fluence, intensity, and lesional area on treatment tolerance. They started

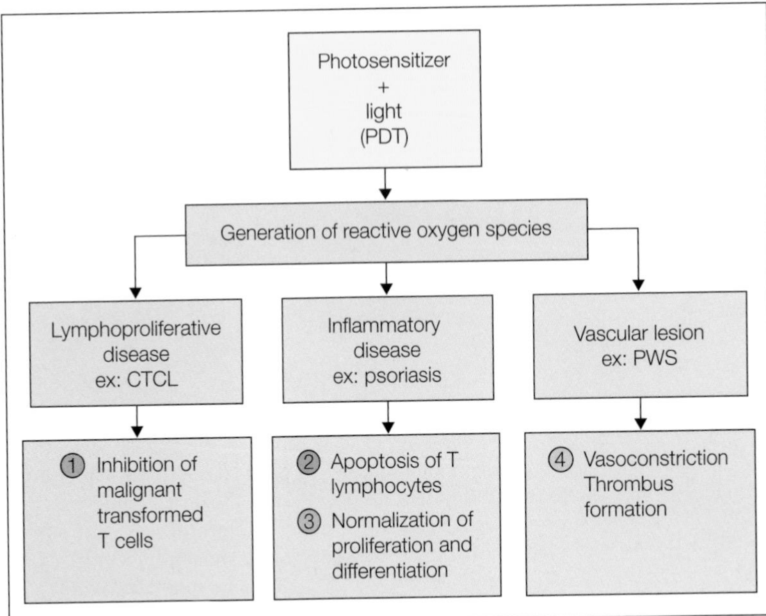

Fig. 10.1 Proposed mechanism for PDT effect in lymphoproliferative, inflammatory, and vascular disorders. 1 = Boehncke et al (1994); 2 = Bissonnette et al (2002); 3 = Fransson & Ros (2005); 4 = Major et al (1997)

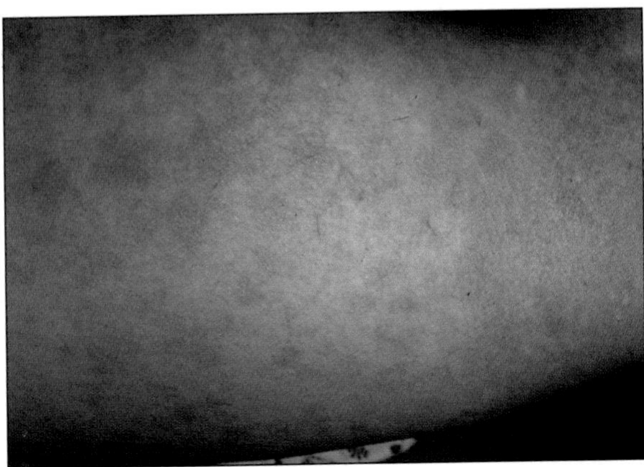

Fig. 10.2 Female with cutaneous T-cell lymphoma on her left leg. Clinical presentation confirmed by biopsy

with a fluence of 180 J/cm^2 but halved this later in their study, secondary to pain. High intensities (200–300 mW/cm^2) were difficult for patients to tolerate, while intensities of 35–125 mW/cm^2 were more comfortable and achieved a good clinical outcome. They also noted that treatment of larger areas resulted in greater pain.

Fractionation may improve results, especially in thick lesions. Orenstein et al used a 30-min irradiation session (580–720 nm, 140 mW/cm^2, 252 J/cm^2) followed by a 1-h dark period and then a second 10–15 min of irradiation (total cumulative dose 340–380 J/cm^2) for 1–4-mm deep tumor stage lesions. Leman et al theorized that fractionation might allow oxygen replenishment and improve the efficiency of the photodynamic process.

Orenstein et al demonstrated the utility of online in vivo fluorescence monitoring as a method to determine optimal light dosing for PDT (Fig. 10.3). For fluorescence detection, they used blue light (400–450 nm, 20 mW/cm^2) delivered by an optical fiber. A CCIR camera was used for imaging and a CCD-based fiberoptic spectrometer (spectral range 570–720 nm, spectral resolution 10 nm) was used for assessment of fluorescence signal intensity. Fluorescence imaging and spectroscopy were performed pretreatment, during treatment, and then 1 h after treatment. Using this imaging technique, re-treatment was considered for lesions for which PpIX fluorescence recurred (most commonly for thicker lesions).

Persistent lesions in difficult-to-treat anatomic locations may provide ideal opportunities for the use of ALA-PDT. Wang et al evaluated the use of ALA-PDT for resistant periocular T-cell lymphoma. One patient had three lesions on the medial canthus and lower eyelids bilaterally and had failed nine cycles of chemotherapy. The eye to be treated was covered with a specially designed intraorbital lead shield. Lesion surface was gently scraped with a scalpel to improve ALA penetration, although significant curetting was not performed (minimizing scarring and limiting discomfort). ALA powder (Porphyrin Products, Logan, Utah) was dissolved in neutral eye ointment (Emulgon®) to achieve a concentration of 20% ALA. Ointment was applied to lesions and a 5-mm margin and covered with a thin adhesive plastic pad (Tegaderm®, 3M, UK). A complete clinical response (CCR) was achieved after three treatments with no recurrence at 33 months. Cosmetic result was excellent, with no scarring.

Coors et al evaluated the use of topical ALA-PDT for difficult-to-treat CTCL lesions resistant to other

Table 10.1 Summary of studies evaluating treatment of cutaneous T-cell lymphoma with topical ALA-PDT

Reference	No. of sites	Application time (h)	Wavelength (nm)	Intensity (mW/cm²)	Fluence (J/cm²)	No. of Rx	Lesion type	Response	Recurrence
Coors & von den Driesch (2004)	7	6	Visible light	60–160	72–144	1–7	5 plaque 2 tumor	CCR all Lesions	None at 14–18 months
Edstrom et al (2001)	12	5–18	600–730	35–300	80–180	2–11	10 plaque 2 tumor	7/10 plaque: CCR 2/10 plaque: Regression 1/10 plaque: No response 2/2 tumor: No response	None in lesions with CCR after 4–19 months
Leman et al (2002)	2	6–24	630	48	100	4	Plaque	CCR all lesions	None at 12 months
Orenstein et al (2000)	6	16	580–720	140	170 patch 380 tumor	1	1 patch 5 tumor	CCR all lesions	None at 24 months
Oseroff et al (1996)	80	Overnight	630	30–150	10–200	1	Not specified	Varied with fluence and intensity	Not reported
Paech et al (2002)	2	4	580–740	Not reported	180	2	Plaque	CCR in all lesions	Not reported
Wang et al (1999)	3	4–6	635	<110	60	3	Periocular	CCR all lesions	None at 33 months

CCR = complete clinical response

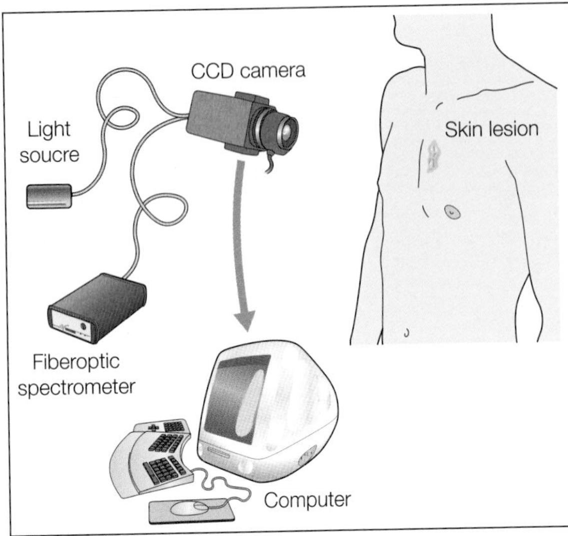

Fig. 10.3 Schematic diagram of fluorescence monitoring during ALA-PDT treatment

therapies. They achieved complete resolution of seven previously resistant lesions after treating them with 20% ALA, under occlusion for 6 h, followed by visible light irradiation.

An HIV-infected patient with CTCL was successfully treated with ALA-PDT by Paech et al. ALA ointment was applied under occlusion to plaques for 4 h, followed by light exposure (580–740 nm) generated by a PDT 1200 irradiation source (Waldmann Medizintechnik, Germany), achieving a dose of 180 J/cm^2. Complete remission was achieved after two cycles of PDT, spaced 4 weeks apart.

• Side effects and complications

Moderate-to-severe discomfort is common during topical PDT treatment of CTCL. Measures to ameliorate some discomfort include the use of intralesional anesthetics, water spray during treatment, liquid nitrogen sprayed repeatedly in the air about 10 cm above the treated lesion, and cold air epidermal cooling. The post-treatment period includes erythema, edema, and epidermal sloughing. Erosion and ulceration may occur. Lesions generally heal with a good cosmetic outcome, although pigmentary changes and scarring can result. It is important to note that light protection practices are important for 48 h following topical ALA-PDT to prevent phototoxicity at treated sites.

• Summary

PDT is an option for treatment of CTCL, although further work is required to optimize treatment parameters. Patients with difficult-to-treat lesions because of localized resistance, location or other health considerations, may be optimal candidates. Careful monitoring for systemic disease or local recurrence is important for all patients with CTCL and must be included in any treatment strategy.

PSORIASIS

Psoriasis is a common inflammatory disorder affecting up to 2% of the population. Characterized by erythematous plaques with silvery white scales, mostly over extensor surfaces, psoriasis is a disease that inflicts significant psychosocial morbidity on those affected.

There are many topical treatments available for psoriasis, including vitamin D derivatives, steroids, and retinoids. Moderate-to-severe psoriasis can be treated using systemic medications such as oral retinoids, methotrexate, cyclosporine, biologic agents or light therapy. Despite these many options, some patients do not achieve complete, long-term control of their psoriasis, or experience unacceptable adverse effects. As such, alternative treatment options are sought.

PDT may offer a treatment alternative for patients with resistant psoriasis (Fig. 10.4). Topical and orally administered ALA has been shown to be taken up selectively into psoriasis plaques and converted to PpIX. Bissonnette et al demonstrated apoptosis in T lymphocytes of some psoriatic plaques after PDT following oral administration of ALA. Fransson and Ros noted normalization of proliferation and differentiation markers, including cytokeratin 16 and filaggrin, in psoriatic plaques after two to five treatments with ALA-PDT. Dermal CD4(+) and CD8(+) T cells were also decreased.

• Patient selection

Optimal candidates are those patients who do not require or want systemic therapies and have localized psoriatic plaques that have been resistant to topical medications.

• Expected benefits

In some patients, rapid control of resistant plaques can be achieved. Prolonged remission may be possible but, as discussed below, treatment strategies will need to be optimized to achieve this on a consistent basis.

• Treatment techniques

Similar to CTCL, a range of strategies has been utilized for ALA-PDT psoriasis treatment (Table 10.2) and the best protocol has yet to be established.

The thick hyperkeratotic scale of psoriatic plaques is a barrier to penetration of topically applied ALA. Therefore, antikeratolytic measures prior to ALA application may be useful, provided these are done cautiously to minimize irritation.

Weinstein et al evaluated topical ALA-PDT for psoriasis utilizing differing ALA concentrations (2%, 10%, and 20%) in combination with UVA light (15 mW/cm^2, 2.5–

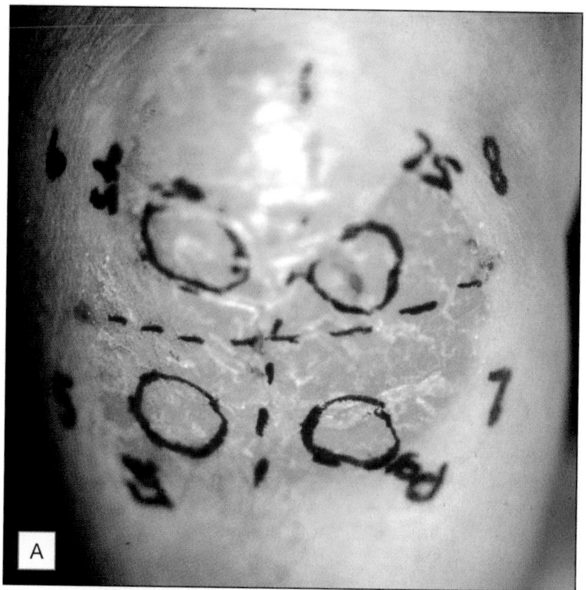

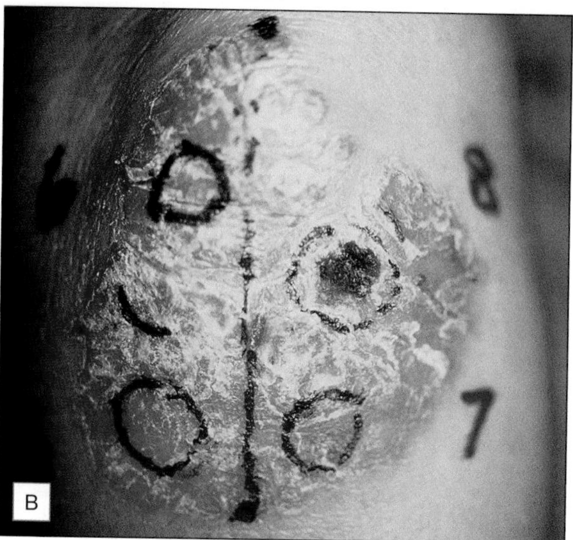

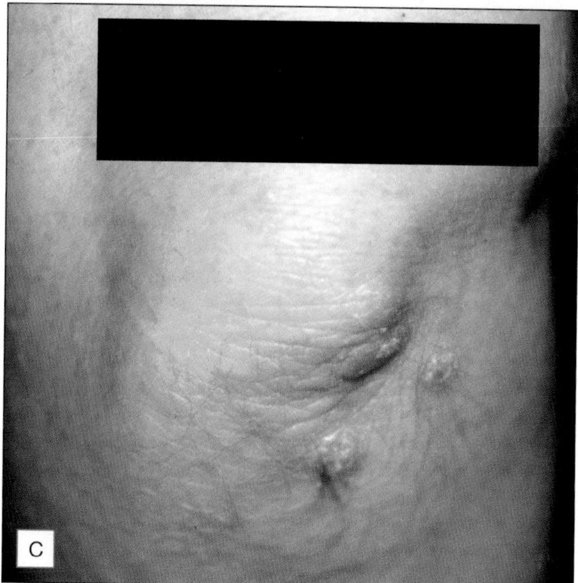

Fig. 10.4 Psoriasis plaque (**A**) before, (**B**) 2-weeks post- and (**C**) 3 months post-PDT treatment (Courtesy of J.S. Nelson, MD, PhD)

3 J/cm^2). Best results were noted with 10% and 20% ALA, achieving greater than 50% improvement after four weekly treatments.

Fritsch et al studied varying application times of topical ALA and concluded that 6 h of application appears to be optimal in terms of the highest porphyrin accumulation in psoriatic lesions; however, they and others found variable PpIX accumulation in psoriatic plaques.

Robinson et al proposed that regimens with multiple planned treatments may achieve greater therapeutic success. They evaluated 19 sites after application of topical 20% ALA for 4 h followed by broadband visible radiation with a modified slide projector (15 mW/cm^2, 2–8 J/cm^2), for up to 12 treatments, one to three times a week. Eight of the 10 patients improved, with four of the 19 sites resolving completely.

Rapid clinical clearance of psoriatic plaques was reported by Collins et al. They treated 36 trunk and extremity sites with 20% topical ALA applied for 4 h and irradiated with 400–650-nm light from a modified slide projector, at 10–40 mW/cm^2, for a total fluence of 2–16 J/cm^2. When evaluated 11–17 days after a single

Table 10.2 Summary of studies evaluating treatment of psoriasis with ALA-PDT

Reference	No. of sites	ALA administration	Wavelength (nm)	Intensity (mW/cm²)	Fluence (J/cm²)	No. of Rx	Response	Recurrence
Bissonnette et al (2002)	180	1, 3, 6 h Oral	417	9–11	1–20	1	0–42%	Not reported
Collins et al (1997)	36	4 h Topical	400–650	10–40	2–16	1	10 lesions clear 4 30–50% reduction 22 no change	5–14 days later
Kim et al (2005)	4	5 h Topical	632	30	15	11	Near complete clearance	Not reported
Radakovic-Fijan et al (2005)	29	Application time not reported Topical	600–740	Not reported	5, 10, 20	Up to 12	Psoriasis severity reduction of: 59% (20 J/cm²) 49% (10 J/cm²) 46% (5 J/cm²)	Not reported
Robinson et al (1999)	19	4 h Topical	Broadband visible	15	2–8	7–12	4 lesions clear, 10 improved, 5 no change	Not reported
Weinstein et al (1994)	84	3 h Topical	Ultraviolet A	15	2.5–3	1–4	Variable Improvement	Not reported

treatment, seven of the 22 test subjects showed improvement, with 10 of the 36 treated lesions clearing completely and four reducing by up to 50%. Lesions began to recur within 2 weeks.

Radakovic-Fijan et al pre-treated 29 patients with a keratolytic consisting of 10% salicylic acid in white petroleum for up to 2 weeks. This was followed by application of 1% ALA (for an unspecified period of time) and irradiation with a filtered halide lamp (Waldmann PDT 1200, 600–740 nm) for a light dose of 5, 10 or 20 J/cm². Treatments were performed twice weekly for a total of 12 sessions or until clearance. Psoriasis severity index (PSI) showed a final reduction of 59% in the group treated with 20 J/cm², as compared to 49% and 46% improvement achieved with light doses of 10 J/cm² and 5 J/cm², respectively. The difference in clinical efficacy between 20 J/cm² and 10 or 5 J/cm² was statistically significant ($P = 0.003$; $P = 0.02$).

Oral administration of ALA may offer advantages over topical application for ALA-PDT treatment of plaque psoriasis. Bissonnette et al had patients ingest ALA (5, 10 or 15 mg) and then after a period of 1–6 h exposed psoriatic plaques to a blue fluorescent lamp at 9–11 mW/cm² using fluences up to 20 J/cm². PpIX fluorescence increased rapidly and significantly in psoriatic plaques, reaching a maximum at 2–3 h. Maximal improvement (42% diminution in PSI at 28 days as compared to baseline) was seen in patients who received 10 or 15 mg of ALA followed after 3 h by 10 J/cm² of blue light.

While most studies have evaluated treatment of plaque psoriasis, PDT has also been used for palmoplantar pustular psoriasis. In a case report by Kim et al, a patient with pustular psoriasis resistant to topical steroids, acitretin, and methotrexate had 20% ALA applied topically for 5 h under occlusion followed by irradiation with a 632-nm diode laser (30 mW/cm², 15 J/cm²). The lesion was almost completely cleared after 11 weekly treatments for a total cumulative dose of 165 J/cm².

• Side effects and complications

Patients undergoing topical ALA-PDT for psoriasis frequently experience pain, burning, and itching, during and up to 72 h post-treatment. Severity of symptoms ranges from mild to severe. Erythema, mild edema, and occasionally erosions may occur post-treatment, especially when higher light doses are used. Post-inflammatory hyperpigmentation often occurs with plaque resolution, although scarring is generally not reported.

While administration of oral ALA has been associated with nausea, vomiting, and hypotension, the 5-, 10- or 15-mg doses used by Bissonnette et al resulted in only one of 12 patients reporting mild nausea. One patient (who received 15 mg) reported a mild burning sensation during light exposure. Asymptomatic erythema and edema lasting 3 days also occurred.

Photosensitivity results post oral or topical administration of ALA, making photoprotection necessary.

• Summary

Pain and unpredictable response are major limitations of topical ALA-PDT treatment of psoriasis. Oral ALA-PDT may be an alternative and facilitates treatment of large body surface areas. Post-treatment photosensitivity is an issue, but may be tolerated if optimization of treatment strategies results in consistent and rapid improvement of resistant plaques. Further research is required to evaluate the psoriatic treatment potential of ALA-PDT and to determine the place of this modality in the psoriatic treatment armamentarium.

PORT WINE STAIN BIRTHMARKS

PWS birthmarks are congenital, vascular malformations of the skin found in 0.3% of the population. While they may be located anywhere on the body, they are most commonly found on the face and can have serious psychological consequences. Additionally, these lesions may be associated with medical complications, including glaucoma, hypertrophy, or local bleeding.

The pulsed-dye laser (PDL) is the standard of care for treatment of PWS but achieves complete clearance in less than 20% of lesions. Therapeutic efficacy of PDL for PWS is affected by a variety of factors, including energy limitations secondary to risk of thermally induced epidermal injury and the inability of PDL to destroy microvessels (diameter < 20 μm).

PDT has been evaluated for PWS birthmarks and may offer an alternative treatment option. PDT uses a continuous wave (CW) light source to provide photons at a desired wavelength, driving photochemical reactions without heat generation. Milliwatt light exposure used during PDT does not cause the epidermal thermal injury produced by high peak power PDL. Further, PDT can destroy vessels of all sizes that contain the photosensitizer, including microvessels spared by PDL.

PWS treatment requires careful design of PDT to achieve selective destruction of PWS vessels without full thickness vascular elimination, which is likely to result in skin necrosis. While topical ALA-PDT has been considered by some for the treatment of PWS and other vascular lesions, this approach is unlikely to result in significant success, due to an inability to achieve vascular compartmentalization. PDT with systemically administered photosensitizers has been evaluated in PWS patients.

• Patient selection

Use of PDT for PWS is currently investigational but may one day offer an option for those with resistant PWS.

• Treatment techniques

Early evaluations from China and the USA (JS Nelson, personal communication) using blue and red light,

Table 10.3 Summary of studies evaluating treatment of PWS birthmarks with PDT

Reference	No. of sites	Photosensitizer	Wavelength (nm)	Intensity (mW/cm²)	Fluence (J/cm²)	No. of Rx	Response*
Evans & Kurwa (2004)	8	30 mg/kg Oral ALA	585	N/A	6.5	3	No significant difference between PDL alone vs. PDL + ALA
Lin et al (1997)	118	4–7 mg/kg Intravenous PSD-007	578	40–90	NR	1	27.1% excellent results 46.6% good results 24.6% fair results 1.7% poor results
Tournas et al (2006)	8	Verteporfin 6 mg/m²	576	100	Up to 75	1	Variable

respectively, resulted in a relatively high incidence of scarring and prolonged photosensitivity (30 days or more).

Lin et al (Table 10.3) evaluated 118 PWS patients who received a purified mixture of six kinds of porphyrin molecules (PsD-007; intravenous 4–7 mg/kg) followed within 30 min by exposure to 578-nm light (40–90 mW/cm^2). Up to 70 cm^2 were treated per session which took 1–2 h. After one treatment, 27.1% of patients had excellent results, 46.6% had good results, 24.6% had fair results, and 1.7% had poor results. Patients were photosensitive for 2 weeks. No hypertrophic scarring or permanent dyspigmentation was reported.

Evans and Kurwa used orally administered ALA (30 mg/kg) and PDT for PWS treatment. Each lesion was divided into three equal areas: (1) PDL alone (1.5 ms; 6.5 J/cm^2); (2) PDL 1 h after administration of ALA; or (3) PDL 2 h after administration of ALA. Patients received three treatments at 4-weekly intervals but no significant difference was found between the three areas. It is possible that the relatively short pulse duration of the PDL (1.5 ms) did not allow adequate generation of cytotoxic species to achieve prolonged vascular effect. Moreover, currently available forms of ALA are not vascular specific, making it difficult to find optimal treatment parameters which allow selective and significant vascular destruction without epidermal injury.

We have proposed combining PDT-induced photochemical and PDL-induced photothermal injuries to achieve a synergistic effect. Initial subtherapeutic PDT exposure makes PWS blood vessel walls, especially smaller vessels (potentially not affected by PDL alone), more vulnerable to subsequent photothermal damage. Subsequent PDL irradiation heats vessels compromised by PDT. Careful parameter selection for both PDT and PDL confine therapeutic effects to the upper 1000 μm of the dermis, containing ectatic PWS venules, while reducing the risk of possible skin infarction which could result from destruction of the lower vascular plexus.

In our protocol, benzoporphyrin derivative monoacid ring A (BPD; Visudyne, QLT, Inc, Vancouver, Canada) is administered intravenously at a dose of 6 mg/m^2, over a 10-min infusion period. Starting 15 min after the infusion onset, PDT irradiation is performed using a CW argon pumped dye laser (rhodamine 560; λ = 576 nm) and a power density of 100 mW/cm^2. This is followed immediately by PDL (585 nm; pulse duration 1.5 ms; 8 J/cm^2). This approach demonstrated significant promise in early animal studies in which PDT + PDL resulted in a statistically greater reduction in vascular perfusion (56%) as compared to either PDT or PDL alone.

Preliminary clinical studies using the PDT + PDL approach were recently reported. In order to increase safety of the study, PDT light dose was initiated at the very low light dose of 15 J/cm^2 and increased by 15 J/cm^2 over the course of the study, to a maximum of 75 J/cm^2. No significant adverse effects related to treatment were noted. PDT + PDL sites demonstrated increased purpura as compared to the PDL-alone test sites (Fig. 10.5). Purpura is a sign of vascular damage and increased purpura has been associated with improved PWS response. Two patients demonstrated improved blanching in the PDT + PDL sites (Fig. 10.6). It is important to note that preliminary animal experiments were conducted using a CW light dosage of 96 J/cm^2. Based on these results, greater effect can be expected to be seen in the PDT and PDT + PDL sites as CW light dosage is increased.

• Side effects and complications

PDT for treatment of vascular lesions must be approached cautiously as there is potential for total vascular destruction and subsequent scarring. Careful design of protocols may help avoid this potential pitfall. Post-treatment patients are photosensitive for variable duration depending on the photosensitizer and must be counseled about photoprotective measures.

• Summary

Further research is required but PDT alone or in combination with PDL may offer an approach for resistant cutaneous vascular lesions.

CONCLUSION

PDT has been used as an alternative treatment option for CTCL and psoriasis and is under investigation for PWS birthmarks. PDT is not first-line therapy for these indications but may offer a treatment option for those who have failed conventional treatments.

ACKNOWLEDGMENT

We would like to thank Dr Ronald J. Barr for his contribution to this chapter.

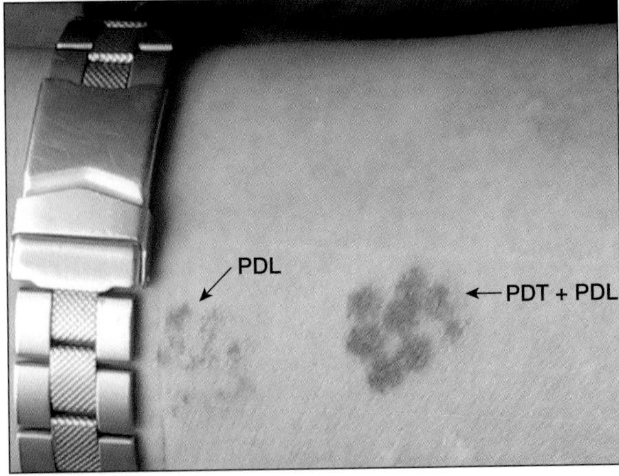

Fig. 10.5 Increased post-treatment purpura noted after PDT + PDL as compared to PDL alone utilizing a CW light dose of 45 J/cm^2 for the PDT spot.

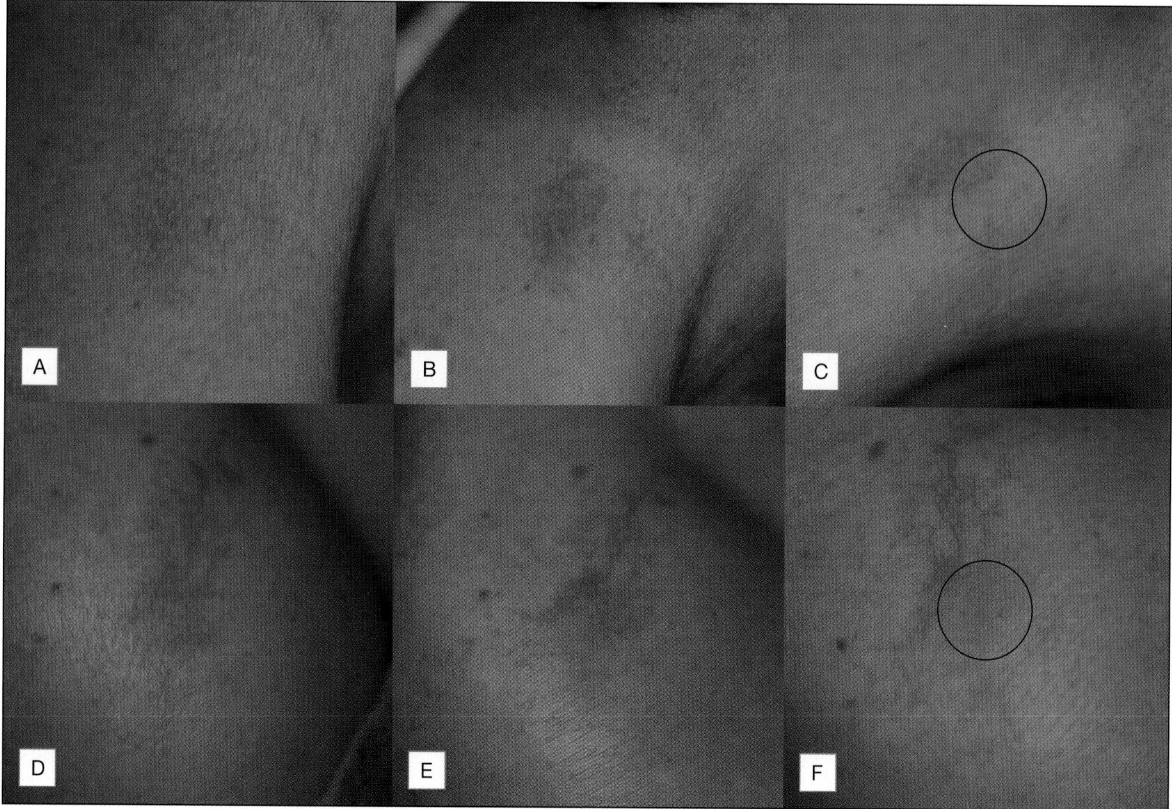

Fig. 10.6 PDL spot (**A**) before, (**B**) 4 weeks post, and (**C**) 8 weeks post intervention. PDT (45 J/cm^2) + PDL spot (**D**) before; (**E**) 4 weeks post, and (**F**) 8 weeks post intervention. Treatment area is outlined in **C** and **F**. Note improved PWS blanching in the PDT + PDL test spot as compared to PDL alone. No PWS blanching was noted in the control or PDT spots. Mild hyperpigmentation is noted in the PDT + PDL test

FURTHER READING

Cutaneous T-cell lymphoma

Boehncke W-H, Konig K, Ruck A et al 1994 In vitro and in vivo effects of photodynamic therapy in cutaneous T cell lymphoma. Acta Dermato-Venereologica 74:201–205 (In vivo fluorescence was used to document the ability of PDT to inhibit proliferation of malignant T cells)

Coors EA, von den Driesch P 2004 Topical photodynamic therapy for patients with therapy-resistant lesions of cutaneous T-cell lymphoma. Journal of the American Academy of Dermatology 50:363–367 (This study evaluates treatment of resistant cutaneous T-cell lymphoma lesions with topical ALA-PDT)

Edstrom DW, Porwit A, Ros A-M 2001 Photodynamic therapy with topical 5-aminolevulenic acid for mycosis fungoides: clinical and histological response. Acta Dermato-Venerologica 81:184–188 (This is an investigation of 5-ALA-PDT for treatment of plaque and tumor lesions of mycosis fungoides)

Leman JA, Dick DC, Morton CA 2002 Topical 5-ALA photodynamic therapy for the treatment of cutaneous T-cell lymphoma. Clinical and Experimental Dermatology 27:516–518 (Case report of topical ALA-PDT for plaque stage cutaneous T-cell lymphoma)

Orenstein A, Haik J, Tamir J et al 2000 Photodynamic therapy of cutaneous lymphoma using 5-aminolevulinic acid topical application. Dermatologic Surgery 26:765–770 (Evaluation of PP accumulation and results of ALA-PDT treatment in patients with cutaneous T-cell lymphoma)

Oseroff AR, Whitaker J, Conti C et al 1996 Effects of fluence and intensity in PDT of cutaneous T-cell lymphoma with topical ALA: High intensities spare the epidermis. Journal of Investigative Dermatology 100:602 (An abstract evaluating the efficacy and epidermal toxicity of ALA-PDT for cutaneous T-cell lymphoma)

Paech V, Lorenzen T, Stoehr A et al 2002 Remission of a cutaneous Mycosis fungoides after topical 5-ALA sensitization and photodynamic therapy in a patient with advanced HIV-infection. European Journal of Medical Research 7:477–779 (Case report of topical ALA-PDT for plaque stage cutaneous T-cell lymphoma in an HIV-infected individual)

Pagliaro J, Elliott T, Bulsara M et al 2004 Cold air analgesia in photodynamic therapy of basal cell carcinomas and Bowen's disease: an effective addition to treatment: a pilot study. Dermatologic Surgery 30:63–66 (Evaluation of the use of cold air analgesia during PDT for superficial skin malignancies)

Wang I, Bauer B, Andersson-Engels S 1999 Photodynamic therapy utilizing topical aminolevulinic acid in non-melanoma skin malignancies of the eyelid and the peri-ocular skin. Acta Ophthalmologica Scandinavia 77:182–188 (Evaluation of topical ALA-PDT for periocular skin malignancies)

Psoriasis

Bissonnette R, Tremblay J, Juzenas P et al 2002 Systemic photodynamic therapy with aminolevulinic acid induces apoptosis in lesional T cell lymphocytes of psoriatic plaques.

Journal of Investigative Dermatology 119:77–83 (Treatment of psoriasis with oral ALA (varying dosage and absorption time) and blue light followed by post-treatment biopsies demonstrating T cell lymphocyte apoptosis)

Boehnke W, Sterry W, Kaufmann R 1994 Treatment of psoriasis by topical photodynamic light therapy with polychromatic light. Lancet 343:801 (Treatment of psoriasis with topical ALA and polychromatic light compared to contra lateral plaques treated with dithranol)

Collins P, Robinson D, Stringer M, Stables G, Sheehan-Dare R 1997 The variable response of plaque psoriasis after a single treatment with topical 5-aminolevulenic acid photodynamic therapy. British Journal of Dermatology 137:743–749 (Evaluation of a single topical ALA and polychromatic light treatment of psoriatic plaques)

Fransson J, Ros A 2005 Clinical and immunohistochemical evaluation of psoriatic plaques treated with topical 5-aminolaevulinic acid photodynamic therapy. Photodermatology, Photoimmunology & Photomedicine 21:326–332 (Evaluation of the clinical and immunohistochemical changes in psoriatic plaques in response to topical ALA-PDT)

Fritsch C, Lehmann P, Stahl W et al 1998 Optimum porphyrin accumulation in epithelial skin tumours and psoriatic lesions after topical application of delta-aminolevulinic acid. British Journal of Cancer 79:1603–1608 (Evaluates the time course of porphyrin metabolite formation after topical application of delta-aminolevulinic acid to epithelial skin tumors and psoriasis, in order to determine the optimal application time)

Kim YC, Lee ES, Chung PS, Phee CK 2005 Recalcitrant palmoplantar pustular psoriasis successfully treated with topical 5-aminolaevulinic acid photodynamic therapy. Clinical and Experimental Dermatology 30:723–724 (Case report of topical ALA-PDT for palmoplantar pustular psoriasis)

Radakovic-Fijan S, Blecha-Thalhammer U, Schleyer V et al 2005 Topical aminolaevulinic acid-based photodynamic therapy as a treatment option for psoriasis? Results of a randomized, observer-blinded study. British Journal of Dermatology 152:279–283 (Report of the results of an observer-blinded study investigating use of topical ALA-PDT for psoriasis)

Robinson D, Collins P, Stringer M et al 1999 Improved response of plaque psoriasis after multiple treatments with topical 5-delta aminolevulinic acid photodynamic therapy. Acta Dermato-Venerologica 79:451–455 (Multiple treatment approach of topical ALA and polychromatic light for psoriasis)

Stringer M, Collins P, Robinson D et al 1996 The accumulation of protoporphyrin IX in plaque psoriasis after topical application of 5-aminolevulinic acid indicates a potential for superficial photodynamic therapy. Journal of Investigative Dermatology 107:76–81 (Psoriatic plaques show increased fluorescence after topical 5-ALA application)

Weinstein G, McCullough J, Jeffes E et al 1994 Photodynamic therapy (PDT) of psoriasis with topical delta aminolevulinic acid (ALA): a pilot dose-ranging study. Photodermatology, Photoimmunology & Photomedicine 10:92 (Treatment of psoriasis with varying concentrations of topical ALA and ultraviolet A light)

Vascular lesions

Edstrom DW, Hedblad M-A, Ros A-M 2002 Flashlamp pulsed dye laser and argon-pumped dye laser in the treatment of port-wine stains: a clinical and histological comparison. British Journal of Dermatology 146:285–289 (Report of the clinical and histological changes observed in port wine stains after treatment with pulsed dye laser and argon-pumped dye laser)

Evans AV, Kurwa HA 2004 Treatment of port wine stains using photodynamic therapy with systemic 5-aminolaevulinic acid as an adjunct to pulsed dye laser therapy. Lasers in Surgery and Medicine S16:19 (Evaluation of PWS blanching after treatment with oral ALA and PDL compared to PDL therapy alone)

Gu Y, Jun-heng L 1992 The clinical study of argon laser PDT for port wine stain. 40 case reports. Chinese Journal of Laser Medicine 1:1–4 (Evaluation of argon laser PDT for the treatment of port wine stains)

Smith TK, Choi B, Ramirez-San-Juan J, Nelson JS, Osann K, Kelly KM 2006 Microvascular blood flow dynamics associated with photodynamic therapy, pulsed dye laser irradiation and combined regimens. Lasers in Surgery and Medicine 38:532–539 (Evaluation of vascular effects after combined PDT + PDL as compared to PDT alone or PDL alone in a chick chorioallantoic model)

Lin XX, Wang W, Wu SF, Yang C, Chang TS 1997 Treatment of capillary vascular malformation (port-wine stains) with photochemotherapy. Plastic Reconstructive Surgery 99:1826–1830 (A retrospective study evaluating PDT using a porphyrin mixture and yellow light as a treatment for port wine stains)

Lou W, Geronemus R 2001 Treatment of PWS by variable pulse width pulsed dye laser with cryogen spray: A preliminary study. Dermatologic Surgery 27:963–965 (A preliminary study on the use of variable pulse width pulse dye laser with cryogen spray in the treatment of port wine stains)

Major AL, Kimel S, Mee S et al 1999 Microvascular photodynamic effects determined *in vivo* using optical Doppler tomography. IEEE Journal of Selected Topics in Quantum Electronics 5:1168–1175 (Animal study to evaluate the role of the microvasculature in tumor destruction as a result of PDT)

Morelli JG, Weston WL, Huff JC, Yohn JJ 1995 Initial lesion size as a predictive factor in determining the response of port-wine stains in children treated with the pulsed dye laser. Archives of Pediatrics and Adolescent Medicine 149:1142–1144 (Study evaluating the effect of PWS lesion size as a predictor of response to PDL treatment)

Tournas JA, Choi B, Kelly KM 2006 Combined photodynamic and pulsed dye laser treatment of port wine stains. Presented at the American Society for Laser Medicine and Surgery Annual Meeting, Boston, MA (Poster presentation on the use of PDT and combined PDT + PDL for the treatment of port wine stains)

Van der Horst CMAM, Koster PHL, deBorgie CAJM, Bossuyt PMM, van Gemert MJC 1998 Effect of timing of treatment of port-wine stains with the flash-lamp-pumped pulsed dye laser. New England Journal of Medicine 338:1028–1033 (Prospective study evaluating effects of age on PDL treatment of port wine stain birthmarks)

11 Prevention of Skin Cancer

Catherine Maari, Robert Bissonnette

INTRODUCTION

• Squamous cell and basal cell carcinoma

Basal cell carcinoma (BCC) and cutaneous squamous cell carcinoma (SCC) are the most frequent cancers in Caucasians. These tumors can invade adjacent structures causing local destruction, which can lead to significant cosmetic impairment. In addition, SCCs and more rarely BCCs can metastasize. The incidence of both BCC and SCC is on the rise. It is estimated that almost one in three Caucasians born in the USA after 1994 will develop a BCC in their lifetime. The cost of treating these tumors has been estimated at $400 million per year for the US Medicare population alone. Sunlight exposure is the major cause of BCC and SCC. Ultraviolet B radiation (UVB) (280–320 nm) is highly mutagenic and can induce actinic keratoses (AKs) and SCC in hairless mice, as well as BCC in the PTCH heterozygous mouse.

The incidence of nonmelanoma skin cancer (NMSC) has been increasing by 2–3% per year in the USA. It is therefore a priority to develop strategies to prevent BCCs and SCCs. This will not only reduce morbidity and mortality rates, but will also decrease the financial burden on health care systems created by treating these lesions.

• Current strategies for skin cancer prevention

Current skin cancer prevention strategies mostly rely on sun avoidance and sun protection with sunscreens and clothing. Much effort has been made to educate the public about the importance of protecting their skin against excessive UV light. Despite this effort, the incidence of skin cancer continues to increase. Clearly, other strategies are needed in order to prevent these common neoplasms. Frequent medical visits for patients at higher risk, such as fair-skinned individuals, patients with a previous history of BCC or SCC, and organ transplant recipients, are also performed to detect and treat early lesions. Treatment of AKs is of utmost importance in order to stop progression into invasive SCCs (see Ch 6). Prospective studies suggest that the regular use of sunscreens can decrease the number of new AKs and SCCs.

Small open studies with patients at high risk of developing NMSC suggest that high-dose oral retinoids can reduce the risks of developing SCC. However, patients often do not tolerate these high doses because of secondary mucocutaneous and musculoskeletal side effects. A study conducted on 981 subjects with a history of at least two BCCs showed no difference in occurrence of new BCC after 3 years of low-dose isotretinoin (10 mg/day) compared to placebo. These lower doses were much better tolerated but lacked efficacy in NMSC prevention. A large randomized placebo controlled trial by Levine et al comparing retinol and low-dose isotretinoin did not demonstrate a significant chemopreventive effect in the high-risk group, defined as patients with a history of at least four BCCs or SCCs. The same authors enrolled 2297 patients with a history of more than 10 AKs and at most two SCCs or BCCs (moderate-risk group) and randomized them to receive either 25 000 IU of retinol or placebo. The subjects in the retinol group had a significantly lower risk of developing a first new SCC than those in the placebo group. This same group did not show a difference in the risk of first BCC compared with the placebo group.

Studies of the use of acitretin for chemoprevention in renal transplantation patients have shown a significant reduction in the development of new NMSCs compared to placebo. Based on these studies, retinoids can be effective as a chemopreventive agent in certain subgroups of patients but would need to be continued indefinitely to maintain their protective benefits.

T4 endonuclease V is an enzyme that repairs damaged DNA in bacteria and has been shown to accelerate the repair of DNA in human cells when it is delivered intracellularly. This molecule is currently being investigated as a chemopreventive agent and is delivered via encapsulated liposomes that are applied topically. The murine model showed a lower incidence of skin tumors in treated mice compared with control mice after repeated UVB exposure. Human studies in patients with xeroderma pigmentosum reported that topical T4 endonucleases V reduced the rate of development of BCCs and AKs. Further investigation with this molecule is thus warranted.

A number of animal studies have suggested that the use of oral and/or topical antioxidants such as green tea and grapeseed polyphenols, and vitamins C and E can prevent the development of UV-induced AKs and SCCs. A large cohort study has shown that oral supplementation with vitamins A, C, and E, folate, and carotenoids did not provide protection against the development of SCCs. A randomized trial involving more than 1000 patients showed that supplements not only failed to prevent BCC and SCC, but actually increased the risk of developing SCC.

Chemoprevention of skin cancer is a very active research field. A currently pursued strategy is targeting of key molecules in the UV-light signal-transduction pathway, such as the activator protein-1, cyclooxygenase-2 (Celecoxib), and difluoromethylornithine. Additional preventive measures for NMSCs are needed in view of the limited number of options currently available. Large-surface photodynamic therapy (PDT) with 5-aminolevulinic acid (ALA) or the methyl ester of ALA (MAL) has the potential to become an important skin cancer prevention modality for BCCs and SCCs.

SKIN CANCER PREVENTION USING PDT IN ANIMAL MODELS

• Squamous cell carcinoma

Prospective clinical studies designed to evaluate skin cancer prevention strategies are difficult to perform because of the delay between carcinogenesis induction and actual lesion appearance, ethical issues related to voluntary exposure to carcinogenic agents, as well as the low incidence of new skin cancers in most populations. This situation explains why animal models, such as the hairless mouse, are frequently used to explore new skin cancer prevention methods. This immunocompetent mouse is characterized by an almost complete absence of hair, which combined with its small size and easy availability makes it ideal for skin cancer prevention studies.

Following daily UV radiation exposure, hairless mice develop skin tumors within 2–4 months. The first lesions are AKs and these evolve with time into invasive SCC. The appearance of these tumors is influenced by daily UV radiation dose, UV exposure frequency, as well as the wavebands of UV radiation generated by the UV source.

In skin cancer prevention experiments performed with ALA- or MAL-PDT, mice are usually exposed 5–7 days a week to UV radiation from fluorescent lamps. In addition they also receive weekly to monthly large-surface ALA-PDT treatments. ALA is applied to the back of mice, with subsequent activation by a visible light source. Pink–red porphyrin fluorescence can be seen on hairless mouse skin after ALA application (Fig. 11.1). Light sources are placed on top of cages so that the mice are free to move during both UV and light exposure. Mice are carefully examined weekly for the presence of skin tumors.

Using the hairless mouse, Stender et al showed that weekly topical ALA-PDT can delay the appearance of AKs and SCC induced by chronic UV radiation exposure. However, in this original report, it was observed that more ALA-PDT-treated mice were withdrawn because of large tumors as compared to mice exposed to UV radiation only. Our group subsequently studied systemic (intraperitoneal) weekly ALA-PDT sessions. They showed that this therapy could delay the appearance of AKs and SCCs and reduce the number of tumors per mouse, without inducing large tumors (Fig. 11.2).

In order to perform a study that was as close as possible to the clinical situation, we exposed a group of hairless mice to UV radiation for only 8 weeks followed by weekly ALA-PDT sessions. In this experiment PDT was performed with topical ALA in the commercially available vehicle and with the BLU-U tubes. Chronic UV exposure took place before weekly ALA-PDT sessions were started in order to create a more clinically relevant situation, as patients diagnosed with skin cancer tend to avoid additional sun exposure. A delay in the appearance of both AKs and invasive SCC was observed (Fig. 11.3). We have also repeated Stender's protocol as best as could be done, using similar UV and visible light sources, but failed to see any increase in incidence of large tumors. Similar prevention studies were performed with topical application of MAL and it was again shown that mice exposed chronically to UV radiation and treated weekly with MAL-PDT showed a delay in appearance of both AKs and SCC.

• Basal cell carcinoma

The search for strategies to prevent BCCs has long been hindered by the lack of an appropriate animal model. BCCs are not observed when the hairless mouse is exposed chronically to UV radiation. The transgenic mouse heterozygous for the PTCH gene has provided the first animal model to study prevention strategies for BCC. The PTCH protein, which is a membrane glycoprotein, binds to and inactivates smoothened, another membrane protein. Mutations in the PTCH or smoothened genes activate the Sonic-Hedgehog (SHH) signaling pathway, which culminates in transformation.

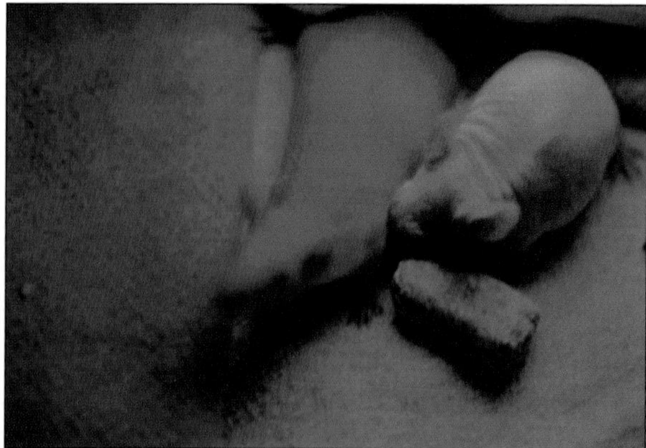

Fig. 11.1 Pink–red fluorescence can be seen with a Wood's lamp on the back of a hairless mouse (right) following ALA administration. The mouse on the left did not receive ALA

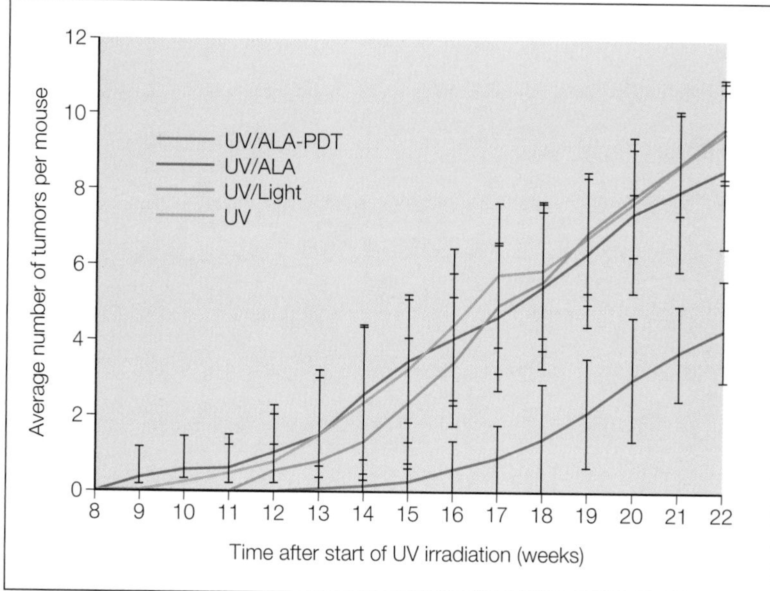

Fig. 11.2 Number of skin tumors per mouse according to time after the start of UV irradiation. Mice were exposed for 5 days per week to UV radiation and treated weekly with ALA-PDT. Weekly ALA-PDT induces a delay in tumor appearance as well as a decrease in the average number of tumors per mouse (Reproduced with permission from Sharfaei S, Viau G, Liu H et al 2001 Systemic photodynamic therapy with aminolevulinic acid delays the appearance of ultraviolet-induced skin tumours in mice. British Journal of Dermatology 144:1207)

The PTCH$^{+/-}$ mouse develops neoplasms resembling BCC-like tumors when chronically exposed to UV or ionizing radiation. In addition, this mouse model presents several developmental abnormalities found in basal cell nevus syndrome patients, namely polydactyly, medulloblastoma, and jaw cysts.

We conducted a study on the ability of PDT with topical MAL to prevent UV-induced BCCs using the PTCH$^{+/-}$ mouse model. In this study, 35 PTCH heterozygous mice were exposed for 5 days per week to UV radiation for a total of 20 weeks. Of these mice, 15 were also treated weekly with topical MAL-PDT. MAL is cleaved into ALA, which subsequently enters the porphyrin biosynthetic pathway and leads to protoporphyrin IX (PpIX) accumulation. The PTCH$^{+/-}$ mice were sacrificed 8 weeks after the end of UV exposure, and multiple skin biopsies were performed to identify microscopic BCCs. A total of 19 microscopic BCCs were found in nine of the mice exposed to UV radiation only, whereas no BCCs were seen in mice exposed to UV radiation and treated weekly with MAL-PDT. To our knowledge, this is the first study looking at the ability of large-surface PDT to prevent BCC in PTCH$^{+/-}$ mice. As MAL is transformed into ALA, we believe that large-surface ALA-PDT will also be able to prevent BCCs in this mouse model.

MECHANISMS OF ACTION OF ALA-PDT AS A SKIN CANCER PREVENTIVE MODALITY

The mechanisms of action involved in the ability of ALA-PDT to delay skin cancer appearance are currently under study. We conducted experiments with topical MAL where the photosensitizer was only applied to one half of the back of mice: the delay in skin cancer appearance was only observed on the side where MAL was applied, suggesting a local rather than a systemic effect .

Investigations conducted in the hairless mouse model have shown that chronic UV exposure induces islands of epidermal cells bearing mutations in the p53 gene. This event occurs as early as 17 days after initiation of daily UV exposure and well before any visible lesions are present on mouse skin. Subsequent investigations have shown that patients with chronic sun exposure also exhibit the same type of islands of epidermal cells harboring p53 mutations, suggesting that these clones of epidermal cells are precursors of visible AKs. Therefore, destruction of these clones by ALA-PDT might prevent the appearance of AKs and, eventually, the appearance of skin cancer. In a further effort to understand the underlying mechanisms of action of ALA-PDT, we used immunohistochemistry with a p53 monoclonal antibody to determine whether an ALA-PDT session would induce a preferential phototoxic reaction in these islands of mutated epidermal cells. Twenty-four hours after ALA-PDT in the hairless mice, the number of keratinocytes showing signs of phototoxicity from light exposure was no higher on the islands of mutated epidermal cells compared to adjacent epidermis, suggesting that these cells are not directly targeted by a phototoxic reaction following ALA-PDT (Fig. 11.4). It is, however, possible that the cellular photodamage generated by ALA-PDT induces specific toxicity in these islands of mutated epidermal cells by an indirect phenomenon. Other possible mechanisms for skin cancer prevention by ALA-PDT include a cytokine-mediated effect that could either delay tumour growth or reverse UV-induced immunosuppression, as well as specific antitumoral immune-mediated effects.

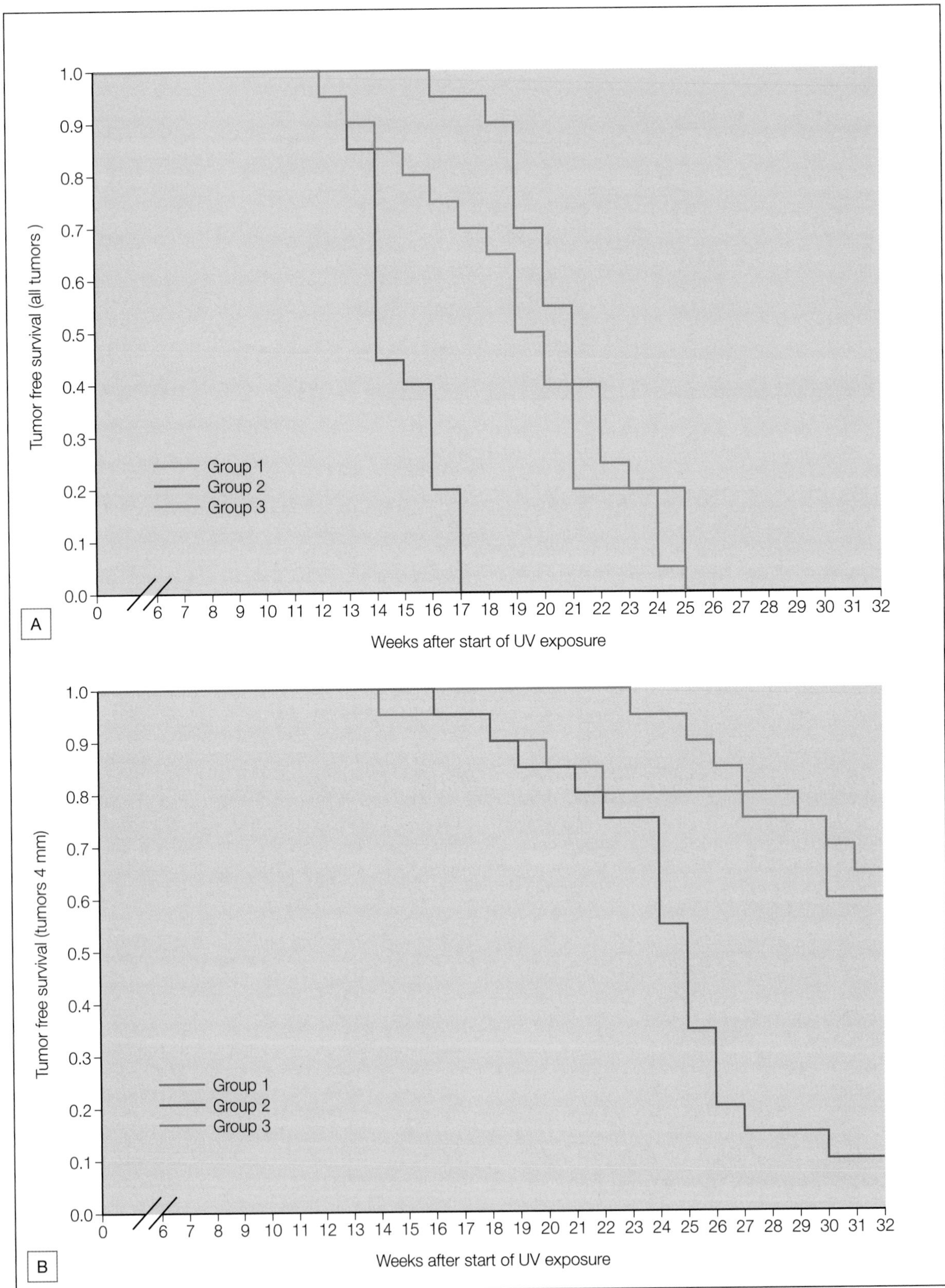

Fig. 11.3 Kaplan–Meier curve showing a delay in all tumors as well as SCC (tumors ≥4 mm) induced by topical ALA-PDT in hairless mice. Group 1 was only exposed to UV radiation for 5 days per week for 8 weeks. Group 2 was also treated weekly with ALA-PDT, which was started at the same time as UV exposure. Group 3 was exposed to UV radiation for 8 weeks followed by weekly topical ALA-PDT (Reproduced with permission from Liu Y, Viau G, Bissonnette R. Multiple large-surface photodynamic therapy sessions with topical or systemic aminolevulinic acid and blue light in UV-exposed hairless mice. J Cutan Med Surg. 2004 Mar–Apr; 8(2):131–9)

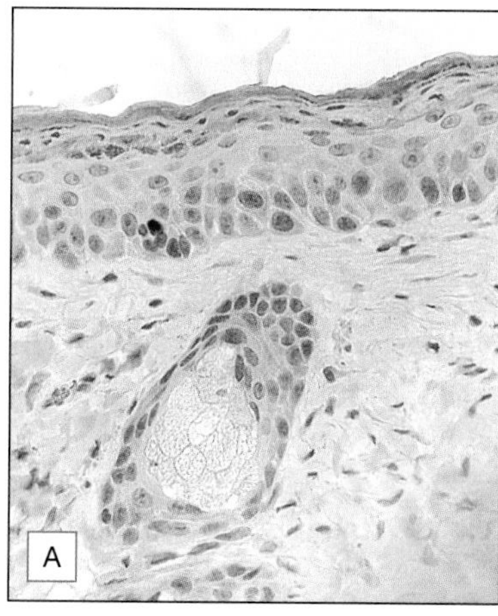

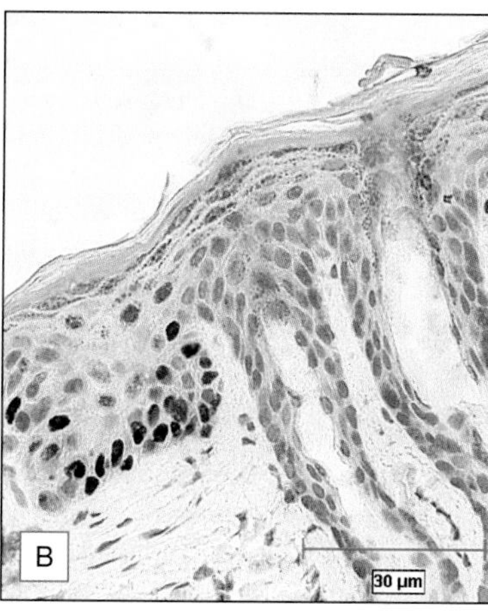

Fig. 11.4 Micrographs from a hairless mouse exposed weekly to UV radiation and treated once with ALA-PDT. 24-h post-PDT the photodamage induced by ALA-PDT is mostly located in the upper epidermis (**A**), whereas clusters of cells with mutated p53 (induced by chronic UV exposure) are present in the lower epidermis (**B**)

SKIN CANCER PREVENTION WITH PDT IN THE CLINIC

Strictly speaking, the use of ALA or MAL-PDT for the treatment of AKs can be considered a skin cancer prevention intervention as AKs are premalignant lesions. However, for the purpose of this chapter, prevention of skin cancer with ALA or MAL-PDT will be defined as the treatment of skin areas devoid of visible malignant or premalignant lesions with the intention of preventing the appearance of such lesions. The use of PDT as a skin cancer preventive modality is still considered experimental. The only approved indication for ALA-PDT in the USA and Canada is the treatment of nonhypertrophic AKs on the face and scalp.

Despite the lack of official approval, some dermatologists have started to use large-surface ALA-PDT as a skin preventive strategy in their practice. This action is based on the animal studies discussed above, as well as the preliminary safety and efficacy results from studies conducted with large-surface ALA-PDT for treatment of extensive AKs and photoaging.

• Patient selection

Patients with only a few AKs are best treated with one or two spot ALA-PDT sessions, or with another treatment modality such as liquid nitrogen. Patients who can benefit from ALA-PDT for skin cancer prevention include those (1) with numerous ill-defined AKs; (2) with frequent new AKs, SCCs or BCCs despite standard treatment; and (3) who are at higher risk of developing skin cancer.

The efficacy of this approach in treating numerous ill-defined AKs has been confirmed in a pilot study. The long-term prevention of recurrences following large-surface ALA- or MAL-PDT remains to be studied.

Multiple ALA-PDT sessions can also be used in patients with a history of frequent new AKs or invasive skin cancer despite standard care. Many immunocompetent AK patients will show a complete response following initial therapy, whether with ALA-PDT or another modality, with very few new lesions on subsequent follow-up visits. These patients may be managed with photoprotection and yearly skin examinations. However, some patients will develop numerous new AKs and sometimes even invasive SCC. For these patients, a more aggressive approach might be beneficial. Following treatment of all lesions, either with PDT or another modality, it is possible to perform regular ALA-PDT sessions to try to prevent the appearance of new lesions. The same strategy could by used in patients with basal cell nevus syndrome. Itkin and Gilchrest performed full-face ALA-PDT on two patients with Gorlin's syndrome to decrease the number of new BCCs. Oseroff and colleagues also published on the efficacy of large-surface ALA-PDT under general anesthesia in the treatment and prevention of BCC in children with Gorlin's syndrome.

Multiple ALA-PDT sessions could also be performed in patients without a history of skin cancer but with a very high risk of developing BCC, SCC or AK, including patients with genetic disorders that predispose to skin cancer such as basal cell nevus syndrome (Gorlin's syndrome) and xeroderma pigmentosum (XP), as well as organ transplant recipients. Our unpublished study on the prevention of skin cancer in a mouse model for Gorlin's syndrome suggests that multiple PDT sessions can delay photocarcinogenesis if started before the appearance of the first BCC. There are no data yet available for XP. XP patients have an impaired ability to repair DNA, which makes their epidermal cells highly sensitive to transformation following DNA strand breaks induced by UV radiation. As some in vitro studies have suggested that ALA-PDT can be genotoxic, a cautious approach is suggested for XP patients.

Two studies have shown that large-surface MAL-PDT can prevent the appearance of new AKs in immunosuppressed transplant patients. However, de Graff et al in a recent study failed to show any benefit from one or two courses of ALA-PDT in transplant patients. The reason for the different outcome in this last study is currently unknown. This study included patients with at least a 5-year history, or organ transplant with a history of previous cancer, or at least 10 keratotic lesions in the treatment field. It is possible that only one to two ALA-PDT sessions was not enough to generate a clinical effect. Differences between the de Graff study and the other studies include the use of blue instead of red light and the absence of skin preparation technique before ALA application.

Some physicians prefer to wait for studies confirming the efficacy of this preventive therapy before using multiple large-surface ALA-PDT sessions in patients who have never previously presented with malignant or pre-malignant lesions.

• ALA-PDT sessions

ALA APPLICATION

Before large-surface ALA application, a careful skin examination is mandatory to exclude the presence of malignant lesions such as melanoma, lentigo maligna, SCC or BCC. The response of invasive SCC to ALA-PDT has been reported to be disappointing, although some investigators have had success when multiple ALA-PDT sessions are used. The treatment of BCC with MAL is currently approved in several European countries and ALA-PDT has been used with success for the treatment of BCC. However, the method has never been standardized and centers often use different protocols, vehicles, and/or light sources. The main risk in performing ALA-PDT for BCC or SCC using suboptimal conditions is tumor recurrence. As the initial superficial clinical response is usually very good, these recurrences may arise more deeply and may eventually require extensive surgery. We therefore suggest biopsy of any lesion suspicious of skin cancer before initiating ALA-PDT for skin cancer prevention.

ALA should be applied to all areas where skin cancer prevention is required. Most often this is to the face. Our strategy using the commercially available ALA solution (Levulan) is to first apply ALA to all visible AKs and to let the solution dry. This is followed by a broad application of the solution to the areas to be treated and finally by a second application on all visible AKs. The total volume of ALA solution provided by one commercially available applicator is sufficient to completely cover the face. It is important that care be taken to completely crush both the ALA and the vehicle vials in order to have enough solution available for a full-face application. There are currently no studies available on the influence of the applied hydro-alcoholic solution volume on PpIX synthesis in the skin. As many European dermatologists compound ALA at 5% with good results for the treatment of AKs and BCCs, a single application of ALA at 20% in the commercially available vehicle should be sufficient. However, this remains to be studied.

After broad-area application, we keep patients in a subdued-light environment (closed ambient lighting in an examination room). Again, studies are not available to confirm if this is necessary. It is probably not essential if light exposure takes place at 1 h after application as little PpIX is generated by the epidermis in the first 30 min after ALA application. Exposure to low-energy output from ambient lighting may even be beneficial in enhancing the efficacy of the ALA-PDT treatment.

LIGHT SOURCE AND TIME OF LIGHT EXPOSURE

The BLU-U fluorescent light source is currently the only light source approved for the spot treatment of AKs. In theory any light source providing sufficient output in the spectral range of one of the excitation peaks of PpIX could be used. We favor the use of the BLU-U as two multi-center randomized, controlled studies have defined parameters for good efficacy in the treatment of AKs with this source. Small opaque plastic eyeshields are used to cover the eyes during light exposure. In the FDA-approved protocol for the treatment of AK with ALA-PDT, light exposure takes place 14–18 h after ALA application. A recent small pilot study suggested that good efficacy for the treatment or AK can also be obtained when light exposure takes place as early as 1 h after ALA application. The authors of that study did not find a significant difference in clinical response of AK when light exposure took place either 1 or 3 h after ALA application. We use 10 J/cm^2 (the approved light dose for the treatment of AKs) at 1 h after ALA application. Other physicians are using a lower fluence with apparently good results.

In our experience, inter-patient variability was noted in both the response in AK clearance and the magnitude of the phototoxic reaction following ALA-PDT performed with light exposure at 1 h. For some patients, it seems that 1 h is not enough. Increasing the incubation time to 2 or 3 h on subsequent exposures will induce AK clearance and a mild-to-moderate phototoxic response. It is unknown if the intensity of the phototoxic response present 24 h after ALA-PDT influences the efficacy of the skin preventive strategy. In hairless mice we have shown that ALA-PDT performed using suberythematous or erythematous fluences are both efficacious in inducing a delay in skin cancer appearance. In their current approach, effort is made to obtain a mild-to-moderate erythema on all treated areas of patients at 24 h after light exposure. Further studies will need to be conducted to evaluate the importance of the phototoxic reaction for long-term prevention of skin cancer.

We sometimes use a pulsed-dye laser (PDL) as a light source (V-Star, Cynosure, Chelmsford, MA) to try to prevent skin cancer development with ALA-PDT. The main advantage of the PDL in our experience is a decrease in pain during treatment. In addition, a full-face treatment can be performed in only a few minutes as compared to 16 min 40 s using the BLU-U at 10 mW/cm^2. We use the following parameters: 595 nm with a 10-mm spot size at 40-ms pulse duration and subpurpuric fluences of 7–8 J/cm^2. An open-label study of the treatment of AKs with PDT performed with ALA and a PDL showed a high clinical response rate using similar settings. Intense pulsed-light sources have also been used for the treatment of AKs with ALA-PDT as the red excitation peaks of PpIX are included in their spectral output.

NUMBER OF SESSIONS

Topical ALA-PDT sessions performed on hairless mice weekly, every 2 weeks or every month, have all decreased the appearance of skin cancer. Unfortunately, as such studies have not been performed in patients, it is not possible to use evidence-based data to determine the ideal frequency for performing preventive ALA-PDT sessions. For some patients whole-face ALA-PDT as frequently as every 2 weeks may be required to prevent AKs and SCCs (Iltefat Hamzavi, personal communication), whereas others may be treated only once or twice a year. Immunosuppressed patients may require more frequent treatments. Our approach is to first perform large-surface ALA-PDT sessions once or twice a year and to then increase treatment frequency should many AKs or SCC lesions develop between treatments. As there is great variability in patient response following PDT performed at 1–2 h after ALA application, we often perform a second PDT session 2–4 weeks after the first if patients did not exhibit a sufficient erythematous reaction following the initial treatment.

SIDE EFFECTS

Pain is the most frequent side effect of ALA-PDT. All patients in the pilot study using broad area PDT at 1 h and more than 90% of patients in the multicenter studies using spot treatment of AK at 14–18 h reported pain during light exposure. The pain usually begins shortly after the light source is turned on and then increases gradually to reach a plateau, often followed by a decrease in pain intensity towards the end of exposure. This pain is believed to be caused by PpIX activation during light exposure and can be easily alleviated by a pause in light exposure. Pain has been reported to be less intense when light exposure takes place at 1 h as compared to 14–18 h. We found that the Smart Cool device sold to be used in conjunction with the Cynosure PDL (Cynosure Chelmsford, MA) provides an excellent method of alleviating pain during light exposure with the Blue-U. Other strategies to manage pain include the use of a fan, spraying of water on the area that is exposed to light, as well as stopping light exposure and applying ice packs. Infiltration with lidocaine can be used if one or two lesions (AKs) are more painful but this is of limited usefulness when a full face is treated. Some patients also experience post-treatment pain which usually subsides within 24–48 h.

Erythema and edema following large-surface ALA-PDT for skin cancer prevention can be considered a desirable phenomenon. Patients have to be warned that they will undergo a moderate sunburn-like reaction on the exposed area. The intensity of the reaction is highly variable with some patients showing almost no erythema, while others show severe erythema (Fig. 11.5), sometimes even with focal crusting. This reaction probably depends on the amount of PpIX present in the skin at the time of light exposure.

From a practical standpoint, working with 20% ALA in hydroalcoholic solution, the main factors that could influence PpIX formation are the time between ALA application and light exposure, the speed of ALA penetration through the stratum corneum barrier, and the extent of photodamage. Therefore, care must be taken when modifying the incubation time. For example, a patient who is usually exposed to light 1 h after ALA application can have a much severer erythematous phototoxic reaction if light exposure takes place inadvertently at 2 or 3 h on that day.

Care should also be taken when treating patients who are using topical retinoids, alpha hydroxyl acids or other keratolytic agents. These agents may enhance ALA penetration and increase post-treatment erythema and edema. Wood's lamp provides an easy and accessible tool for evaluating PpIX levels in the skin. PpIX exhibits a characteristic pink–red fluorescence when viewed under long-wave UVA and blue light radiation. The human skin is usually devoid of such fluorescence except for follicular (1 mm) dot fluorescence on facial skin that is believed to be from bacterial origin, as well as large red fluorescent areas on psoriasis plaques that are generated by PpIX present in the scales. In our practice, the skin is always examined 1 h after ALA application with a UVA lamp (Black-Ray long model B-100, UVP, Upland, CA). We aim to perform light exposure at a time where red–pink fluorescence is seen with the UVA lamp. As the UVA output of these lamps varies according to the model being used, this strategy should be used with caution by physicians who have never used their UVA lamp to assess the presence of porphyrin in the skin after ALA application. In cases where red–pink fluorescence is seen at the time of light exposure, patients have all had at least a moderate phototoxic reaction the day following PDT

There is always the option to expose only a small skin area for the first treatment if PpIX fluorescence is present 1 h after ALA application. As the sensitivity of a Wood's lamp to detect PpIX fluorescence depends on its exact spectral and power outputs, it is suggested that the same Wood's lamp is always used. Patients with extensive sun damage have been observed to often present a more important phototoxic reaction 24 h following PDT. This could relate to the higher cellular levels of PpIX accumulated by sun-damaged keratinocytes, as demonstrated by us in hairless mice chronically exposed to UV radiation .

Post-PDT erythema usually recedes within 7–10 days. Patients should expect at least moderate desquamation starting 2–3 days after the PDT session. This situation is completely different from that seen in patients treated with 5-fluorouracil where erythema often persists for weeks and sometimes months after therapy. The intensity

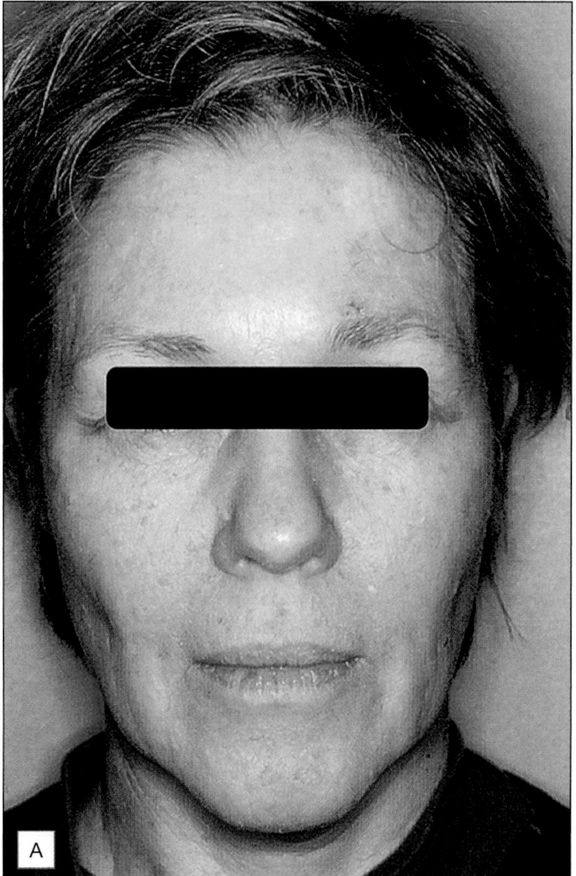

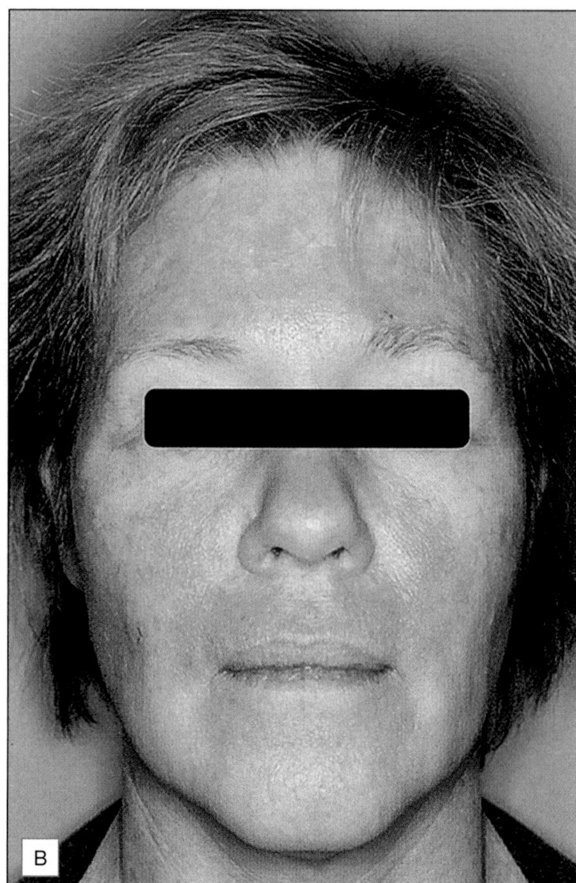

Fig. 11.5 Patient with extensive photodamage and numerous ill-defined AKs (**A**) before and (**B**) 24 h after large-surface ALA-PDT

of the reaction is not as severe as that usually seen when imiquimod is used in patients with AKs and extensive sun damage. The erythema generated by ALA-PDT is very similar to a sunburn and we have never seen the pur-pura-like reaction that can sometimes be observed in imiquimod-treated patients.

All patients should be warned about potential phototoxic reactions following sun exposure, especially when facial treatments are performed. This is particularly important when light exposure takes place 1 h after ALA application as skin PpIX levels will not reach their maximum until after light exposure. Patients should be advised to avoid spending time outdoors for 2 days after ALA application. They should also avoid intense broad-spectrum light, such as dentist or operating room lights, on areas where ALA was applied. Patients should be instructed that current sunscreens do not protect well against visible light.

Hyper- and hypo-pigmentation can occur after ALA-PDT. This is usually not seen in patients with phototype II–III when the treatment is performed on the face. The risks are higher with the treatment of extrafacial regions, especially the legs. We have never seen scarring following large-surface ALA-PDT for skin cancer prevention. Scarring is sometimes seen after the treatment of tumors with ALA-PDT but it could be argued that it arises from previous destruction of normal tissue by the original tumoral process.

BENEFITS

Large-surface ALA-PDT performed 1 h after ALA application has been shown to induce a good complete response rate in patients with multiple AKs (Fig. 11.6). These authors have also had good success with the treatment of AKs using this strategy. Preliminary, human data on the prevention of skin cancer with repeated large-surface MAL-PDT sessions in transplant patients suggest that large-surface PDT could prevent AK and skin cancer. The pilot study of full-face ALA-PDT performed in patients with multiple AKs has also shown improvement in signs of photoaging, which is an additional benefit for patients.

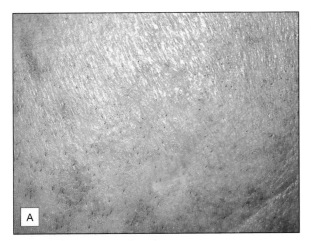

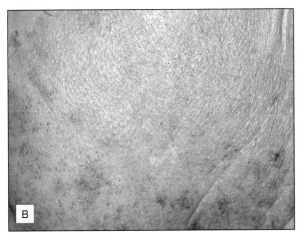

Fig. 11.6 Patient with AKs (**A**) before and (**B**) after large-surface ALA-PDT

FUTURE DIRECTIONS

Long-term clinical studies are needed to assess the efficacy of ALA- and MAL-PDT as a skin cancer prevention modality. Separate studies should be performed for different populations, such as patients with a history of multiple AKs and/or SCC, immunosuppressed patients, and Gorlin's syndrome patients. These studies should aim to assess the ability of multiple ALA-PDT sessions to prevent skin cancer, as well as to study the influence of different parameters such as light fluence, ALA incubation time, and frequency of treatments. In addition, DUSA Pharmaceuticals is currently sponsoring a multicenter split-face study comparing the efficacy of multiple ALA-PDT sessions in photoaging to light alone. As a secondary efficacy measure the number of new AKs appearing on treated sites during the trial will be monitored. Results of these trials could provide clinical evidence of the ability of large-surface PDT to prevent skin cancer.

CONCLUSION

Multiple large-surface ALA-PDT sessions have been shown to delay the induction of AKs, SCCs, as well as BCCs in mice. A pilot study has shown that large-surface ALA-PDT, with a short incubation time, is safe and can induce rapid clearing of AKs. MAL-PDT has also been shown to delay the appearance of AKs in transplant patients. Based on these findings, repeated large-surface ALA-PDT is currently used by many physicians to try to prevent skin cancer. Future studies are needed to confirm and measure the efficacy of multiple ALA-PDT sessions in preventing skin cancer in different patient populations.

FURTHER READING

Bavinck JN, Tieben LM, Van der Woude FJ et al 1995 Prevention of skin cancer and reduction of keratotic skin lesions during acitretin therapy in renal transplant recipients: a double-blind, placebo-controlled study. Journal of Clinical Oncology 13:1933–1938

Bissonnette R, Bergeron A, Liu Y 2004 Large surface photodynamic therapy with aminolevulinic acid: treatment of actinic keratoses and beyond. Journal of Drugs in Dermatology 3:S26–31

Caty V, Liu Y, Viau G et al 2006 Multiple large surface photodynamic therapy sessions with topical methylaminolaevulinate in PTCH heterozygous mice. British Journal of Dermatology 154:740–742

de Graaf YG, Kennedy C, Wolterbeek R et al 2006 Photodynamic therapy does not prevent cutaneous squamous-cell carcinoma in organ-transplant recipients: results of a randomized-controlled trial. Journal of Investigative Dermatology 126:569–574

Duffield-Lillico AJ, Slate EH, Reid ME et al 2003 Nutritional Prevention of Cancer Study Group. Selenium supplementation and secondary prevention of nonmelanoma skin cancer in a randomized trial. Journal of the National Cancer Institutes 95:1477–1481

Fung TT, Spiegelman D, Egan KM et al 2003 Vitamin and carotenoid intake and risk of squamous cell carcinoma of the skin. International Journal of Cancer 103:110–115

Kuchide M, Tokuda H, Takayasu J et al 2003 Cancer chemopreventive effects of oral feeding alpha-tocopherol on ultraviolet light B induced photocarcinogenesis of hairless mouse. Cancer Letters 196:169–177

Levine N, Moon TE, Cartmel B et al 1997 Trial of retinol and isotretinoin in skin cancer prevention: a randomized, double-blind, controlled trial. Cancer Epidemiology Biomarkers & Prevention 6:957–961

McKenna DB, Murphy GM 1999 Skin cancer chemoprophylaxis in renal transplant recipients: 5 years of experience using low-dose acitretin. British Journal of Dermatology 140:656–660

Oseroff AR, Shieh S, Frawley NP et al 2005 Treatment of diffuse basal cell carcinomas and basaloid follicular hamartomas in nevoid basal cell carcinoma syndrome by wide-area 5-aminolevulinic acid photodynamic therapy. Archives of Dermatology 141:60–67

Piacquadio DJ, Chen DM, Farber HF et al 2004 Photodynamic therapy with aminolevulinic acid topical solution and visible blue light in the treatment of multiple actinic keratoses of the face and scalp: investigator-blinded, phase 3, multicenter trials. Archives of Dermatology 140:41–46

Sharfaei S, Juzenas P, Moan J et al 2002 Weekly topical application of methyl aminolevulinate followed by light exposure delays the appearance of UV-induced skin tumours in mice. Archives of Dermatological Research 294:237–242

Sharfaei S, Viau G, Lui H et al 2001 Systemic photodynamic therapy with aminolevulinic acid delays the appearance of ultraviolet-induced skin tumours in mice. British Journal of Dermatology 144:1207–1214

Stege H 2001 Effect of xenogenic repair enzymes on photoimmunology and photocarcinogenesis. Journal of Photochemistry and Photobiology. B—Biology 65:105–108

Stender IM, Beck-Thomsen N, Poulsen T et al 1997 Photodynamic therapy with topical delta-aminolevulinic acid delays UV photocardinogenesis in hairless mice. Photochemistry and Photobiology 66:493–496

Tangrea JA, Edwards BK, Taylor PR et al 1992 Long-term therapy with low-dose isotretinoin for prevention of basal cell carcinoma: a multicenter clinical trial. Isotretinoin-Basal Cell Carcinoma Study Group. Journal of The National Cancer Institutes 84:328–332

Touma D, Yaar M, Whitehead S et al 2004 A trial of short incubation, broad-area photodynamic therapy for facial actinic keratoses and diffuse photodamage. Archives of Dermatology 140:33–40

Wennberg AM, Keohane S, Lear JT October 2005 A multicenter study with MAL-PDT cream in immuno-compromised organ transplant recipients with non-melanoma skin cancer. Poster presented at the European Academy of Dermatology and Venereology Meeting, London

Wulf HC, Pavel S, Stender I et al 2006 Topical photodynamic therapy for prevention of new skin lesions in renal transplant recipients. Acta Dermato-Venerologica 86:25–28

Yarosh D, Klein J, O'Connor A et al 2001 Effect of topically applied T4 endonuclease V in liposomes on skin cancer in xeroderma pigmentosum: a randomised study. Xeroderma Pigmentosum Study Group. Lancet 357:926–929

12 Photodynamic Rejuvenation with Methyl-Aminolevulinic Acid

Ricardo Ruiz-Rodriguez, Laura Lopez-Rodriguez

INTRODUCTION

Nonablative lasers and light sources have been used for the past few years to improve the visible signs of photoaging. The benefits of these nonablative procedures include quicker patient recovery time and low risk of unwanted pigmentary and textural abnormalities. However, the results usually are not comparable to ablative treatment, such as laser resurfacing. In this chapter the role of photodynamic rejuvenation among the armamentarium of nonablative facial rejuvenation is assessed.

NONABLATIVE REJUVENATION

Nonablative rejuvenation describes technologies which improve aging structural changes in the skin without disruption of cutaneous integrity, minimize downtime, and have a low-risk profile.

One category is visible light lasers or light sources that have greater absorption by hemoglobin and melanin, and therefore greater influence on the telangiectatic and melanotic components of photoaging. These sources can be subdivided into vascular (Table 12.1) and pigmented lasers. Intense pulsed light (IPL) is a broadband light source with filters used to limit the emitted spectrum (Table 12.2).

Another category is infrared lasers with absorption predominantly by water. Infrared wavelengths are used to create thermal dermal and collagen injury. The most commonly used devices are 1320-nm Nd:YAG laser, 1450-nm diode laser, and 1540-nm erbium:glass laser (Table 12.3).

A nonlaser radiofrequency device delivering high energy was developed to remodel and tighten collagen in the deeper dermis and subcutaneous tissue to improve lax or aging skin.

Fractional resurfacing produces multiple columns of thermal damage, referred to as microthermal treatment zones, and might be included in the group of nonablative technologies. Finally, a skin rejuvenation modality using high-energy plasma (plasma skin rejuvenation) is a promising new nonablative procedure.

• Photodynamic rejuvenation

The primary goal of such nonablative procedures is a long-lasting, effective rejuvenation without major side effects or a long period of recuperation. Among the novel methods for maximizing the efficacy of nonablative treatments is the concurrent use of a photosensitizing agent.

In 2002 Ruiz-Rodriguez et al studied the use of IPL as a light source for photodynamic treatment (PDT) in patients with actinic keratoses (AKs), and the technique was called "photodynamic photorejuvenation". They treated 17 patients with a combination of AKs and diffuse photodamage. They applied 20% 5-aminolevulinic acid (ALA) mixed in an oil-in-water emulsion and under occlusion for 4 h before treatment (0.2 g/cm^2) with the pulsed-light device (Lumenis, Inc), using a 615-nm cut-off filter and a total fluence of 40 J/cm^2 in a double-pulse mode of 4 ms, with a 20-ms interpulse delay.

The results were extended by Alexiades-Armenakas and Geronimus, who showed that PDT treatment of AK could be accomplished not only with IPL but also with a 595-nm pulsed-dye laser (PDL). This device offered the benefits of rapidity of treatment and the comfort and protective epidermal effects associated with cryogen spray cooling. The ALA incubation time was 3 h, and nonpurpuric PDL settings (4.0–7.5 J/cm^2; 10-ms pulse duration; 10-mm spot size; and 30-ms cryogen spray with a 30-ms delay) were used. In this study the authors were focused on AKs.

Goldman and Avram in 2004 studied the use of ALA-IPL in treating both AKs and signs of photodamage in 17 patients. ALA was applied for 1 h before a single treatment with an IPL device using a 560-nm filter Vasculite Elite (Lumenis Corporation) at 28–32 J/cm^2 with a doubled pulse of 3.0 and 6.0 ms and a 10-ms delay. Their study showed that ALA-IPL is a safe, effective way to treat both AKs and photodamage with little downtime.

In 2005 Dover et al showed the superior efficacy of IPL-PDT over IPL alone in a prospective, randomized, split-face study. Twenty subjects participated in a series of three split-face treatments 3 weeks apart, in which half of the face was pre-treated with ALA followed by IPL treatment, while the other half was treated with IPL alone. The ALA incubation time was 30–60 min. The adjunctive use of ALA in the treatment of facial photoaging with IPL provided significantly greater improvement in global photodamage, mottled pigmentation, and fine

Table 12.1 Pulsed-dye lasers

Product name	Wavelength (nm)	Type	Supplier	Pulse width (ms)
C-Beam V-Beam	585 595	PDL	Candela	0.45 0.45–40
Photogenica V V star	585 585–595	PDL	Cynosure	0.5 0.5–40
N Lite	585	PDL	ICN	0.35

Table 12.2 IPL comparison chart

Product name	Wavelength (nm)	Type	Supplier
ProLite	550–900	IPL	Alderm
Quantum SR/Lumenis 1	560–1200	IPL	Lumenis
Estelux	525–1200	IPL	Palomar
Ellipse	530–950	IPL	DDD
Spa Touch	400–1200	IPL	Radiancy
SpectraPulse	510–1200	IPL	Primary Tech.
Aurora SR	580–980	IPL + RF	Syneron

Table 12.3 Infra-red laser comparison chart

Product name	Wavelength (nm)	Type	Supplier
Cool Touch III	1320	Nd:YAG	New star lasers
Smoothbeam	1450	Diode	Candela
Aramis	1540	Erbium Glass	Quantel

lines than treatment with IPL alone. They showed that this combination treatment enhances the results of photorejuvenation and improves patient satisfaction. Adverse effects and tolerability did not differ significantly between the IPL-only treated areas and the areas treated with ALA-IPL.

Marmur and Goldberg published in 2005 a small pilot study about the ultrastructural changes seen after ALA-IPL photorejuvenation. They found a greater shift toward type I collagen synthesis in the ALA-IPL treatment group compared to the IPL-only treatment group.

Therefore, a wide range of light sources can be used in photodynamic rejuvenation. Blue light is the most potent wavelength for activation of the PDT effect. The absorption maximum of protoporphyrin IX (PpIX) is around 410 nm, and this makes blue light 40 times more potent that red light and significantly greater than yellow light in terms of a photochemical effect. However, for cosmetic skin conditions, blue light ALA-PDT is limited by a lack of cutaneous penetration and superficial melanin absorption. Despite these limitations, nonablative rejuvenation has been reported using blue light. Therefore, although blue light is more effective at photoactivating porphyrins than other light sources, red light shows a better tissue penetration (Fig. 12.1).

The two devices currently most used for photodynamic rejuvenation are IPL and PDL. Deeper penetrating visible wavelengths produced by IPL and PDL not only have enough energy to activate the photochemical process but also have long enough wavelengths to effectively reach and thermally target multiple chromophores, including hemoglobin, melanin and, to a less selective degree, collagen.

We are still far from having a thorough understanding of the molecular mechanism of photodynamic rejuvenation, although the activation of a nonspecific immune response could be involved. It is likely that surface texture and pigmentation are improved through mild desquamation. Histologic studies have also demonstrated increased fibrosis and new collagen formation in the dermis several months after ALA-PDT for the treatment of basal cell (BCC) and squamous cell carcinoma (SCC).

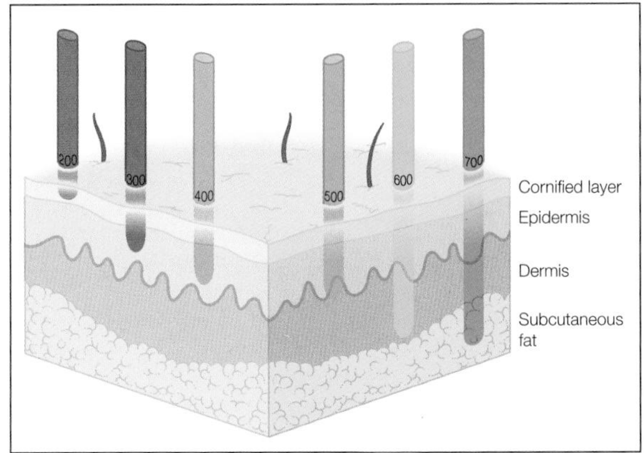

Fig. 12.1 Tissue penetration depth in relation to light wavelength

TOPICAL METHYL AMINOLEVULINATE

In the USA, the ALA hydrochloride (Levulan Kerastick) is approved for photodynamic treatment of AK in combination with blue light. Currently, in most European countries, New Zealand and Australia, Metvix is approved for the treatment of BCC, AK, and Bowen's disease in combination with red light.

Metvix cream contains methyl-aminolevulinate (MAL) as the hydrochloride salt in a 20% solution. The optimal regimen for MAL-PDT (as used in all clinical trials) is MAL 160 mg/g applied for 3 h before illumination with red light (570–670 nm) at a total light dose of 75 J/cm^2, as determined in dose-finding trials.

Topically applied MAL penetrates the skin and induces a high production of porphyrin metabolites in cells, leading to intracellular accumulation of photoactive porphyrins. The underlying mechanism of this induction is not fully understood. However, there is evidence that MAL may enter the heme biosynthetic pathway without hydrolysis to ALA, an endogenous precursor of PpIX. If photoactive porphyrin-loaded cells are exposed to appropriate wavelengths of light, reactive oxygen species are generated that irreversibly oxidize cellular components and cause cell death, tissue injury, and necrosis.

Local phototoxicity reactions were the most common local adverse events in all clinical trials using MAL-PDT, mainly burning sensation, erythema, crusting, and pain. Most of the local events resolved quickly on the day of treatment and all of them within 2 weeks. There was no increase in the incidence of local adverse events after the second cycle of MAL-PDT.

The higher lipophilicity of esterified forms of ALA permits more effective penetration of the cutaneous tissue. Comparison of ALA and MAL in patients with AK revealed that Metvix cream induced higher accumulation of the porphyrins in tumor than in normal tissue. Furthermore, ALA induced a higher porphyrin level than MAL; however, MAL was more selective for lesional skin than ALA 6 h after application. This might have been due to different cellular uptake and feedback mechanisms. Higher lipophilicity, penetration depth, and selectivity for neoplastic lesions are its desirable characteristics compared with ALA. However, there is no comparison study of these two molecules in rejuvenation.

In a study by Wiegell et al, 20 patients were their own controls for pain in tape-stripped normal skin of the forearms treated with ALA or MAL. ALA generated significantly more pain than MAL during and after illumination. The authors hypothesized that ALA and not MAL may be transported by γ-aminobutyric acid receptors into peripheral nerve endings, explaining the higher pain scores.

MAL-induced contact eczema has been described in a case who demonstrated strong reaction after a patch test with MAL but not with ALA. However, it should be noted that many thousands of patients have been treated with MAL without experiencing allergic reactions.

• Metvix–red light rejuvenation study

In Europe the most widely used PDT protocol is Metvix and red light. We have studied full-face Metvix-PDT rejuvenation using red light and comparing 1 h and 3 h exposure time. As far as we know, there has been no split-face study of Metvix and red light in rejuvenation and comparing exposure time.

Our study was a prospective, randomized, full-face, side-by-side comparison study in 10 patients with moderate photodamage and no AK. Two tubes of Metvix were applied to the whole face. Red light was administered to one side of the face 1 h later using the Aktilite lamp in a dose of 37 J/cm^2, and to the other side 3 h after the Metvix application. Aktilite is a light-emitting diode (LED) lamp which emits an average wavelength of 630 nm. A statistically significant moderate improvement was seen in skin quality and fine wrinkling. Neither improvement in mottled pigmentation nor in telangiectasias was observed. The improvement was superior on the 3 h side (Fig. 12.2) than on the 1 h side (Fig. 12.3) in most patients.

Regarding side effects, more erythema, edema, and scaling was seen on the 3 h side (Fig. 12.4) compared to the 1 h side. UVB photos were taken and greater fluorescence was observed on the 3 h side compared to the 1 h side (Fig. 12.5).

Histologic results correlated with the clinical improvement. Using blue alcian dye to stain mucopolysaccharides, a major deposit was observed in the dermis and between the keratinocytes (Fig. 12.6). Using CD44, which binds to the receptor for hyaluronic acid, a major expression was seen not only throughout the epidermis but also in the follicle (Fig. 12.7). Van Geison stain demonstrated a major deposit of elastic fibers in the dermis in a more homogeneous distribution (Fig. 12.8).

In conclusion, Metvix-PDT using red light is effective for skin rejuvenation (fine lines and skin tightness), and 3 h exposure produces better results than 1 h exposure,

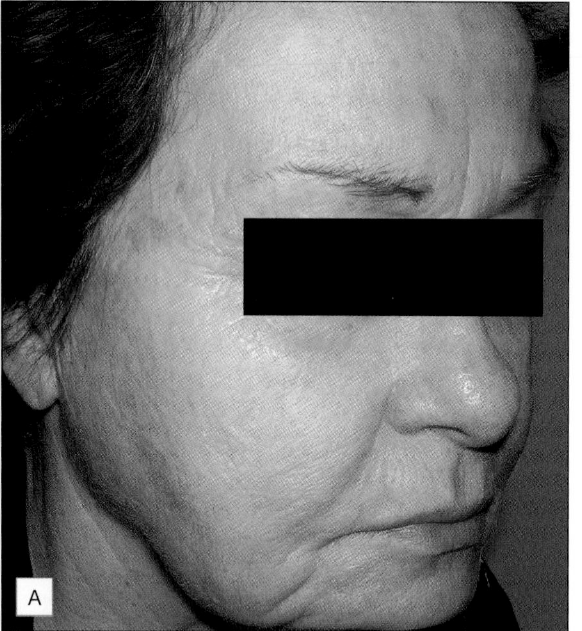

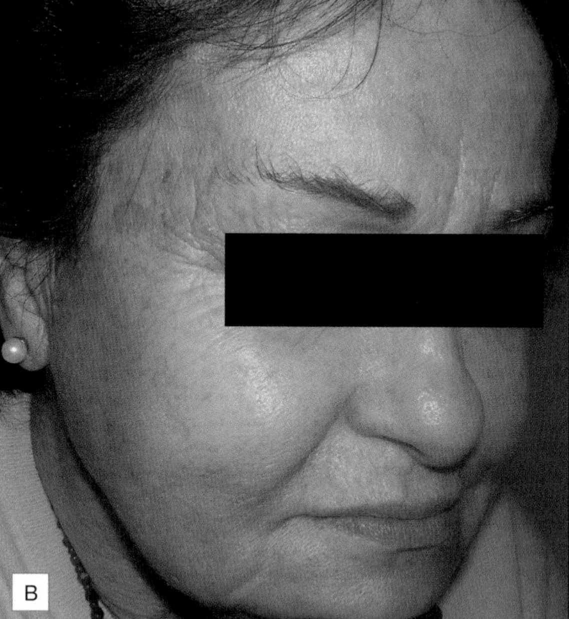

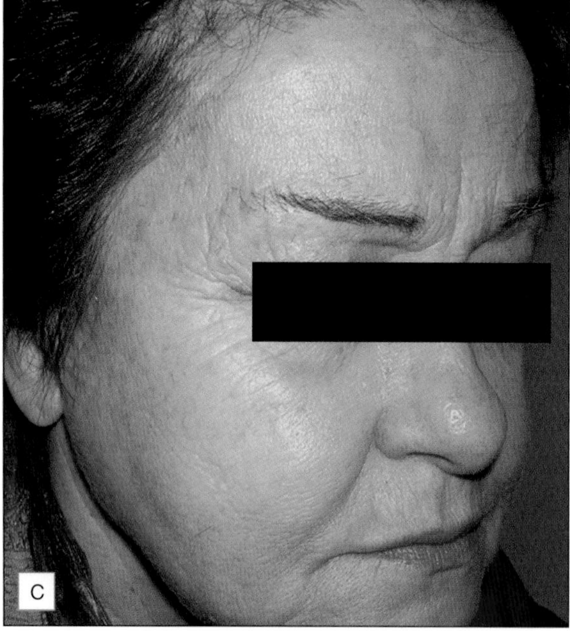

Fig. 12.2 Results for the 3-h incubation-time side of the face at baseline (**A**), 2 weeks after the third and last treatment (**B**), and 2 months after the third treatment (**C**). Improvement was seen 2 months after the last treatment

but with a significant increase in adverse effects (erythema and edema).

OVERVIEW OF TREATMENT STRATEGY

The patient requesting nonablative rejuvenation needs to have a realistic expectation of outcome. Also, the patient should understand that maintenance treatments once to twice a year are necessary in order to maintain positive effects.

As public demand grows for less invasive, yet highly effective, modalities to address common cosmetic skin concerns, dermatologists must use the right technique for each patient. Understanding the laser–tissue interactions associated with PDT is crucial in selecting patients who are most likely to benefit. Shorter wavelengths are more valuable in the management of pigmented dyschromia, vascular ectasias, and pilosebaceous irregularities, while longer, more deeply penetrating wavelengths are more effective in wrinkle reduction and prophylaxis. Depending

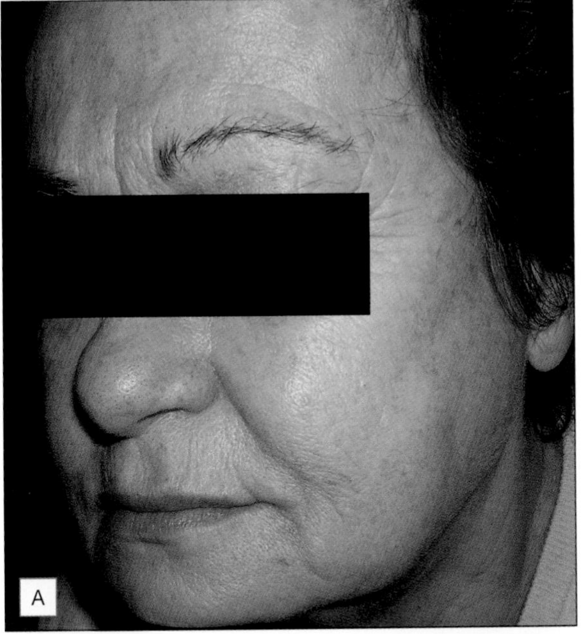

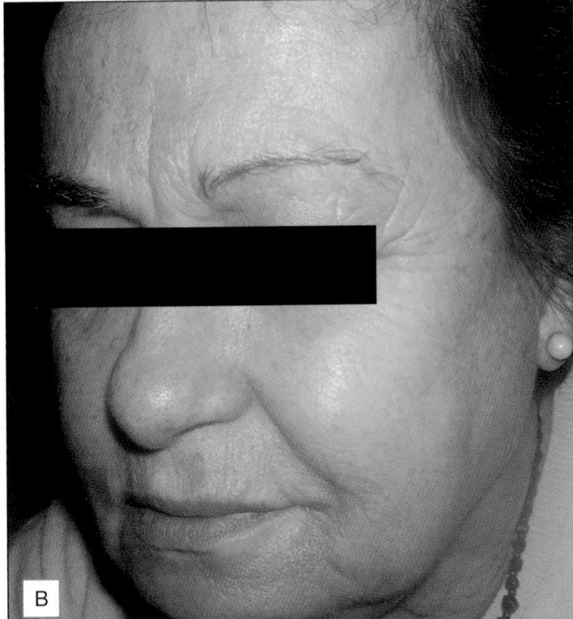

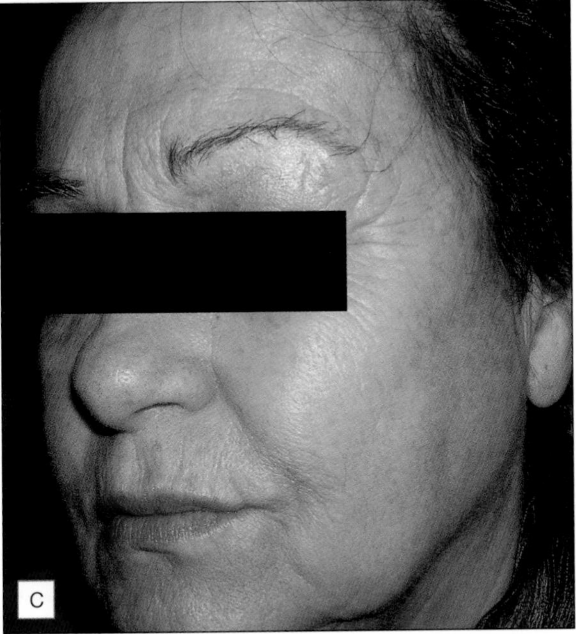

Fig. 12.3 Results for the 1 h incubation-time side of the face at baseline (**A**), 2 weeks after the third and last treatment (**B**), and 2 months after the third treatment (**C**). Improvement was seen 2 months after the last treatment

on the type of photodamage the patient has, different procedures should be used (Fig. 12.9):

1. Type I: Lentigines, telangiectasias, increased coarseness, symptoms of rosacea. In these cases, IPL and/or a combination of Q-switch and vascular lasers can be used.
2. Type II: Wrinkles, laxity, dermatochalasis. We have been using mid-infrared lasers for these patients, although their current treatments of choice are Fraxel laser and plasma skin rejuvenation. Radiofrequency technology can produce tightening of dermal collagen and can be combined with other procedures that improve the more superficial changes associated with photoaging.
3. Type III: AK, nonmelanoma skin cancers. Photodynamic rejuvenation is the treatment of choice, sometimes in combination with other nonablative

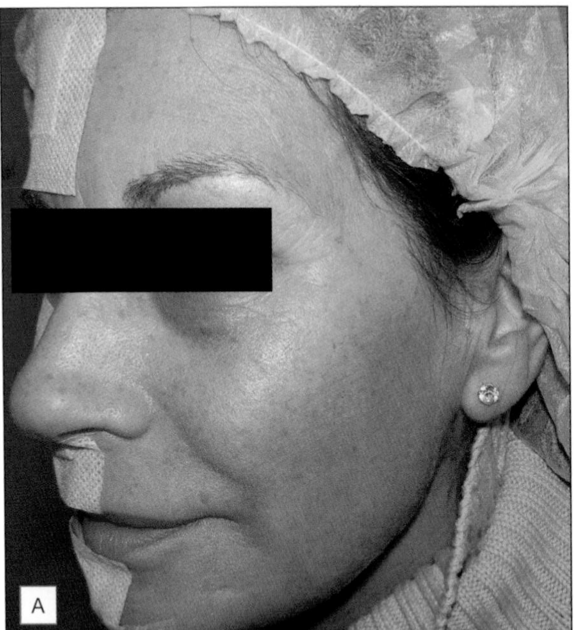

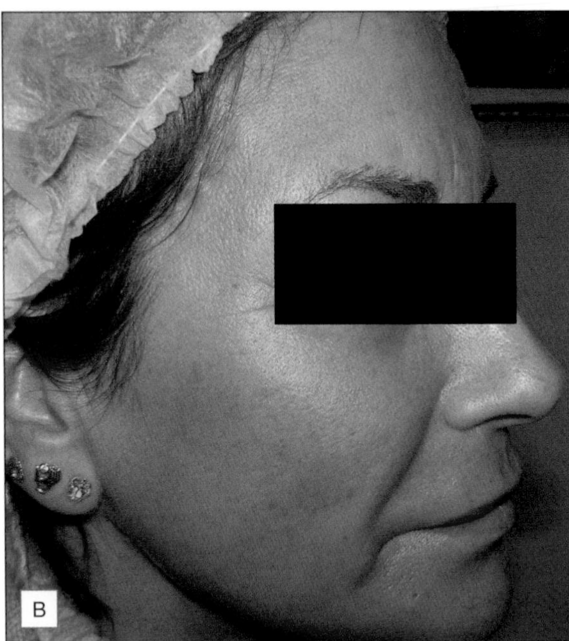

Fig. 12.4 Erythema, edema, and scaling on the 3 h incubation-time side of the face (**B**) compared to the 1 h side of the face (**A**)

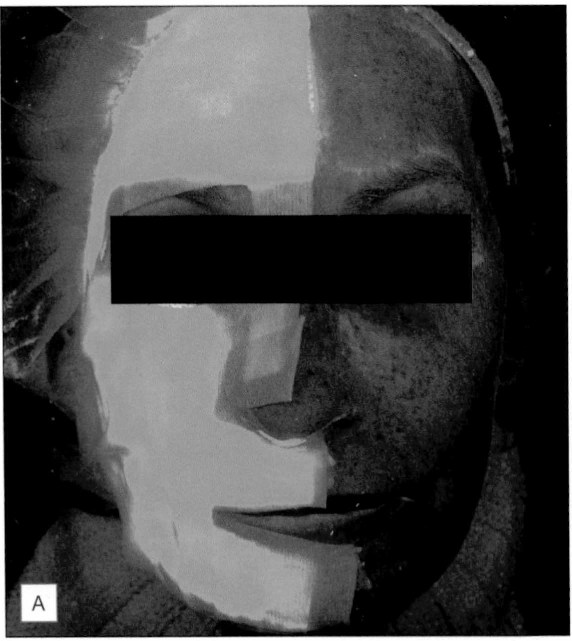

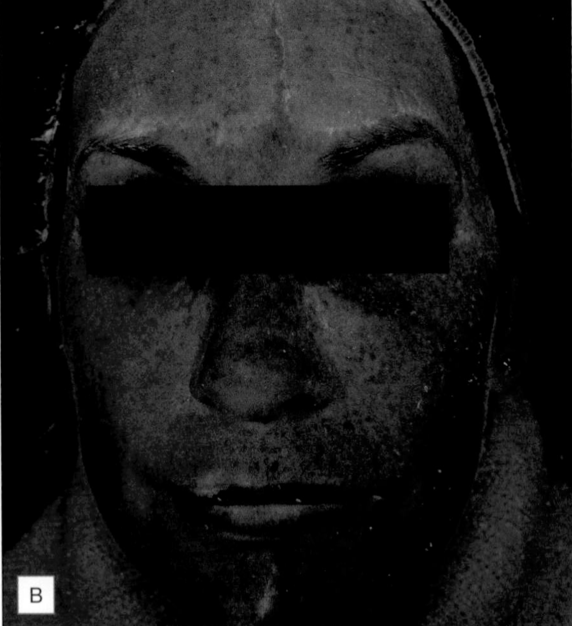

Fig. 12.5 Fluorescence of the 3 h incubation-time side of the face (**B**) compared to the 1 h side of the face (**A**) Both photographs were taken after Metvix incubation and prior to illumination with the red light

treatments. The risk of temporarily masking non-melanoma skin cancer makes it prudent to maintain a low threshold to biopsy any suspicious lesions. The approach in the type III group of patients can be further divided:

- Patients with multiple AKs and diffuse facial redness: PDT rejuvenation using PDL as the preferred light device, purpura-free fluences of 5–7.5 J/cm^2, 10-ms pulse width, and a 10-mm spot. The ideal immediate treatment endpoint

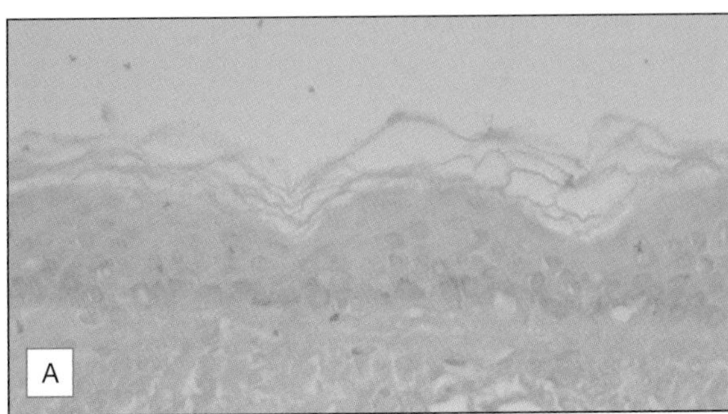

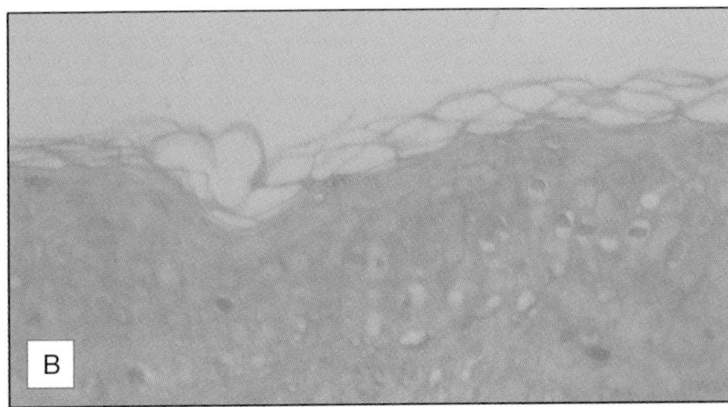

Fig. 12.6 Results of the biopsy study at baseline (**A**) and 2 weeks after the third treatment (**B**). Staining with Blue Alcian dye revealed a major deposit of mucopolysaccharides in the dermis and between the keratinocytes

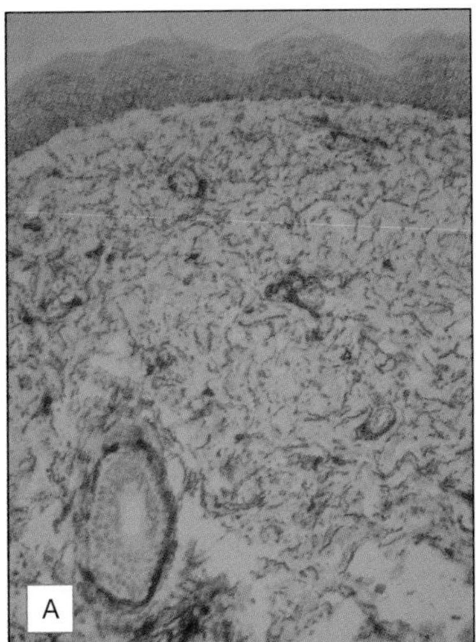

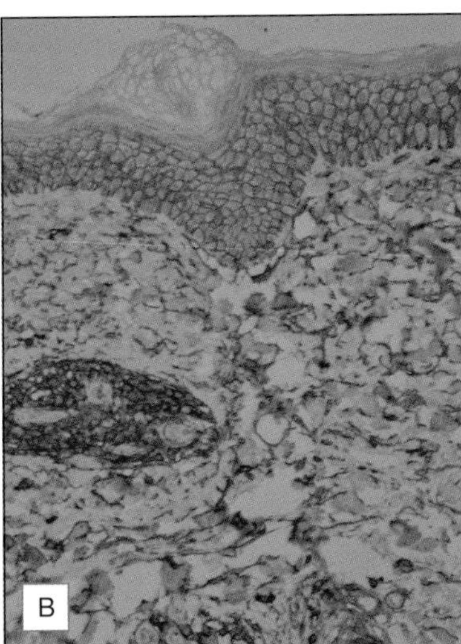

Fig. 12.7 Results of the biopsy study at baseline (**A**) and 2 weeks after the third treatment (**B**). Staining for CD44, which binds the receptor for hyaluronic acid, revealed an abundant expression not only throughout the epidermis but also in the follicle

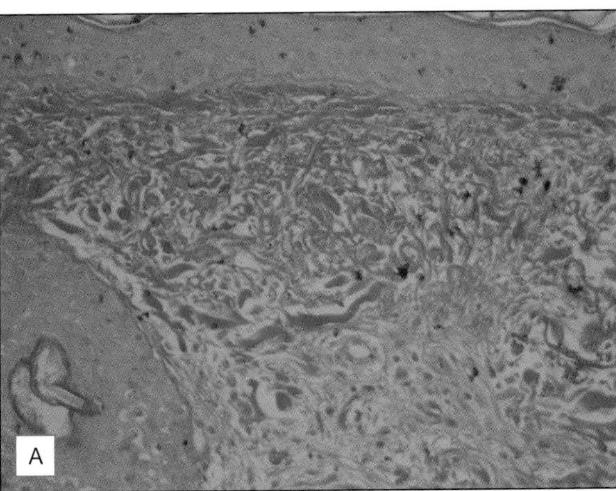

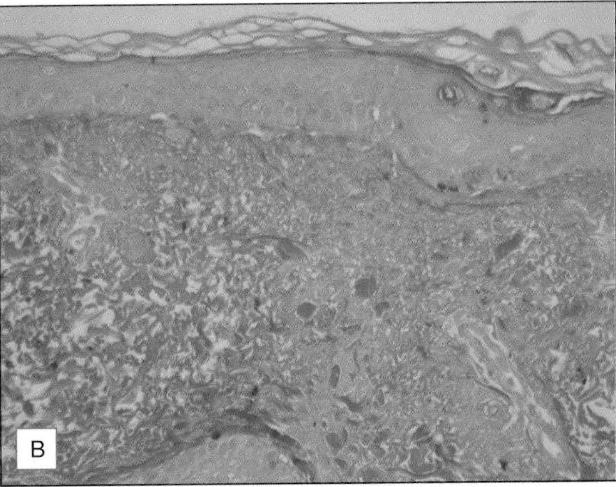

Fig. 12.8 Results of the biopsy study at baseline (**A**) and 2 weeks after the third treatment (**B**). Van Gieson staining revealed a major deposit of elastic fibers in the dermis in a homogeneous distribution

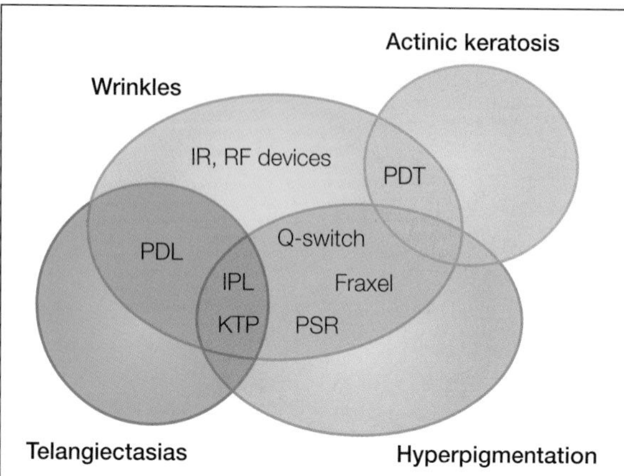

Fig. 12.9 Treatment applications. IPL = intense pulse light; IR = mid-infrared lasers; KTP = potassium titanyl phosphate vascular laser; PSR = portrait plasma skin regeneration; RF = radiofrequency devices; PDL = pulsed-dye lasers; PDT = photodynamic thearpy

is visible spasm of vessels without purpura, sometimes using two or three passes.

- Patients with multiple AKs, multiple lentigines, and telangiectasias: IPL is the light of choice for PDT in these patients. When using the Quantum IPL, a 560-nm cut-off filter and parameters between 24 and 32 J/cm^2, with a pulse duration setting of 2.4 and 4.0 ms for the first and second pulses in the pulse sequence, respectively, should be applied.
- According to our study described above, Metvix-PDT using red light is effective for skin rejuvenation (fine lines and skin tightness). Patients with AK can benefit cosmetically from this technique. If telangiectasias or lentigines are present, these lesions might be treated additionally with PDL or Q-switch laser, respectively, as red light-PDT has no effect on these conditions. We have found that the results for AK are much better using red light than using IPL or PDL as a light source for PDT.

THERAPEUTIC PEARLS IN PHOTODYNAMIC REJUVENATION

Some therapeutic pearls can be useful when performing photodynamic rejuvenation:

- Some authors recommend microdermabrasion immediately before treatment to remove stratum corneum and allow more uniform and rapid penetration of the photosensitizer. Other techniques that improve absorption of the photosensitizer are vibradermabrasion, urea 40% cream or just cleaning the skin with either alcohol or acetone. Our experience favors the use of fractional resurfacing prior to PDT in skin rejuvenation to enhance the penetration of the photosensitizer. Further studies with different light sources and in vivo fluorescence microscopy analysis are warranted.
- Regarding pain management, we have found that a forced cool-air device (Cryo 5 Zimmer; SmartCool, Cynosure) is very helpful in alleviating pain in patients who find pain during light exposure difficult to bear, especially on the scalp with multiple AKs.
- Application of topical analgesics like eutectic mixtures of lidocaine/prilocaine prior to irradiation is not recommended as their high pH can chemically inactivate the photosensitizer.
- Strict avoidance of sun and bright lights is essential to limit the redness, swelling, and crusting associated with phototoxicity. Invariably a certain amount of PpIX remains in situ following treatment. Careful patient selection, patient education, and sun avoidance for up to 2 days after treatment is essential for successful photodynamic rejuvenation.
- When treating the full face, sometimes it is necessary to divide the face in two or more areas for illumination (with the Aktilite lamp we divide the face into two areas). It is very important to cover the side that is not being treated during the illumination, so as not to activate the photosensitizer before the treatment.
- Treatment frequency is determined by the device that is used. At least 4 weeks should separate treatments with the IPL, PDL or red light for complete healing of the deeper photothermal effects. The blue-light devices can be used again as soon as 1–2 weeks following a treatment as the thermal effects are negligible.
- A downside of photodynamic rejuvenation is the cost of the treatment. However, cost-effectiveness analysis indicates that with relatively low costs for permanent equipment, this technique is probably no more expensive than conventional therapy when its lower side-effect profile is considered. The use of a photosensitizer appears to enhance the effectiveness of IPL, PDL or other light sources for treating facial photodamage, reducing the number of treatments required for significant clinical improvement.

FUTURE DIRECTIONS

It is our opinion that photodynamic rejuvenation is a promising technology for treating skin aging resulting from UV exposure. With further clinical and basic research to determine suitable target structures, optimal wavelengths, and adequate exposure times, this may become one of the best methods in treating photoaging. In future, photodynamic rejuvenation may be combined with other nonablative procedures. This should be done judiciously and at minimum risk to the patient. Conservative parameters should be used when more than one treatment is provided at the same time.

Photodynamic rejuvenation could theorically prevent skin cancer appearance by inducing a phototoxic reaction in nonvisible lesions. Weekly large-surface ALA-PDT performed on hairless mice has been shown to delay the appearance of UV-induced AK (see Ch 11). Therefore, photodynamic rejuvenation may provide the bridge between cosmetic and medical dermatology, enabling skin to be not only more beautiful but also healthier.

FURTHER READING

Alexiades-Armenakas MR, Geronimus RG 2003 Laser-mediated photodynamic therapy of actinic keratosis. Archives of Dermatology 139:1313–1320

Avram DK, Goldman MP 2004 Effectiveness and safety of ALA-IPL in treating actinic keratoses and photodamage. Journal of Drugs in Dermatology 3:S32–S39

Bissonette R, Bergeron A, Liu Y 2004 Large surface photodynamic therapy with ALA: treatment of actinic keratosis and beyond. Journal of Drugs in Dermatolory 3:S26–S31

Dover JS, Bhatia AC, Stewart B, Arndt KA 2005 Topical 5-aminolevulinic acid combined with intense pulsed light in the treatment of photoaging. Acta Dermatologica 141:1247–1252

Fink-Puches R, Soyer HP, Hofer A et al 1998 Long-term follow-up and histological changes of superficial nonmelanoma skin cancers treated with topical ALA-PDT. Archives of Dermatology 134:821–826

Manstein D, Herron GS, Sink RK, Tanner H, Anderson RR 2004 Fractional photothermolysis: a new concept for cutaneous remodeling using microscopic patterns of thermal injury. Lasers in Surgery in Medicine 34:426–438

Marmur ES, Phelps R, Goldberg DJ 2005 Ultrastructural changes seen after ALA-IPL photorejuvenation: a pilot study. Journal of Cosmetic Laser Therapy 7:21–24

Nowis D, Makowski M, Stoklosa T, Legat M, Issat T, Golab J 2005 Direct tumor damage mechanisms of photodynamic therapy. Acta Biochimica Polonica 52:339–352

Ruiz-Rogriguez R Photodynamic Rejuvenation. Paper presented at American Academy of Dermatology Annual Winter Meeting; March 3, 2007

Ruiz-Rodriguez R, Sanz-Sanchez T, Córdoba S 2002 Photodynamic photorejuvenation. Dermatologic Surgery 28:742–744

Siddiqui MA, Perry CM, Scott LJ 2004 Topical methyl aminolevulinate. American Journal of Clinical Dermatology 5:127–137

Stender IM, Bech-Thomson M, Poulsen T, Wulf HC 1997 Photodynamic therapy with topical delta-aminolevulinic acid delays UV photocarcinogenesis in hairless mice. Photochemistry and Photobiology 6:493–496

Van den Akker JTHM, de Bruijn HS, Beijersbergen van Henegouwen GMJ, Star WM, Sterenborg HJCM 2000 Protoporphyrin IX fluorescence kinetics and localization after topical application of ALA pentyl ester and ALA on hairless mouse skin with UVB-induced early skin cancer. Photochemistry and Photobiology 72:399–406

Wiegell SR, Stender IM, Na R, Wulf HC 2003 Pain associated with photodynamic therapy using 5-aminolevulinic acid or 5-aminolevulinic acid methylester on tape-stripped normal skin. Archives of Dermatology 139:1173–1177

Wulf HC, Philipsen P 2004 Allergic contact dermatitis to 5-aminolevulinic acid methylester but not to 5-aminolevulinic acid after photodynamic therapy. British Journal of Dermatology 150:143–145

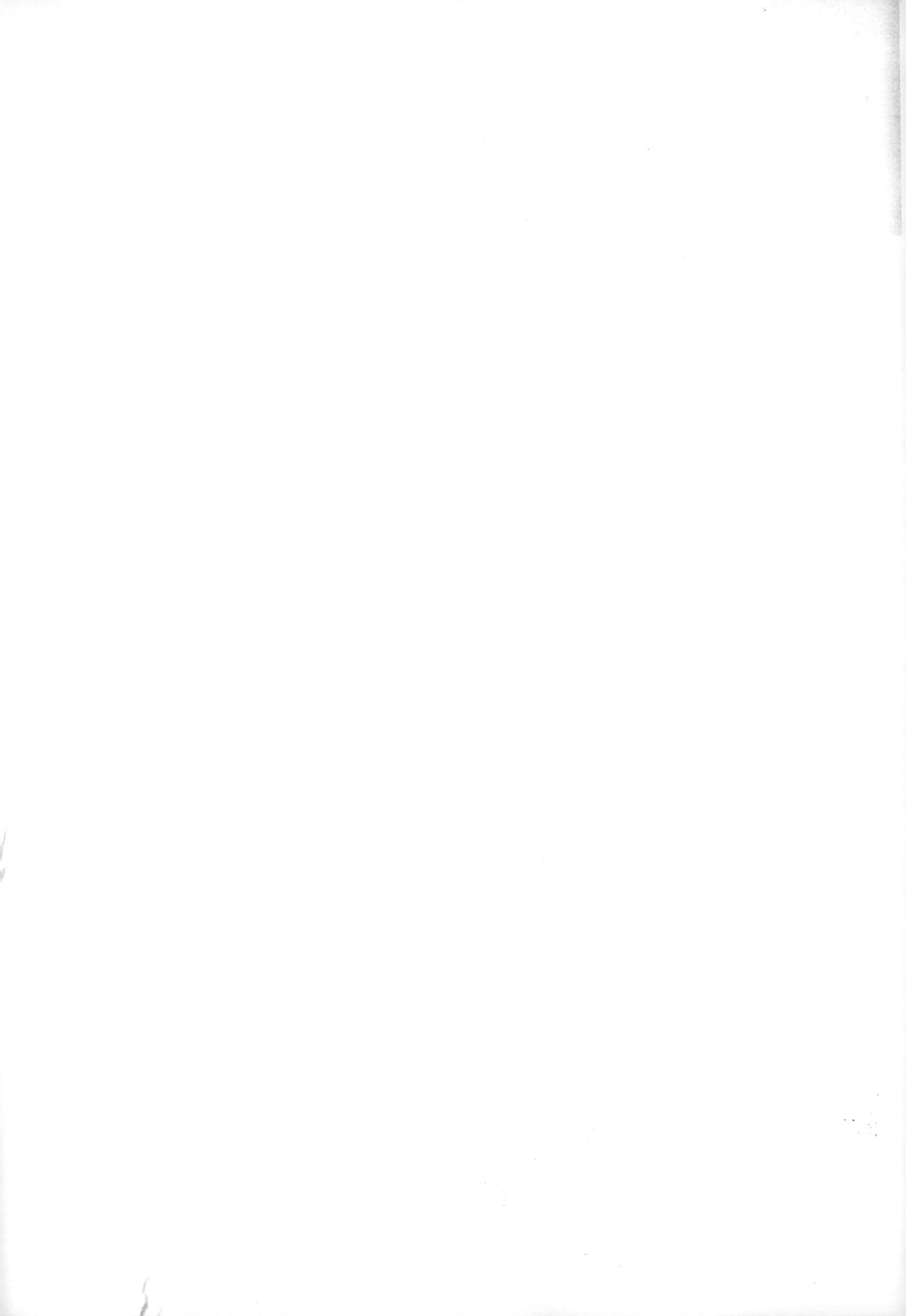

13 Photodynamic Therapy for Photorejuvenation

Pavan K. Nootheti, Michael H. Gold, Mitchel P. Goldman

INTRODUCTION

Light therapy is widely used in dermatology. An enhancement to this therapy is the use of a photosensitizing medication along with light therapy, known as photodynamic therapy (PDT). PDT is primarily used for the treatment of precancerous lesions, acne vulgaris, and nonmelanoma skin cancer, and has also been shown to improve the appearance of photodamaged skin. This chapter reviews the available literature for the treatment of photodamaged skin using PDT.

PHOTOREJUVENATION

Photodamage is not only unsightly, leading to wrinkles, pigmentary unevenness, lentigines, telangiectasias, and textural changes; but it can also lead to precancerous conditions with the development of actinic keratoses (AKs). Numerous light sources have been documented to treat photodamage with PDT, such as blue light, red light, intense pulsed light (IPL), and the pulsed-dye laser (PDL). Blue light sources utilize the maximum absorption peak of photoporphyrin IX (PpIX) at 410 nm; however, the shorter wavelength of blue light provides less tissue penetration. Red light seeks to utilize one of the smaller absorption peaks of PpIX at 630 nm, while maximizing tissue penetration with the longer wavelengths. Several other light sources, such as broadband lamps, activate smaller peaks at 505, 540, and 580 nm. The choice of which light source to use for 5-aminolevulinic acid (ALA)-PDT depends on such factors as the condition being treated, efficacy, and cost of use. Red light can penetrate 6 mm into the skin and is the desirable light source when deeper lesions are being treated. Light sources in the 400–500-nm range (blue light) are best used for superficial lesions as photon penetration is only up to 1–2 mm.

• With blue light

Photorejuvenation studies using blue light have been conducted by Goldman et al, where a blue light source was used to illuminate the face after the topical application of ALA. Thirty-two patients with photodamage and AKs were treated with topical ALA for one session with a blue light source. ALA was applied to the whole face for 1 h before the blue light treatment. AKs showed a 90% improvement, and skin also showed a 72% improvement in texture and a 59% improvement in pigmentation. Gold documented that the use of a blue light source for ALA-PDT in the treatment of nonhyperkeratotic facial AKs also resulted in an improvement of skin elasticity and reduced skin thickening in patients with photodamaged skin. Touma et al studied the effectiveness of ALA and blue light illumination in the treatment of AKs and diffuse photodamage. Eighteen patients with facial nonhypertrophic AKs and mild-to-moderate facial photodamage were evaluated. ALA was applied for 1–3 h with subsequent exposure to blue light. After 1- and 5-month intervals, there was a significant reduction in AKs and significant improvement in photodamage parameters such as skin quality, fine wrinkling, and sallowness. Mottled pigmentation showed borderline improvement, but coarse wrinkling showed no improvement. Satisfaction was rated as good to excellent in more than 80% of the patients. It was also suggested in the study that the use of microdermabrasion just before application of ALA leads to a more uniform and rapid penetration of ALA. In addition to proving the effectiveness of ALA-PDT using blue light, the study by Touma's group also emphasized the utility of an 1-h incubation for the ALA versus the traditional 14–18-h ALA incubation times. Figure 13.1 demonstrates the natural course of erythema and inflammation caused by treatment with PDT using blue light. The marked improvement in reduction of erythema can be visualized from baseline to the day 8 visit.

• With red light

The use of red light sources for ALA-PDT has also been documented to provide excellent cosmetic results. A study was performed to investigate the photodynamic efficacy of irradiation with coherent light at wavelengths ranging from 622 to 649 nm; it was suggested that irradiation of human keratinocytes in vitro at 635 nm provided the best cell-killing effects. Szeimies et al investigated PDT with the methyl ester of ALA (MAL) in the treatment of AKs using a noncoherent red light source

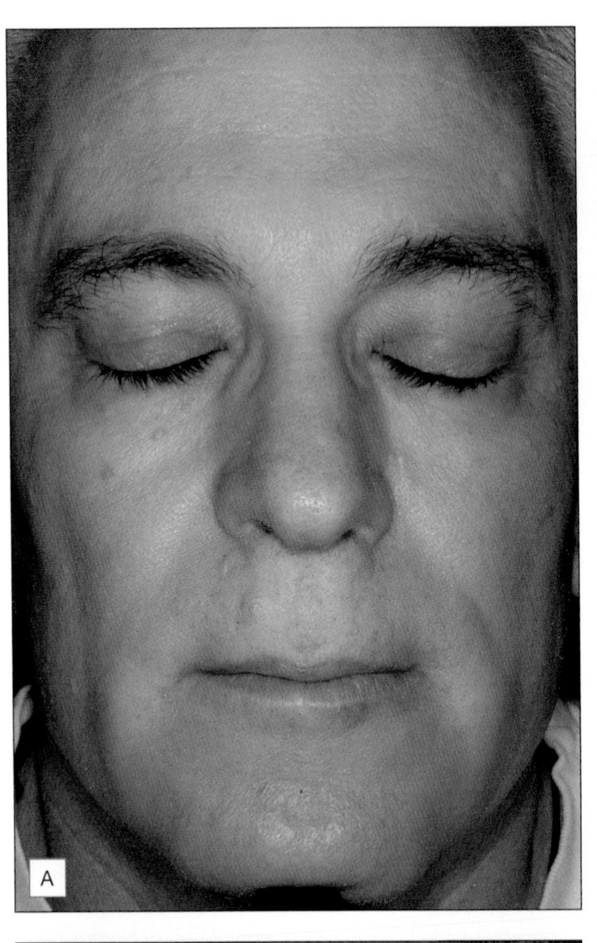
A

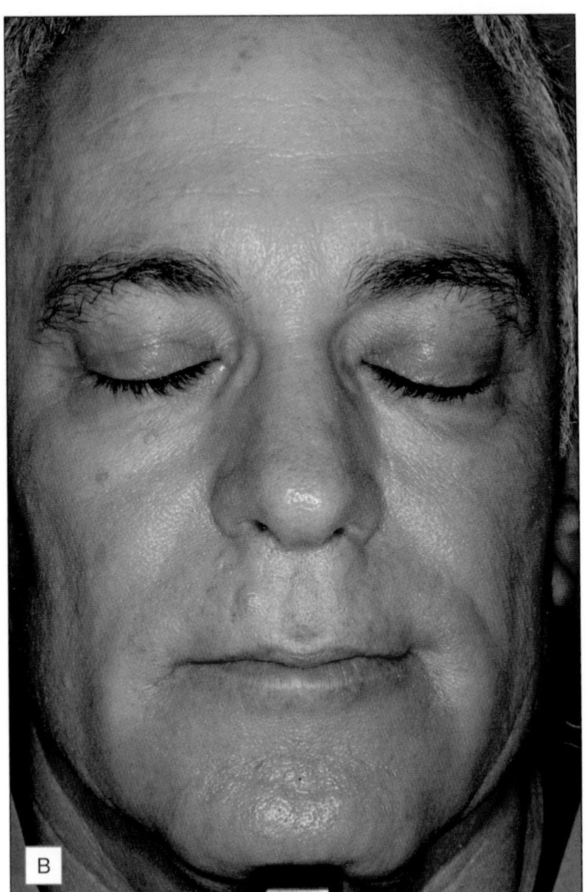
B

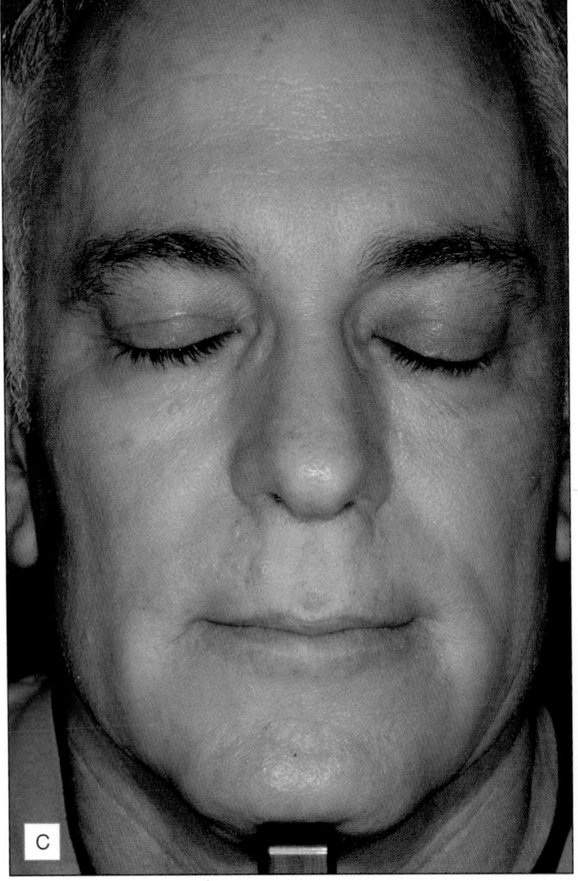
C

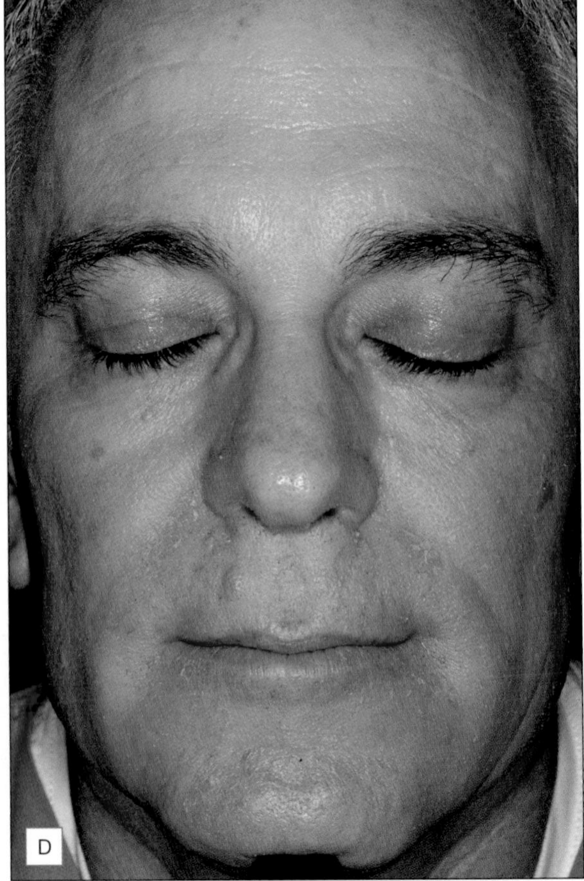
D

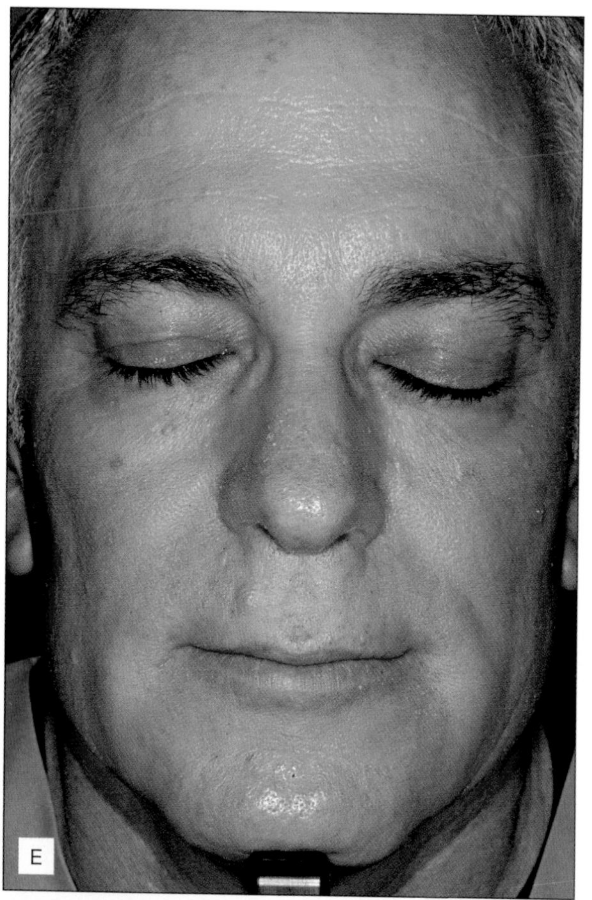

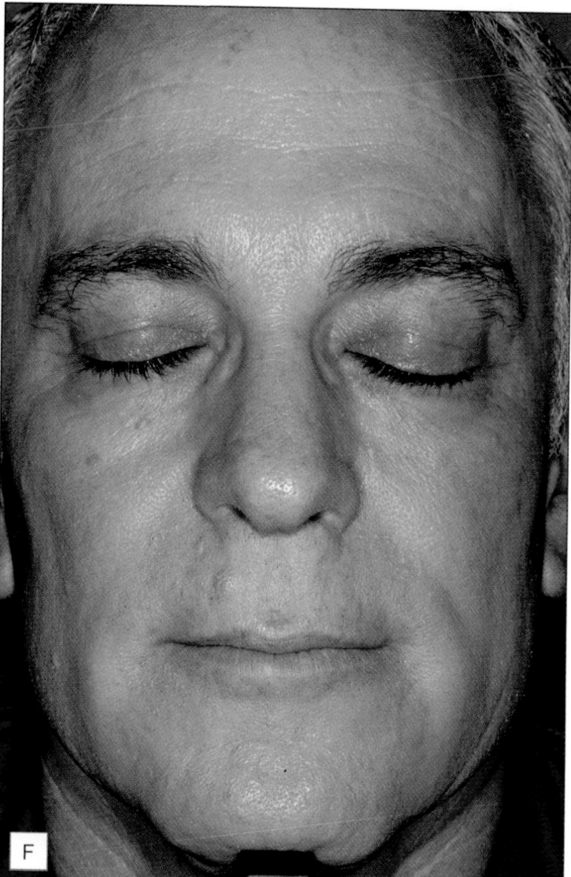

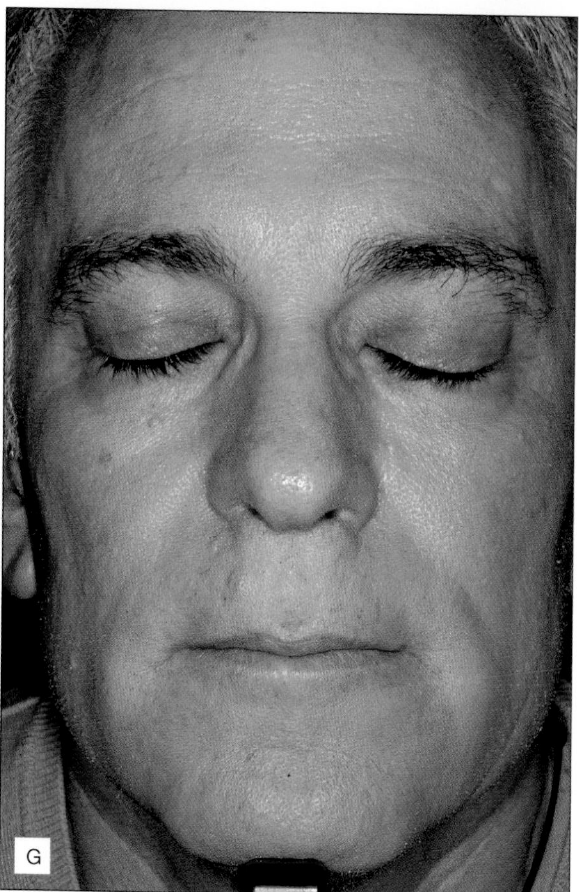

Fig. 13.1 (**A**) Frontal view of a male with photodamage consisting of marked erythema. Levulan PDT treatments with BLU-U. Levulan incubation was for 50 min followed by 10 min of exposure to BLU-U. (**B**) 1 day after PDT treatment; note the erythema of treated skin. (**C**) 2 days after PDT treatment, erythema persists in areas of treated skin. (**D**) 3 days after PDT treatment, resolution of erythema begins along with peeling of dry skin. (**E**) 4 days after PDT treatment, resolution of erythema continues. (**F**) 5 days after PDT treatment, erythema has resolved with minimal peeling. (**G**) 7 days after PDT treatment, there is complete resolution of erythema and peeling

(570–670 nm) versus cryotherapy. They demonstrated that MAL-PDT is a valuable treatment option for patients with AKs. PDT had a response rate similar to that of cryotherapy, but the cosmetic results were superior with high patient satisfaction. In a similar study, Pariser et al used a noncoherent red light source (570–670 nm) to illuminate AKs after application of MAL and found that it was a safe and effective treatment of AKs, again with excellent cosmetic results.

• With intense pulse laser

IPL is a light source that emits noncollimated, noncoherent light with wavelengths in the range of 500–1200 nm, which corresponds to the visible light and near-infrared spectrum. Various filters can be used to block certain wavelengths below the cut-off point of the desired filter. Although IPL alone has proven effectiveness in the treatment of photodamage, the addition of ALA to IPL treatment (ALA-IPL) appears to be more effective in treating photodamaged skin.

Ruiz-Rodriguez at al investigated the treatment of photodamage and AKs using ALA-PDT with IPL as the light source for photorejuvenation. Seventeen patients with various degrees of photodamage and AKs (38 in total) underwent therapy with ALA-IPL. Two treatments were performed with a 1-month interval and a follow-up evaluation at 3 months. Thirty-three of the 38 (87%) AKs disappeared and the treatment was well tolerated. Good cosmetic results were noted in the areas of wrinkling, coarse skin texture, pigmentary changes, and telangiectasias.

Avram and Goldman evaluated the use of ALA-IPL for the treatment of photorejuvenation with one treatment session: 69% of the AKs responded to the use of ALA-IPL and there was an improvement in photorejuvenation parameters of 55% for telangiectasias, 48% for pigment irregularities, and 25% for skin texture. Figure 13.2 shows the clinical improvement in pigment irregularities and skin texture after one PDT treatment with the IPL and BLU-U, and it allows the natural progression of healing after PDT to be visualized. Figure 13.3 also demonstrates the

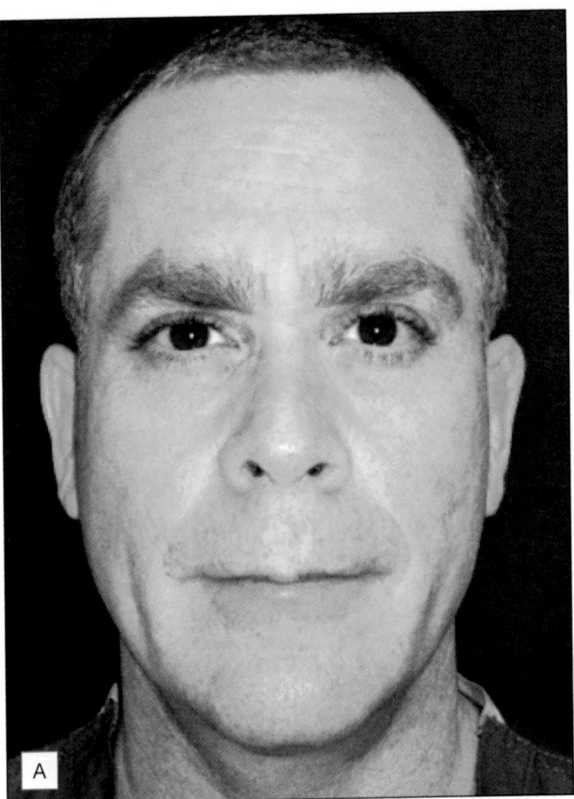

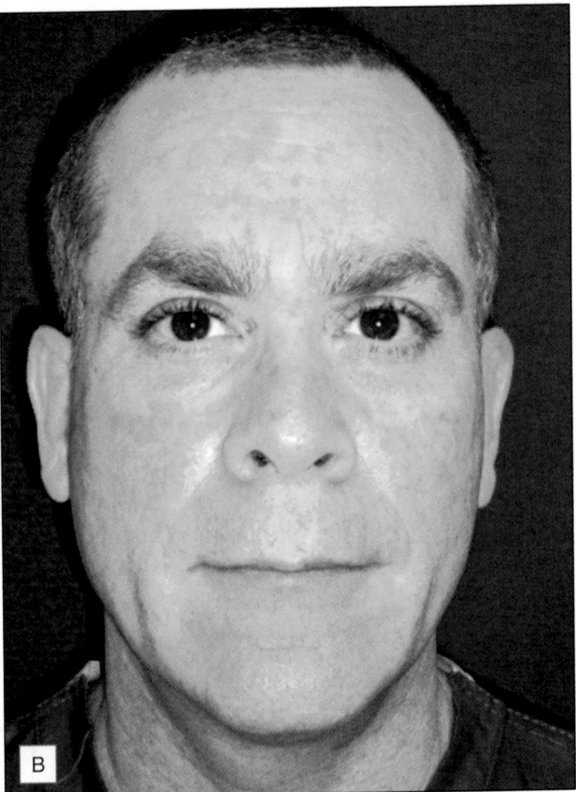

Fig. 13.2 (**A**) Frontal view of a 51-year-old male with photodamage consisting of numerous solar lentigos. (**B**) 1 day after PDT treatment. Levulan ALA was applied to the entire area (not spot treatment) for 1 h. IPL treatment with Lumenis One using a 560-nm cut-off filter, double pulse of 4 and 4 ms with a 10-ms delay at 18 J/cm^2 followed by 10-min exposure with the BLU-U. Note the erythema and crusting of all actinically damaged skin. (**C**) 2 days after PDT treatment, further increase in erythema is seen in areas of actinically damaged skin. (**D**) 3 days after PDT treatment, resolution of erythema begins. (**E**) 4 days after PDT treatment, further resolution of erythema. (**F**) 7 days after PDT treatment, complete resolution of erythema

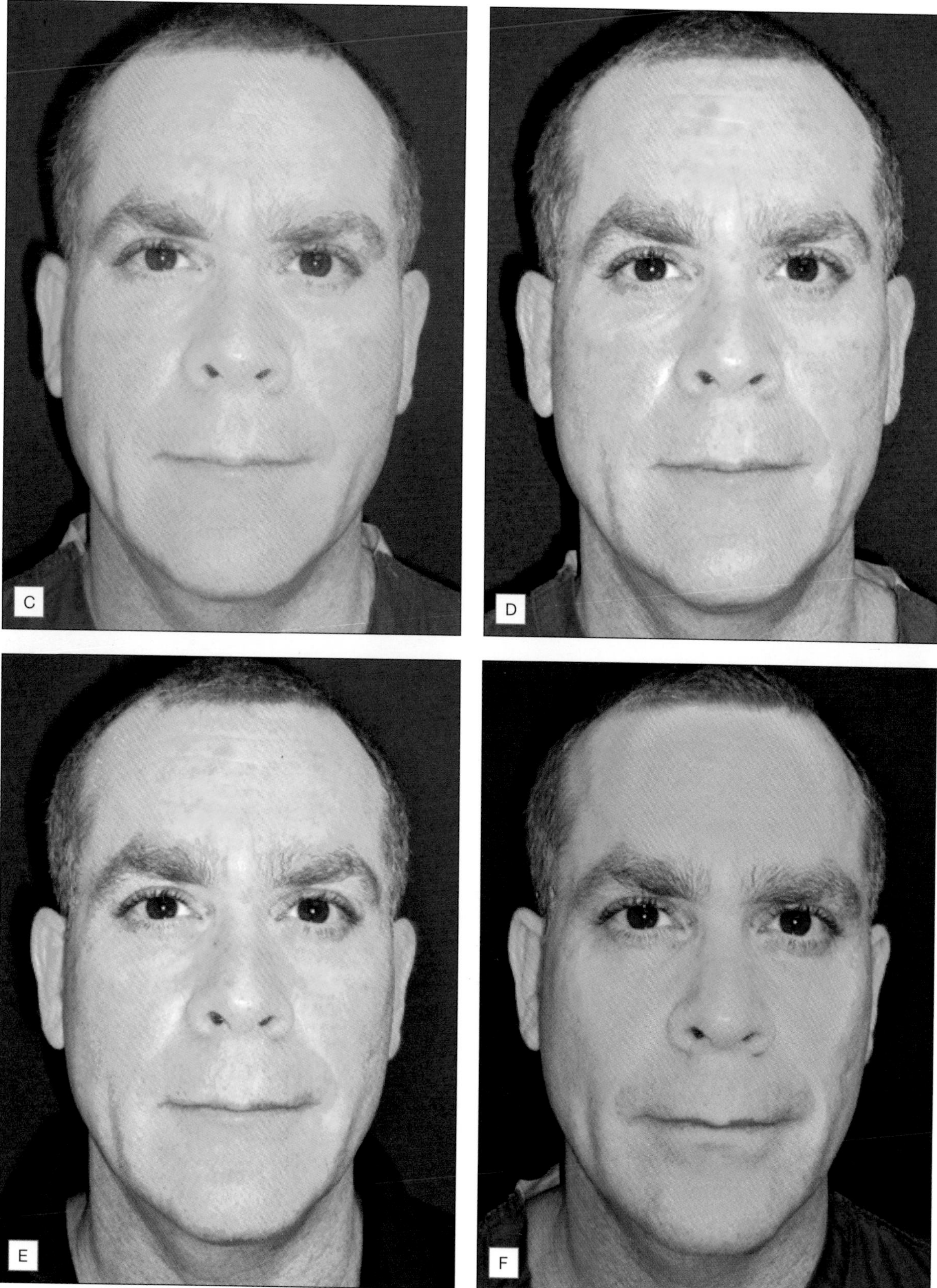

Fig. 13.2 *Continued*

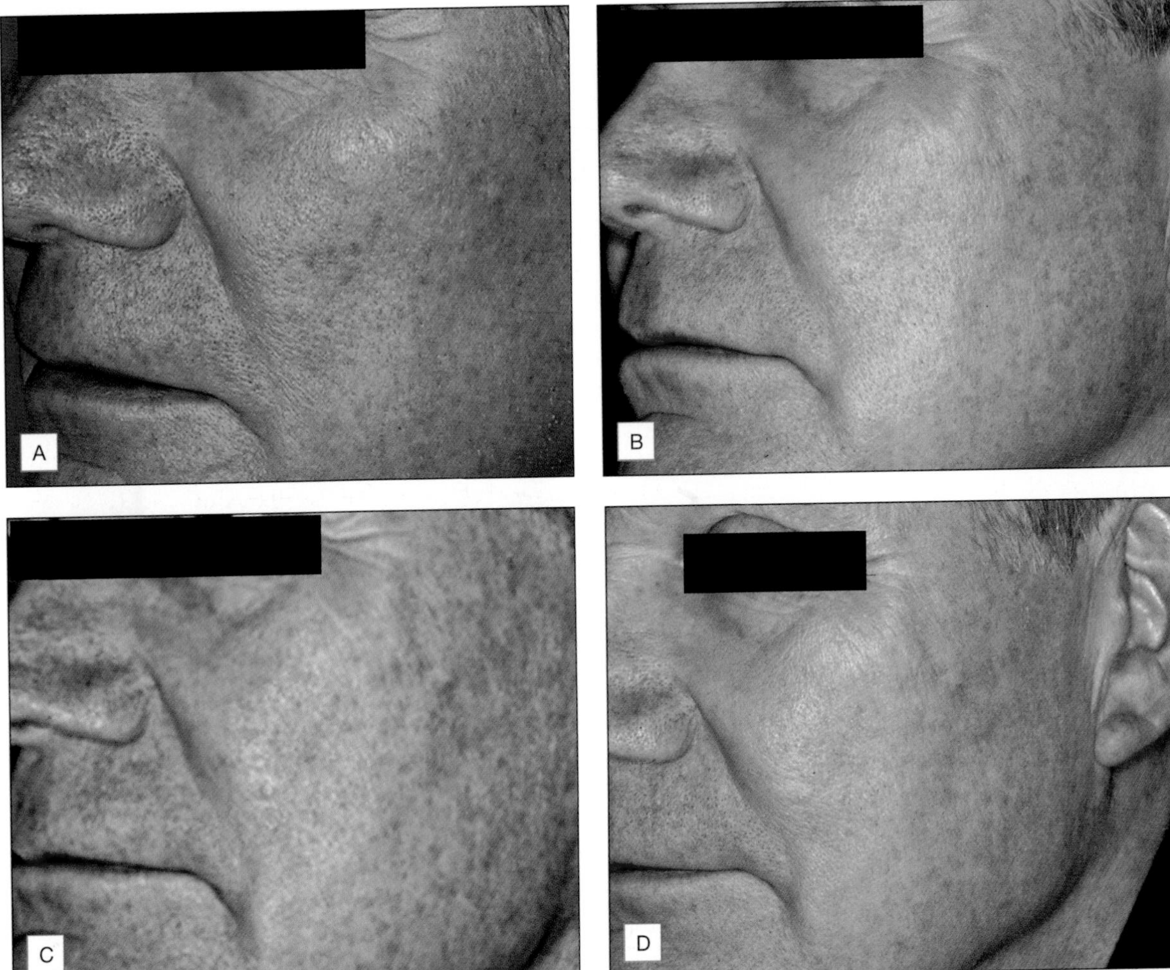

Fig. 13.3 (**A**) Before two Levulan PDT treatments with Vasculight activation, followed by BLU-U. Two IPL Levulan treatments: Vasculight 560-nm filter 31–35 J/cm^2, double pulse: 2.4/10/4.0 followed by BLU-U 6 min (time in BLU-U was decreased due to patient discomfort). Levulan incubation was 60 min for the first treatment and 90 min for the second treatment. (**B**) 1 year after the PDT treatments with good resolution of the erperhema and dyspigmentation. (**C**) 2 years and (**D**) 3 years after the PDT treatments; note the natural progression of photodamage to the skin

clinical improvement in pigment irregularities and skin texture after two PDT treatments with the IPL and BLU-U, as well as the natural progression of photodamage 3 years after the PDT treatment.

Table 13.1 summarizes the recent peer-reviewed reports of split-face ALA-PDT in the evaluation of photorejuvenation. One of these, by Alster et al, evaluates the effectiveness of ALA-IPL compared to IPL treatment alone. Ten patients received two treatments with ALA-IPL on one side and IPL alone on the contralateral side at 4-week intervals. Clinical improvement scores were noted to be higher on the side of the face treated with ALA-IPL. They concluded that the combination of topical ALA + IPL is safe and more effective than IPL alone for the treatment of facial rejuvenation.

Marmur et al conducted a pilot study to assess the ultrastructural changes seen after ALA-IPL photorejuvenation. Seven adults were treated with a full-face IPL treatment, but half received only IPL and the other half was pre-treated with topical ALA before the IPL treatment. Pre- and post-treatment biopsies were reviewed by electron microscopic ultrastructural analysis for changes in collagen. A greater increase in type I collagen was noted in the subjects who were pre-treated with topical ALA and treated with the IPL as opposed to the group treated with IPL alone. They concluded that the addition of ALA-PDT using IPL could be superior to IPL alone.

Dover et al also performed a randomized split-face study to assess the benefit of using ALA-PDT with IPL versus IPL alone. Twenty subjects had three split-face

Table 13.1 Summary of recent peer-reviewed reports of ALA-PDT in AKs and measurement of photorejuvenation

Reference	Sensitizer/light source	Results
Alster et al (2005)	ALA-IPL	ALA-IPL more effective than IPL alone
Marmur et al (2005)	ALA-IPL	ALA-IPL could be superior to IPL alone Greater type I collagen increase with ALA-IPL
Dover et al (2005)	ALA-IPL	Significantly better results and fewer treatment sessions with ALA-IPL than IPL
Gold et al (2006)	ALA-IPL	ALA-IPL better than IPL alone

treatments, 3 weeks apart, with half of the face treated with ALA followed by IPL treatment and the other half was treated with IPL alone. Two more additional full-face treatments were then performed to both sides of the face, 3 weeks apart. A blinded investigator was used to evaluate the global photodamage, fine lines, mottled pigmentation, tactile roughness, and sallowness during the study. They concluded that pre-treatment with ALA followed by IPL treatment resulted in greater improvement in global score for photoaging (80% vs 50%) and mottled pigmentation (95% vs 65%). Successful results were also noted for fine lines for the ALA-IPL side compared to the IPL-alone side (55% vs 20%). Although tactile roughness and sallowness were noticeably better, pre-treatment with ALA did not enhance the results of using IPL alone. It was important to note that both modes of treatment were well tolerated and that no significant differences in the side-effect profiles were observed. They concluded that ALA-PDT using IPL for the management of photodamage provided results that were significantly better for global photodamage, mottled pigmentation, and fine lines in contrast to IPL alone, without an increase in side effects. Thus, fewer treatment sessions and better cosmetic results would be provided with ALA-IPL versus IPL alone.

Another split-face comparative study of ALA-PDT with IPL on one side and IPL alone on the other side was performed by Gold to evaluate photorejuvenation. Subjects were treated with three IPL sessions at 1-month intervals. Results showed that skin texture, mottled hyperpigmentation, facial telangiectasias, and associated AKs all showed better response on the side of the face treated with ALA-PDT. It could be clearly shown that ALA-IPL showed enhanced efficacy in photorejuvenation, as well as being an effective treatment of AKs.

• With pulsed-dye laser

PDLs as the light source for photorejuvenation with ALA have also been studied. Sterenberg and Gemert entered various numerical data on hematoporphyrin excitation and de-excitation into a mathematical model to test the effectiveness of PDT using different PDL sources. It was noted that commonly used PDLs using either a copper vapor or a frequency doubled Nd:YAG laser had a PDT effectiveness identical to a continuous wave (CW) laser source. Karrer et al investigated the efficacy of PDT both in vitro and in vivo using ALA with a long-pulse (1.5 ms) PDL (LPDL). Human keratinocytes were incubated in ALA, then exposed to the LPDL at either 585, 595, or 600 nm, or an incoherent light source (580–740 nm). Twenty-four patients were treated with topical ALA and then exposed to the LPDL or an incoherent light source. They demonstrated that cytotoxic effects in vitro were maximized using the LPDL at 585 nm or the incoherent lamp. AKs treated on the forehead with ALA-LPDL achieved 79% clearance, whereas ALA combined with the incoherent lamp achieved 84% clearance. This study demonstrated both the in vitro and in vivo benefits of ALA-PDT using the PDL.

Alexiades-Armenakas et al found ALA-PDT with the 595-nm PDL was successful in treating AKs and in improving photorejuvenation. Their study included 2561 AKs on the face and scalp treated with ALA-PDT using a PDL. Clearance rates of 99.9% at 10 days, 98.4% at 2 months, and 90.1% at 4 months were noted. Lesions on the extremities and torso also showed improvement, although the rates were not as high as for the face and neck. A second study utilizing the PDL also showed its benefits in the treatment of actinic chelitis.

These results show the potential usefulness of a variety of lasers and light sources in the treatment of AKs and in the improvement of photodamage and photorejuvenation utilizing ALA-PDT treatments. Beyond the active treatment of AKs, photodamage, nonmelanoma skin cancers, and beneficial cosmetic outcome for photorejuvenation, ALA may hopefully prevent or delay the onset of nonmelanoma skin cancers.

Some dermatologists are already using ALA-PDT as a skin cancer preventative mechanism, although its use for this purpose has to be considered experimental at present (see Chapter 11). Animal studies have been preformed by Sharfaei et al to examine this subject. Topical MAL-PDT was applied to half of the backs of hairless mice and the other side was treated with vehicle only and then exposed to UV radiation. It was concluded that topical MAL followed by light exposure under suberythematous conditions delayed the appearance of UV-induced skin tumors without increasing mortality or morbidity, and therefore was able to show some benefit in preventing skin tumors. The underlying mechanism of action is yet to be clarified. Some possible mechanisms include toxicity to the islands of mutated epidermal cells by some indirect phenomenon, a cytokine-mediated effect that delays tumor growth, reversal of UV-induced immunosuppression, or other specific antitumoral immune-mediated effects.

TREATMENT TECHNIQUE

As many different techniques can be used to achieve similar results, there is no golden rule to follow with regards to the proper protocol. The following are general guidelines and principles that could maximize treatment benefits for ALA-PDT and which we use in our practice.

• Levulan protocol: Photodynamic photorejuvenation

1. Get the patient to wash skin with soap and water.
2. Perform microdermabrasion with the Vibraderm over the area to be treated.
3. Scrub the skin vigorously with acetone on a 4 × 4 gauze.
4. Break the two glass ampules in the Kerastick as per instructions on the stick. Shake the stick for about 2 min. If you would like to see how the powder mixes with the solvent you can remove the plastic Levulan Kerastick from the cardboard sleeve by pushing a pen or needle driver into the end of the stick and the plastic sleeve will extrude from the cardboard sleeve.
5. Apply the contents to the area you wish to treat by painting the Levulan on the entire area. Do not worry about applying too much Levulan solution (applying two coats of the solution is recommended). It is important to get close to the eyes, as it will be apparent that the periorbital skin was not treated adequately if you fail to do this.
6. Allow the Levulan to incubate for 60 min on the skin indoors.
7. Wash the face prior to any treatment to remove the Levulan.
8. Activate the Levulan with the appropriate light source. We use an IPL followed by the BLU-U light.
9. **It is important to wash the face really well with soap and water after completing light treatments to remove any residual Levulan from the skin surface.**
10. Warn the patient to remain out of direct sunlight for 24 h. We recommend SPA MD ultragentle cleanser and moisturizing night cream for 7 days after treatment. Ideally, patients should begin use of the La Roche-Posay Cicaplast cream and cleanser 4 weeks prior to PDT treatment.
11. Patients are given La Roche-Posay Thermal Spring Water spray to apply to their skin four to six times a day.
12. Repeat the treatment in 2–4 weeks. Increase incubation time if there was little reaction, and re-evaluate your skin preparation technique.

As described above, multiple light sources can be used for ALA-PDT. Table 13.2 summarizes the most common parameters used in our clinic. Boxes 13.1–13.5 show our patient information and consent forms.

SIDE EFFECTS AND COMPLICATIONS

As described above, most of the adverse events of ALA-PDT relate to patient discomfort and phototoxicity. Patient discomfort with complaints of burning, stinging, or itching can be handled with the proper patient education about what to expect and calming reassurance, as these symptoms usually improve on their own within a

Table 13.2 Levulan activation parameters for the most popular light sources. It is not necessary to adjust the parameters downwards with an IPL when used with Levulan

Lumenis One	560 filter, 16–18 J/cm², 4.0/4.0 with 10–40 ms delay, one pass
Vasculight	560 filter; 28–32 J/cm², 2.4/4.0 with 10–40 ms delay, one pass or 35 J/cm², 3.0–6.0 with 10-ms delay
Quantum	560 filter; 24–28 J/cm², 2.4/4.0 with 10–40 ms delay, one pass or 30 J/cm², 3.0–6.0 with 10-ms delay
Aurora	16–22 J, with an RF of 16–22 J, one pass
Estelux	19–30 J at 20 ms, one pass
V-Beam	10-mm spot; 7.5 J; 6-ms pulse width, two passes with 50% overlap
V-Star	10-mm spot: 7.5 J; 40-ms pulse width; two passes with 50% overlap
Clearlight	15 min under the light
BLU-U	15 min under the light (Levulan can stay on the skin during the treatment)

Box 13.1 Client consent for Levulan-PDT

Levulan (aminolevulinic acid 20%) is a naturally occurring photosensitizing compound which has been approved by the FDA to treat pre-cancerous skin lesions called actinic keratosis. Levulan is applied to the skin and subsequently "activated" by specific wavelengths of light. This process of activating Levulan with light is termed Photodynamic Therapy. The purpose of activating the Levulan is to improve the appearance and reduce acne rosacea, acne vulgaris, sebaceous hyperplasia, decrease oiliness of the skin, and improve texture and smoothness by minimizing pore size. Any pre-cancerous lesions are also simultaneously treated. The improvement of these skin conditions (other than actinic keratosis) is considered an "off-label" use of Levulan.

I understand that Levulan will be applied to my skin for 30–60 minutes. Subsequently, the area will be treated with a specific wavelength of light to activate the Levulan. Following my treatment, I must wash off any Levulan on my skin. I understand that I should avoid direct sunlight for 24 hours following the treatment due to photosensitivity. I understand that I am not pregnant.

Anticipated side effects of Levulan treatment include discomfort, burning, swelling, redness, and possible skin peeling, especially in any areas of sun damaged skin and pre-cancers of the skin, as well as lightening or darkening of skin tone and spots, and possible hair removal. The peeling may last many days, and the redness for several weeks if I have an exuberant response to treatment.

I consent to the taking of photographs of my face before each treatment session. I understand that I may require several treatment sessions spaced 2–4 weeks apart to achieve optimal results.

I understand that medicine is not an exact science, and that there can be no guarantees of my results. I am aware that while some individuals have fabulous results, it is possible that these treatments will not work for me. I understand that alternative treatments include topical medications, oral medications, cryosurgery, excisional surgery, and doing nothing.

I have read the above information and understand it. My questions have been answered satisfactorily by the doctor and his staff. I accept the risks and complications of the procedure. By signing this consent form I agree to have one or more Levulan treatments.

____

Signature

____

Print Name

____________________ ____________________

Date Witness

Box 13.2 Therapy (PDT) patient guide

WHAT IS PHOTODYNAMIC THERAPY?

Photodynamic therapy (PDT) is a special treatment performed with a topical photosensitizing agent called Levulan (5-aminolevulinic acid or ALA) activated with the correct wavelength of light. This is also known as "ALA-PDT treatment." These treatments remove sun damaged pre-cancerous zones and spots called actinic keratoses. Sun damage, fine lines, and blotchy pigmentation are also improved because of the positive effect of Levulan and the light treatment. ALA-PDT treatment also has the unique ability to minimize pores and reduce oil glands, effectively treating stubborn acne vulgaris, acne rosacea, and improve the appearance of some acne scars.

HOW MUCH IMPROVEMENT CAN I EXPECT?

Patients with severe sun-damaged skin manifested by actinic keratosis, texture, and tone changes including mottled pigmentation and skin laxity may see excellent results. You may also see improvement of large pores and pitted acne scars. Active acne can improve dramatically.

HOW MANY TREATMENTS WILL IT TAKE TO SEE THE "BEST RESULTS"?

To achieve maximum improvement of pre-cancerous (actinic keratoses) sun damage, skin tone and texture, a series of 2–3 treatments 3 to 4 weeks apart is most effective. Some patients with just actinic keratoses are happy with one treatment. More treatments can be done at periodic intervals in the future to maintain the rejuvenated appearance of the skin.

WHAT ARE THE DISADVANTAGES?

Following PDT, the treated areas can appear red with some peeling for 2–7 days. Some patients have an exuberant response to PDT, and experience marked redness of their skin. Temporary swelling of the lips and around your eyes can occur for a few days. Darker pigmented patches called liver spots can become temporarily darker and then peel off leaving normal skin. (This usually occurs over 7–10 days.) Repeat treatments may be necessary as medicine is not an exact science.

WHAT ARE THE ADVANTAGES?

1. **Easier** for patients than repeated topical liquid nitrogen, Efudex (5-FU), or Aldara because the side effects are minimal, rapid healing, and only 1–3 treatments required.
2. The ALA-PDT treatment at our clinic is nearly **painless** verses liquid nitrogen, 5-FU, and Aldara.
3. **Reduced scarring** and improved cosmetic outcome compared with cautery, surgery, and Efudex. Liquid nitrogen can leave white spots on your skin.
4. Levulan **improves the whole facial area treated** creating one color, texture, and tone rather than just spot treating with liquid nitrogen, cautery, and surgery.

In summary, PDT matches the "**ideal treatment**" for actinic damage:

- Well tolerated (essentially painless)
- Easily performed by a specialty clinic environment
- Noninvasive (no needles or surgery required)
- Excellent cosmetic outcome (particularly in cosmetic sensitive areas of the face)

Box 13.3 Treatment steps

1. Patients who have a history of recurring cold sores (Herpes simplex type I) should start oral Valtrex 500 mg or Famvir 250 mg tablets, one tablet twice daily for 3 days—starting this prescription the morning of your PDT treatment. The prescription for this product will be ordered for you.
2. Make sure your skin is clean and free of all make-up, moisturizers, and sunscreens. Bring a hat, sunglasses, and scarf when appropriate to the clinic.
3. Photography will be done by the staff before the Levulan is applied.
4. You must sign a consent form.
5. An acetone scrub is performed. This will enhance the absorption of the Levulan and give much more even uptake. In some patients microdermabrasion will also be performed immediately prior to the application of Levulan.
6. Levulan is applied topically to the whole area to be treated (such as the whole face, back of the hands, extensor part of the forearms).
7. The Levulan is left on for 30–60 minutes before any light treatment.
8. The Levulan is activated with the BLU-U and/or IPL device. This unique spectrum of light activates the Levulan beginning with low energy levels.
9. Post-treatment instructions will be given to you to care for your improved skin.

Box 13.4 Home care instructions for patients following photodynamic skin rejuvenation

Day of treatment

1. If you have any discomfort, begin applying ice packs to the treated areas. This will help keep the area cool and alleviate any discomfort, as well as help keep down any swelling. Swelling will be most evident around the eyes and is usually more prominent in the morning.
2. Remain indoors and avoid direct sunlight.
3. Spray on La Roche-Posay Cicaplast Thermal Spring Water often.
4. Apply La Roche-Posay Cicaplast moisturizing cream.
5. Take analgesics such as Advil if necessary.

Day 2–7

1. You may begin applying make-up once any crusting has healed. The area may be slightly red for 1–2 weeks. If make-up is important to you, please see one of our estheticians for a complimentary consultation for DYG Mineral Make-up, which is all natural, inert, anti-inflammatory, and acts as a concealer with sunscreen. It is especially effective to mask redness.
2. The skin will feel dry and tightened. La Roche-Posay Cicaplast moisturizer should be used daily.
3. Try to avoid direct sunlight for 1 week. Use a total block zinc oxide based sunscreen with a minimum SPF 30. We recommend Ti-Silc, Spa MD or Cool Clenz.

few hours after the treatment session. Phototoxic events are best prevented by using the proper parameters and the proper laser for the patient and with strict avoidance of the sun for 24 h after the treatment session. If a phototoxic reaction does develop, the use of ice packs and topical corticosteroids will usually suffice as treatment. Cutaneous infections secondary to ALA-PDT therapy are usually low, but they can be managed with the appropriate topical antibacterial or antiviral medications. Patients with a history of herpes simplex should be given the appropriate antivirals to prevent the reactivation of the virus (see Box 13.3).

Box 13.5 Levulan talking points for staff

1. Levulan is all natural and produced by your body to make hemoglobin.
2. Levulan is applied to your skin. There are no internal side effects.
3. Uptake of Levulan is by abnormal cells. Levulan targets these cells (acne oil glands, pre-cancers).
4. Appropriate light wavelength activates the Levulan.
5. Your damaged skin then sheds leaving you with new, revitalized skin.

SUMMARY

A variety of lasers and light sources have been evaluated utilizing ALA-PDT. These include blue light (405–420 nm), red light (635 nm), PDLs (585 and 595 nm), and the IPL source (500–1200 nm). All of these devices have shown safety and efficacy in PDT and can be utilized in treating photodamaged skin. Physicians utilizing these devices should feel confident utilizing PDT in their patients.

The future of ALA-PDT is now. For many years, dermatologists have hoped that ALA-PDT would leave the laboratory setting and become part of everyday practices. Cosmetic improvements have been shown in a variety of cutaneous concerns, including photorejuvenation of photodamaged skin. Short-contact, full-face/broad-area ALA-PDT treatments make this therapy more practical for the dermatologic community and trials have shown that it is safe, efficacious, relatively pain free, and without significant adverse effects. Clinicians should be ready for these new therapeutic approaches to common skin concerns and may need to rethink how they treat photodamaged skin, bridging more closely the worlds of medical dermatology and cosmetic dermatologic surgery.

FURTHER READING

Alexiades-Armenakas M 2006 Laser-mediated photodynamic therapy. Clinical Dermatology 24:16–25

Alexiades-Armenakas MR, Geronemus RG 2003 Laser mediated photodynamic therapy of actinic keratoses. Archives of Dermatology 139:1313–1320

Alster TS, Tanzi EL, Welsh EC 2005 Photorejuvenation of facial skin with topical 20% 5-aminolevulinic acid and intense pulsed light treatment: a split-face comparison study. Journal of Drugs in Dermatology 4:35–38

Avram D, Goldman MP 2004 Effectiveness and safety of ALA-IPL in treating actinic keratoses and photodamage. Journal of Drugs in Dermatology 3 (Suppl):36–39

Dover J, Arndt K, Bhatia A, Stewart B 2005 Adjunctive use of topical aminolevulinic acid with intense pulsed light in the treatment of photoaging. Journal of the American Academy of Dermatology 52 (Suppl):208

Gold MH 2002 The evolving role of aminolevulinic acid hydrochloride with photodynamic therapy in photoaging. Cutis 69 (6 Suppl):8–13

Gold MH 2006 A split face comparison study of ALA-PDT with intense pulsed light versus intense pulsed light alone for photodamage/photorejuvenation. Dermatologic Surgery 32:795–803

Goldman MP, Atkin D, Kincad S 2002 PDT/ALA in the treatment of actinic damage: real world experience. Journal of Lasers in Surgery and Medicine 14 (Suppl):24

Karrer S, Baumler W, Abels C, Hohenleutner U, Landthaler M, Szeimies RM 1999 Long-pulse dye laser for photodynamic therapy: investigations in vitro and in vivo. Lasers in Surgery and Medicine 25:51–59

Marmur ES, Phelps R, Goldberg DJ 2005 Ultrastructural changes seen after ALA-IPL photorejuvenation: a pilot study. Journal of Cosmetic Laser Therapry 7:21–24

Morton CA, Brown SB, Collins S et al 2002 Guidelines for topical photodynamic therapy: report of a workshop of the British photodermatology group. British Journal of Dermatology 146:552–567

Pariser DM, Lowe NJ, Stewart DM et al 2003 Photodynamic therapy with topical methyl aminolevulinate for actinic keratosis: results of a prospective randomized multicenter trial. Journal of the American Academy of Dermatology 48:227–232

Ruiz-Rodriguez R, Sanz-Sanchez T, Cordoba S 2002 Photodynamic photorejuvenation. Dermatologic Surgery 28:742–744; discussion 744

Sharfaei S, Juzenas P, Moon J, Bissonnette R 2002 Weekly topical application of methyl aminolevulinate followed by light exposure delays the appearance of UV-induced skin tumours in mice. Archives of Dermatological Research 294:237–242

Sterenborg HJ, van Gemert MJ 1996 Photodynamic therapy with pulsed light sources: a theoretical analysis. Physics in Medicine and Biology 41:835–849

Szeimies RM, Abels C, Fritsch C et al 1995 Wavelength dependency of photodynamic effects after sensitization with 5-aminolevulinic acid in vitro and in vivo. Journal of Investigative Dermatology 105:672–677

Szeimies RM, Karrer S, Radakovic-Fijan S et al 2002 Photodynamic therapy using topical methyl 5-aminolevulinate compared with cryotherapy for actinic keratosis: A prospective, randomized study. Journal of the American Academy of Dermatology 47:258–262

Touma DJ, Gilchrest BA 2003 Topical photodynamic therapy: a new tool in cosmetic dermatology. Seminars in Cutaneous Medicine and Surgery 22:124–30

Touma D, Yaar M, Whitehead S, Konnikov N, Gilchrest BA 2004 A trial of short incubation, broad-area photodynamic therapy for facial actinic keratoses and diffuse photodamage. Archives of Dermatology 140:33–40

14 Treatment of Vascular Lesions

Zhou Guoyu

INTRODUCTION

According to the 1982 classification by Mulliken and Glowacki, vascular lesions are of two kinds: hemangiomas and vascular malformations.

• Hemangiomas

Hemangiomas are caused by overgrowth of endothelial cells with the marked clinical feature of rapid growth. The pathologic manifestation is capillary generation mixed with mast cells and fibroblasts. Owing to the fast regeneration of endothelial cells, the lack of nutrition of the central part of the tumor will often lead to necrosis, which is the main cause of ulceration. Hemorrhage, infection, and tissue damage are the next most common complications. Airway obstruction and hemorrhage can be severe and even lethal in some hemangioma cases. However, a large number of hemangiomas will undergo spontaneous regression, making clinical management choices difficult. A wait-and-see policy is good management during a period of spontaneous regression, but delayed or mistimed treatment is a common problem. Incorrect treatment can lead to over-treatment, resulting in possible scar tissue formation. Best management of lesions is treatment as early as possible, and laser treatment is a logical approach.

Selective photothermolysis, such as with a pulsed-dye laser (PDL) at a wavelength of 585 nm or 595 nm, gives a good therapeutic result for superficial hemangioma. The mechanism of this laser therapy is dependent on the high absorption of hemoglobin at a wavelength of 577–595 nm. With this range of wavelengths, as the target hemangioma tissue is rich in hemoglobin while the surrounding normal tissue is not, there will be a selectively high absorption of laser energy within the hemangioma tissue, but little light absorbed by the surrounding tissue. The laser energy heats and causes mechanical damage to the hemangioma with little effect on normal surrounding tissue.

Another therapy is selective photocoagulation. It differs from photothermolysis in that it uses heat to selectively destroy the target hemangioma. The long-pulsed Nd:YAG laser 1064 nm achieves a good response with deeper lesions. Severe cases of hemangioma need comprehensive treatments, such as hormone therapy (prednisolone 4–5 mg/kg), combined with laser illumination, and/or surgical resection.

• Vascular malformations

In contrast to a hemangioma, a vascular malformation consists of near-normal structured blood vessels. An example is venous malformation, classically termed cavernous hemangioma. This lesion consists of a large venous sinus-like structure surrounded by normal muscle or normal collagen. Selective photocoagulation using the Nd:YAG laser (1064 nm) or diode laser (980 nm) at continuous wave (CW) will give good results for superficial lesions. Surgical laser therapy after surgical flap raising to coagulate the deep vascular malformation is another means of treatment. Photodymanic therapy (PDT) has little effect on this kind of vascular malformation.

A second example is the venular malformation of a port wine stain (PWS), which consists of a large number of capillaries within the epidermis and dermis. For PWS, even though the capillary may appear contracted or dilated, the high density of capillaries in the skin gives the lesion a reddish color. Clinical investigation often confirms slowly developed dilation of vessels with aging. Treatments such as tattoo, cryosurgery, skin transplantation, and isotope glue were alternated with laser therapy due to adverse effects. With the PDL, high laser energy is transferred to target blood vessels, without significant absorption by surrounding tissue. Selective photothermolysis is carried out to destroy the capillaries. PDL treatment has become the standard treatment for PWS, with many physicians reporting success using this technique. However, the degree of PWS blanching following PDL therapy remains variable and unpredictable. The average success rate for complete blanching is less than 25%, even after multiple PDL treatments. Unfortunately, PDL treatment of skin types IV–V produces more frequent adverse effects, most commonly hyper- and hypo-pigmentation, skin texture changes, and scar formation. For example, in Chinese patients, good result can be achieved for some less serious cases with complete remission, while a large number of cases undergo partial remission accompanied by adverse effects (Fig. 14.1).

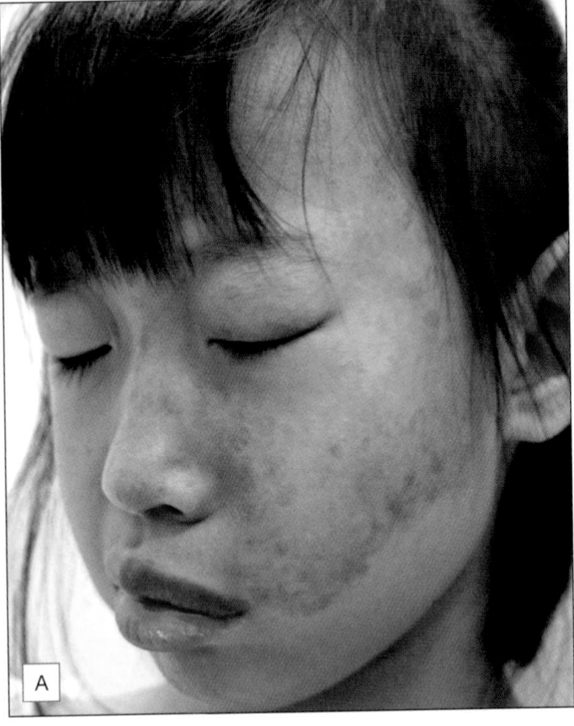

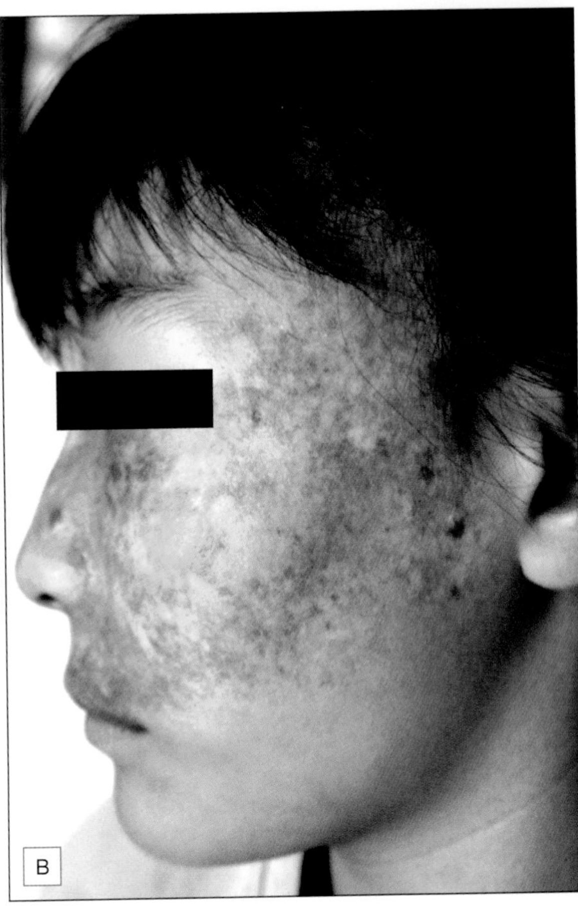

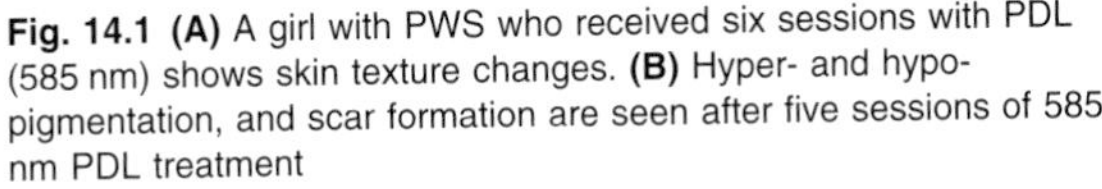

Fig. 14.1 **(A)** A girl with PWS who received six sessions with PDL (585 nm) shows skin texture changes. **(B)** Hyper- and hypo-pigmentation, and scar formation are seen after five sessions of 585-nm PDL treatment

Repeat treatments increase clearance rate but at the expense of increased risk of adverse effects. For a moderate-to-severe lesion, PDL treatment can result in partial remission but is often accompanied by hypopigmentation and skin atrophy. We have compared PDL at 585 nm and 595 nm, and found that the latter gives a slightly better result. Recently, we have used the long-pulsed Nd:YAG laser (Gentle YAG, Candela, Inc, USA), and the immediate reaction is somewhat lighter than the "purple" result achieved with PDL, and more acceptable to the patient. Clinical data reveal deeper effects with the Nd:YAG laser than with the PDL of 585–595-nm wavelength. If PDL is combined with a dynamic cooling device, which decreases skin temperature, the adverse effect of hyperpigmentation is greater with PDL (585–595 nm) therapy alone.

The failure of PDL therapy to remove the PWS completely in the majority of patients has necessitated the search for an alternative therapy.

DEVELOPMENTAL OF PDT FOR PORT WINE STAINS

Apart from photothermolysis therapy, PDT has been used to treat vascular malformations such as PWS. Professor Ma Baozhang noted that after PDT, many specimens of oral or maxillofacial carcinoma revealed destruction of blood vessel structure. Also, histopathology commonly showed local hemorrhage and red blood cell extravasation after PDT, both in animals and humans. This suggested that the effects of PDT are not the result of direct tumor cell kill but could be secondary to vascular effects, such as constriction, thrombosis, endothelial cell damage, and loss of vessel wall integrity with increased permeability, which disrupts the microvasculature structure. This phenomenon stimulated Baozhang to use PDT to treat vascular lesions. As the vascular lesion needing to be destroyed is more superficial than a tumor, she inferred that PDT would be more effective at treating PWS than carcinomas. The

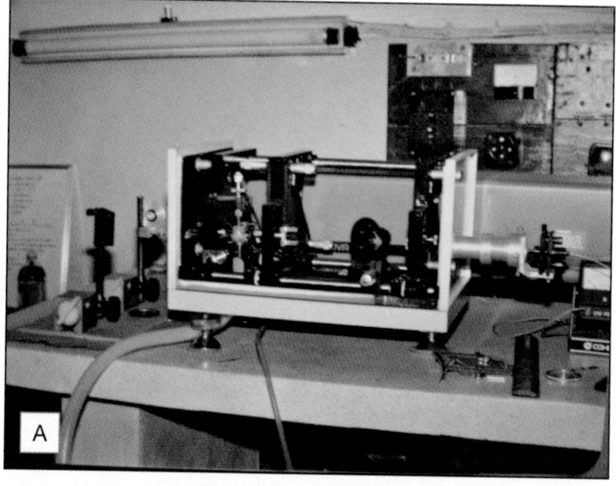

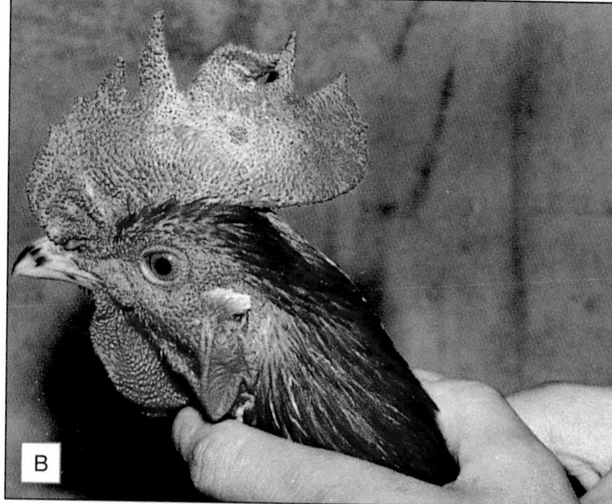

Fig. 14.2 (**A**) Argon pumped dye laser PDT (600 nm) system (Coherent Laser Group, USA). (**B**) Animal experiment using a chicken's comb as a model for PWS shows blanching after one session of dye laser PDT

reddish wavelength of the 600-nm laser can penetrate to a depth of 0.5–1.0 cm, so it is logical to predict that it would be more effective in treating deep vascular lesions.

In 1984, Baozhang performed an experimental PDT study on a chicken's comb using the argon pumped-dye laser (600 nm, CW, 250 mW/cm^2; Fig. 14.2A) and 5 mg/kg of a hematoporphyrin-derivative (HpD) photosensitizer (YHpD; Yangzhou Biochemistry Phamaceutics) administered intravenously immediately before laser illumination. Chicken's comb shares a similar tissue structure to PWS, and can be used as a model to simulate the PWS lesion. The chicken's comb was blanched 3–4 weeks after dye laser PDT (Fig. 14.2B). Histopathology findings confirmed endothelial blood cell damage within the illuminated comb.

Encouraged by the animal experiment, a clinical study using the same dye laser PDT was carried out on Chinese volunteers. Clinical observation found similar tissue reactions as in the animal experiment using the dye laser at settings of 600 nm and 150–250 mW/cm^2. The photosensitizer (YHpD) was injected intravenously before laser irradiation at 5 mg/kg concentration. Skin allergy tests were done for each volunteer before clinical treatment.

The PWS birthmarks went purple immediately, and epidermal necrosis with seeping occurred within 2 weeks. The lesions became paler 1 month after one session of PDT. In fact, all lesions showing blanching of color following treatment underwent skin necrosis and the clinical manifestation was an apparent wound healing process. At follow-up, there were changes in skin texture and some scar formation on treated areas. Decreasing the laser energy would have resulted in less blanching.

In 1988, when guided by Baozhang to carry out further clinical studies, we were faced with the problem that argon pumped dye laser PDT can cause skin necrosis, but we could not explain why this happened or resolve the problem. We tried using the argon laser alone to perform PDT with the photosensitizer YHpD, given intravenously at 5 mg/kg. Laser irradiation was started immediately after YHpD injection. The main light source of the argon laser had a mixed 488/514.5 nm wavelength. These green and blue lights penetrate skin tissue more superficially than the light 600-nm light from the argon pumped dye laser. We hoped to diminish the skin necrosis by using the argon laser, but unfortunately both 488- and 514.5-nm PDT resulted in nearly the same necrosis as with the 600-nm pumped dye laser PDT. For a good blanching result, initial skin necrosis was inevitable (Fig. 14.3).

Although our clinical research progressed slowly, Gu Ying and Li Junhun reported the first successful application of argon laser (mixed spectrum, i.e. 488 and 514.5 nm) PDT to treat PWS in 1992. They used the photosensitizer YHpD, given intravenously at a concentration of 5 mg/kg, the laser parameter 50–100 mW/cm^2, and fluencies of 90–540 J/cm^2. Argon laser illumination was carried out immediately after administration of YHpD. Very good results were reported using this method. Unfortunately, we could not duplicate this success in our clinical trial of argon laser PDT. In particular, we noticed that the skin wound healing process often occurred in well reacted lesions. We tried adjusting both the photosensitizer concentration and laser energy level separately, but neither action helped to avoid skin necrosis. Scar formation and skin texture alterations thus were the key problems impeding the clinical application of PDT for PWS. Another major and indirect problem were the common adverse effects from sun exposure after YHpD administration. Strict avoidance of sunlight exposure and staying in a dark room for 1 month after treatment were recommended.

We noticed a literature report on a physical model of PWS that selectively absorbed 577-nm wavelength light. A new method of PDT for PWS was introduced that used the 578-nm copper vapor laser, and Gu Ying et al reported a clinical study using this laser. They hoped that the photodynamic reaction combined with copper vapor laser coagulation would have a synergistic therapeutic effect.

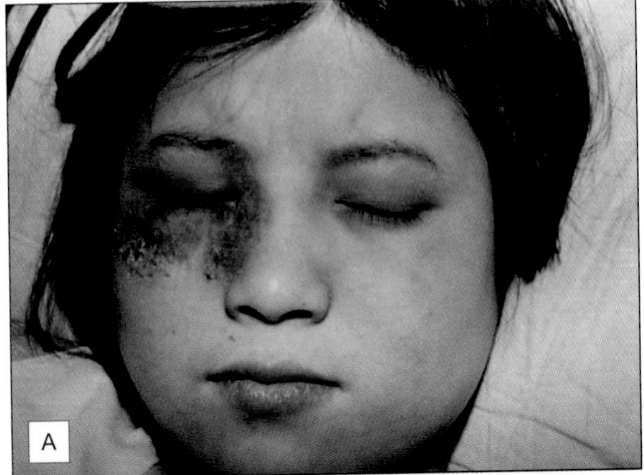

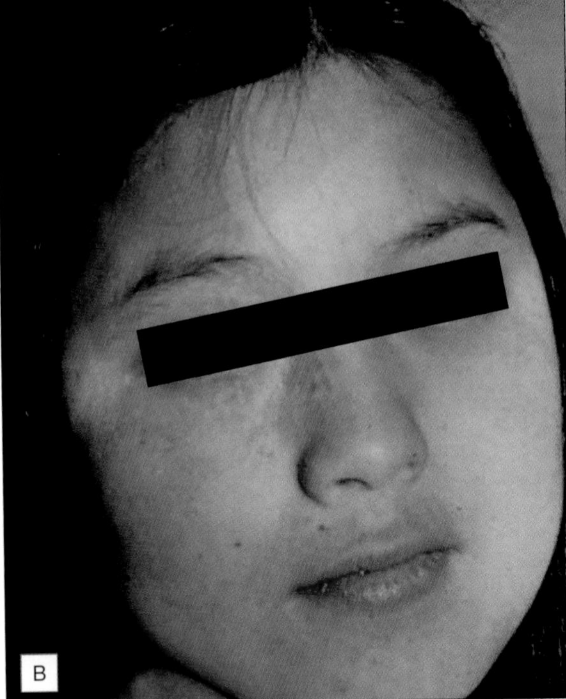

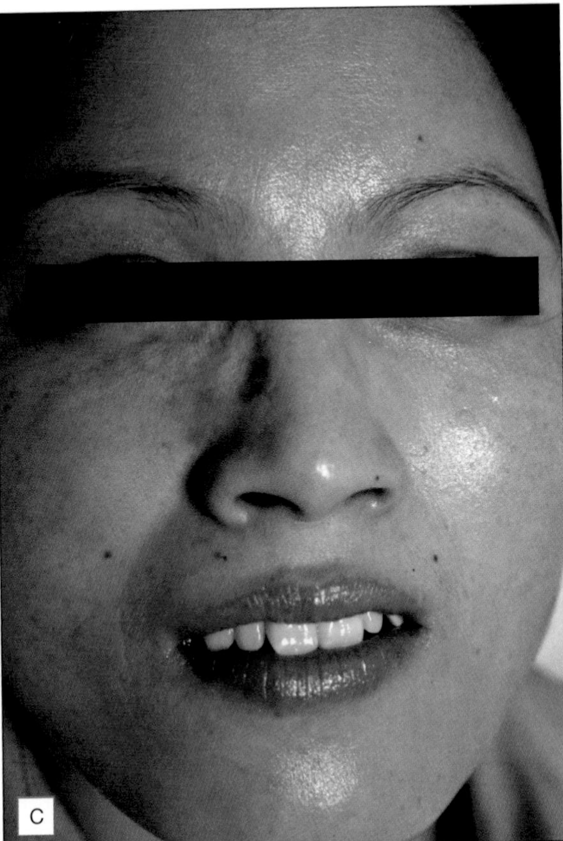

Fig. 14.3 (**A**) 3-day view post argon laser 488-nm PDT of a girl with PWS; there was seeping and blistering on the treated area. (**B**) After six sessions of argon laser PDT, the PWS was clear but with slight scar formation. (**C**) 14 years later

At the same time, we studied argon laser PDT using the photosensitizer PsD-007, which is a mixture of artificially synthesized porphyrin compounds (first manufactured by Shanghai Second Military University in 1984). Clinical trials revealed that this had the advantage of fewer adverse effects from skin sun exposure, but a similar therapeutic effect as YHpD-mediated PDT. Since then, many applications of copper vapor laser PsD-007-PDT have been carried out in different hospitals in China, and clinical results have been the same as for argon PDT.

TREATMENT OF PWS WITH NONTHERMAL EFFECTIVE AND SELECTIVE PDT

We were conscious of the importance of the need to reduce and possibility to avoid the adverse effects seen with earlier laser PDT methods. When we measured the absorption spectrum of PsD-007, it was found to have a maximum peak at 408 nm. This is the characteristic absorption curve of the porphyrin chemical structure, and gave us the idea of matching the wavelength of the laser PDT to the PsD-007 absorption. The theory was that if the therapeutic photodynamic reaction could be made more effective at lower laser energy levels, the laser energy used could be sharply decreased to a level that dimished skin necrosis but that was still sufficient for effective PDT. In 1999 we carried out a study of a 413-nm wavelength krypton laser PDT to treat PWS in Chinese patients.

The ideal treatment of PWS selectively destroys target vessels without causing surrounding dermal tissue damage. Our strategy for selective target vessel destruction is as follows: First, strictly control the duration between photosensitizer administration and laser exposure time. Carry out laser irradiation immediately after intravenous drug injection and perform laser PDT within 40 min. The reason for keeping to this strict time schedule is to ensure that laser PDT is performed during the photosensitizer distribution within the vessels: PsD-007 appears immediately after drug injection in the PWS vessels, but later penetrates surrounding tissue from the endothelial cells. Our previous experimental study using PsD-007 administered to Tca-8113, a cultured human tongue squamous carcinoma cell line, revealed that it distributes to the membrane structure within the cytoplasma and outside the nucleus both in normal and carcinoma cells, with "drainage" of the drug after 30–40 min. Thus, photosensitizer-mediated PDT will cause a phototoxic reaction on the cell's membrane structure, leading to cell apoptosis and target selectivity between tumor and normal cells will depend on the distribution of photosensitizer at the time of laser exposure. So, there is a need to control the time from drug administration to laser exposure in order to prevent drug extravasation. Clinical cases showing skin necrosis from using copper vapor laser PDT over 80-min periods is proof of this effect.

The second way to achieve selective therapy is to choose a photosensitizer whose optimal absorption characteristic is matched to the laser wavelength necessary for PDT. This uses lower laser energy level exposure but still activates the optimal photochemical reaction, so-called real nonthermal effective laser PDT. This is particularly important for the sensitive skin of the Chinese population (skin types IV–V) to avoid laser thermal coagulation of the skin. During the earlier laser PDT trials using dye, argon and copper vapor laser activated methods, the light wavelengths are 600, 488, 514.5, and 578 nm. These are all in the lower absorption range of the photosensitizer porphyrin-typed PsD-007. The clinical dilemma is that using these lasers below 250 mW/cm^2 will not destroy target vessels, but raising the laser energy exposure time directly increases the risk of surrounding tissue damage, which leads to purpura, blistering, and seeping (PBS; incidence close to 50% with argon and copper vapor laser PDT), and in turn to some degree of skin necrosis. Clinical investigations show that adverse effects, such as hypopigmentation, skin texture alteration, and scar formation, then take place. It is very dangerous to use this kind of PDT. Logically, laser therapy needs to be alternated to prevent skin necrosis. From following up patients with an unsatisfactory result from clinical argon and copper vapor laser PDT, the idea of setting up a nonthermal effective and selective PDT came to mind. The krypton laser at the 413-nm wavelength light was chosen to perform the first PDT, followed by PDT with the new photosensitizer which produces a reddish wavelength optimally absorbed with reddish diode laser. New photosensitizer PDT is reasonable but unfortunately difficult to apply. A series of preclinical studies need to be undertaken with the new photosensitizer before it can be used clinically. Further, two questions need to be answered about the krypton laser PDT method: (1) Does the 413-nm wavelength laser, which penetrates skin to a depth of about 0.2 mm, effectively destroy the PWS vessels between the epidermis and dermis?; and (2) Is krypton laser PDT both nonthermal and effective?

KRYPTON LASER 413-NM PDT TREATMENT OF PWS

The first clinical study was carried out on two volunteers with PWS lesions on the arms. The two main factors impacting on the final PDT result are: photosensitizer and laser illumination. For the selected porphyrin photosensitizer PsD-007, concentration is the one variable factor. In general, photodynamic efficacy is related to the concentration, i.e. increasing the drug concentration will improve the therapeutic efficacy. However, above certain concentrations, adverse effects are common and severe. They are caused by the accumulation of photosensitizer remaining in the body after PDT; the incomplete excreted drug residue in the body will be activated by some degree of light exposure, such as sun exposure and strong lamp illumination. The patient's skin will become purpuric and edematous, and bleed. The skin could become hyper- or hypo-pigmented, suffer skin necrosis and texture alteration, and/or even hypertrophic scar formation. Decreasing the concentration of photosensitizer used could reduce these adverse effects but at the expense of therapeutic efficacy. In our study, we set the reasonable concentration of PsD-007 at 5 mg/kg. This concentration had proved safe in a previous study using the argon laser PDT. Adverse effects can be avoided easily by keeping the patient in room lamp illumination conditions for 1 month. In contrast, the photosensitizer YHpD used at the same concentration requires strict adherence to full darkroom conditions for 1 month, as post-treatment the patient's skin can be severely damaged by common sun exposure. With this stringent requirement, YHpD has lost its clinical value.

• Clinical method

Each patient was given intravenous PsD-007 at a concentration of 5 mg/kg, after skin testing showed a negative allergic reaction. The krypton laser (type Serbe R, Coherent Laser Group, USA) at a wavelength of 413 nm was used to illuminate the PWS. Purplish laser light was

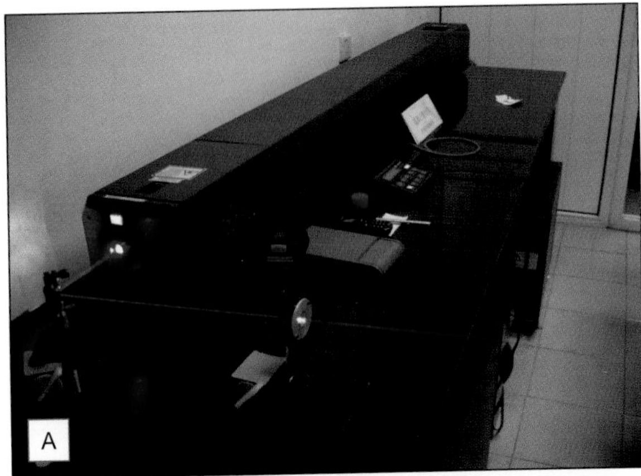

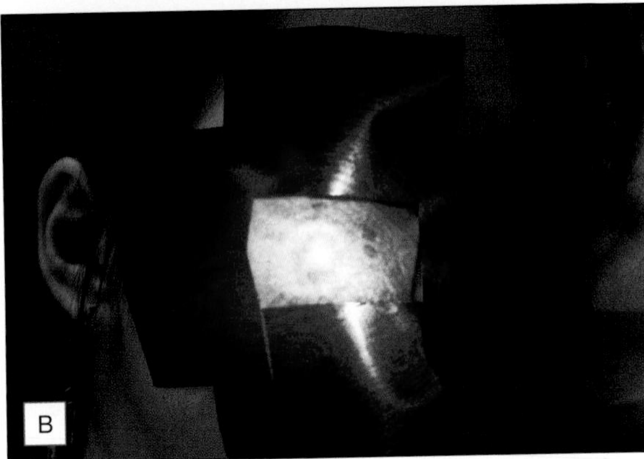

Fig. 14.4 **(A)** Krypton laser 413-nm PDT system (Coherent Laser Group, USA). **(B)** 413-nm laser PDT of PWS

transmitted directly by a mirror with 98.8% reflection (Fig. 14.4). This reflection of the laser beam directly to the lesion produces stable irradiation, and a fixed laser beam on the lesion is needed for even illumination. During our early studies using argon laser PDT, an optic fiber was used to deliver the laser beam to the PWS lesion. We noticed the uneven distribution of light, which often had high energy density on the central part of the beam, while the periphery had lower energy density. Optic fibers not only do not achieve even illumination, but the illumination cannot be duplicated even by the same physician. We believe the scan irradiation technique is important in the early photocoagulation laser therapy of PWS. Robot scanning has become popular in laser ablative therapy, such as ultrapulse CO_2 and Er:YAG laser skin resurfacing. When PDT is carried out, the goal is to evenly irradiate the lesion during the entire treatment period. The diameter of the laser beam was 5–6 cm. Laser output was set at 2 W, and thus the calculated laser energy density was 100–150 J/cm^2. Power density was 100 mW/cm^2. Each session consisted of one to four exposures, and the interval between exposures was 10 min. Before starting PDT, the parent or person accompanying the patient was asked to experience the sensation of laser exposure at therapeutic level. They experienced a lukewarm heat as the laser light was set at the nonthermal effective level. This helps them explain the procedure to the children.

• Clinical results

Immediately post-laser PDT, the lesion color changed to a light purple or white and the irradiated area showed slight edema. Clinical observation revealed a dark purplish color and severe edema on the treated area. During the first week after laser PDT, there was no PBS, which differed from the earlier experience with argon laser PDT. After 3–4 weeks, the treated areas showed wound healing. Gu Ying reported the incidence of scabs as 43% post copper vapor laser PDT (578 nm), i.e. wound healing occurred in nearly 50%, and our earlier study with argon laser PDT showed a similar result. However, after the skin wound healing process, high incidences of skin pigmentation and texture change, and scar formation were also reported in these earlier studies. Clinical krypton laser PDT followed the principle of nonthermal effective and selective PDT. All cases in our group revealed selective target vessel destruction without surrounding tissue damage. No scabs or seeping were found. At 1-month follow-up, lesion color had faded with normal skin texture (Fig. 14.5).

Adverse effects were observed mainly as a result of secondary sun exposure after PDT, with skin hyperpigmentation in the "exposed" body area, such as arms, legs, and face. In some cases an allergic reaction was observed in the exposed skin area, with blister formation. When these patients were asked to stay indoors, spontaneous regression of these photosensitizer-induced skin allergic reactions generally was observed. In rare cases, infected blister formation could lead to scarring. Therefore, post treatment exposure to sun must be avoided, and exposure to television PC screens limited, for 1 month, because the metabolic cycle of PsD-007 is about 1 month. Photosensitizer remaining in the eyes will cause retinal blood vessel damage if exposed to TV or PC screens. No patients developed this complication after 1 month of strictly limited exposure.

After a long period of observation to confirm the safety of krypton laser PDT, a method suitable for use in children was developed in 2004. If concerned about the age of a patient, we focus the tolerance degree of the krypton laser PDT. Patients describe the sensations felt during PDT as "biting", heat and pain. Patients older than 8–10 years of age are capable of tolerating illumination for 10 min at each anatomic site to be treated. It is not necessary to apply anesthesia. We have performed krypton laser PDT using systemic anesthesia (intravenous administration of ketamine), allowing children aged 2–8 years to be treated by this PDT which is very safe for their sensitive skin (Fig. 14.6).

There is no direct adverse effect of nonthermal effective PDT. Secondary sessions can be done after 3 months,

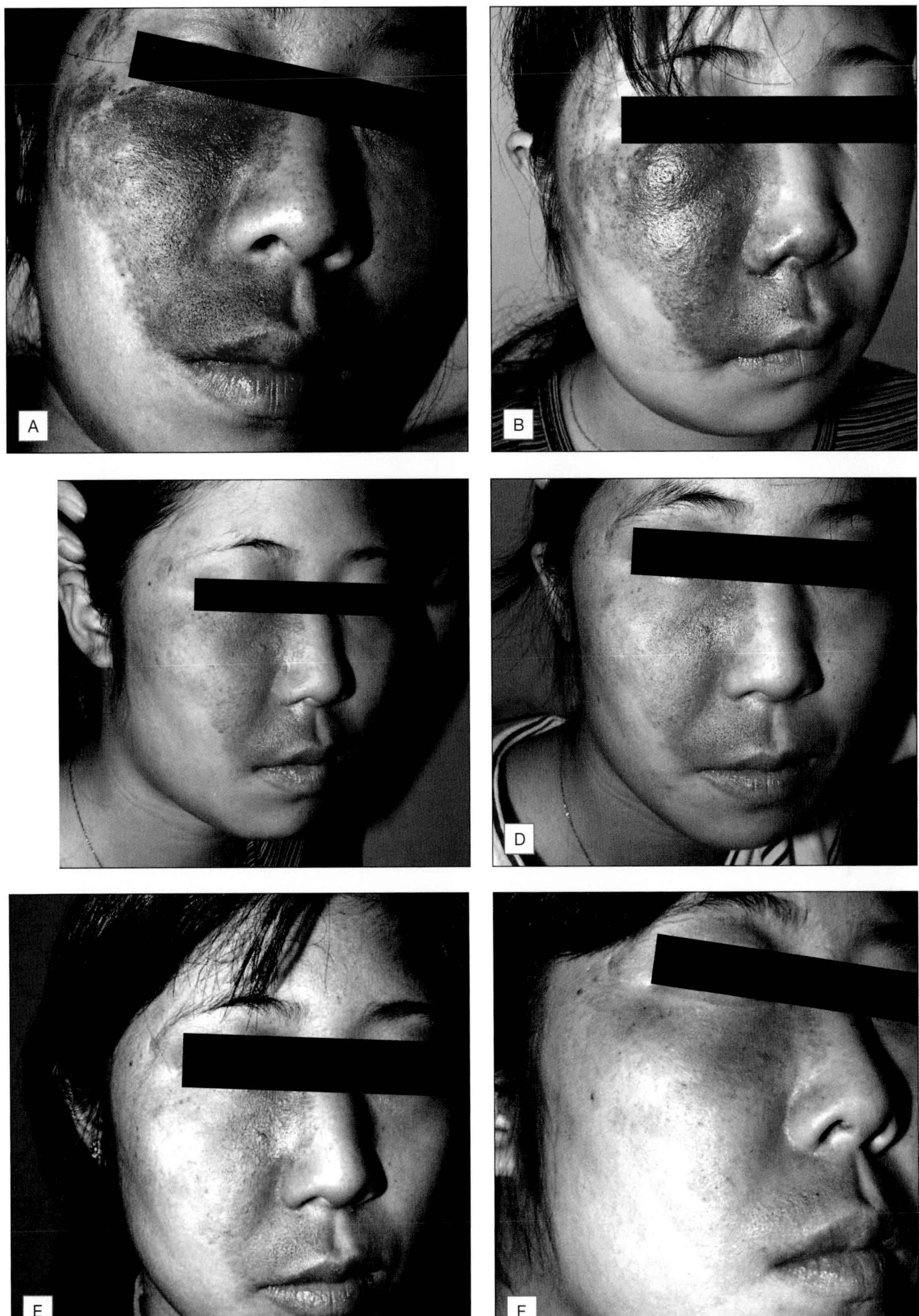

Fig. 14.5 (A–F) Series of views of a female patient with PWS who received five sessions of krypton laser PDT, before treatment and after each treatment session

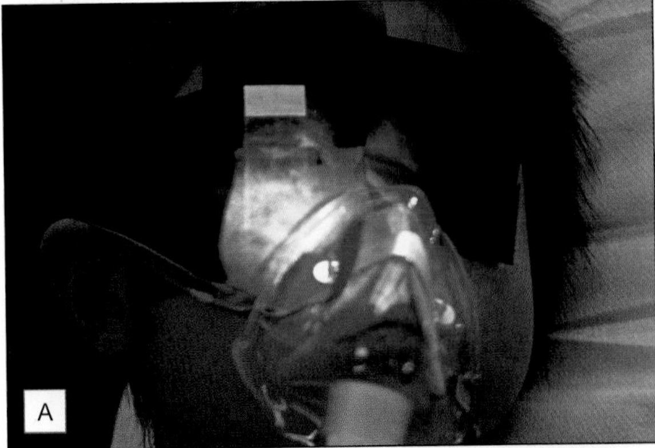

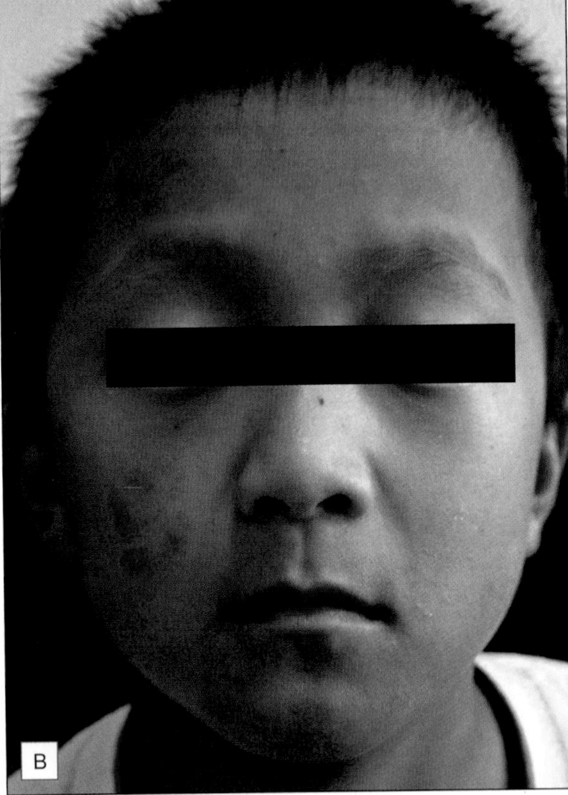

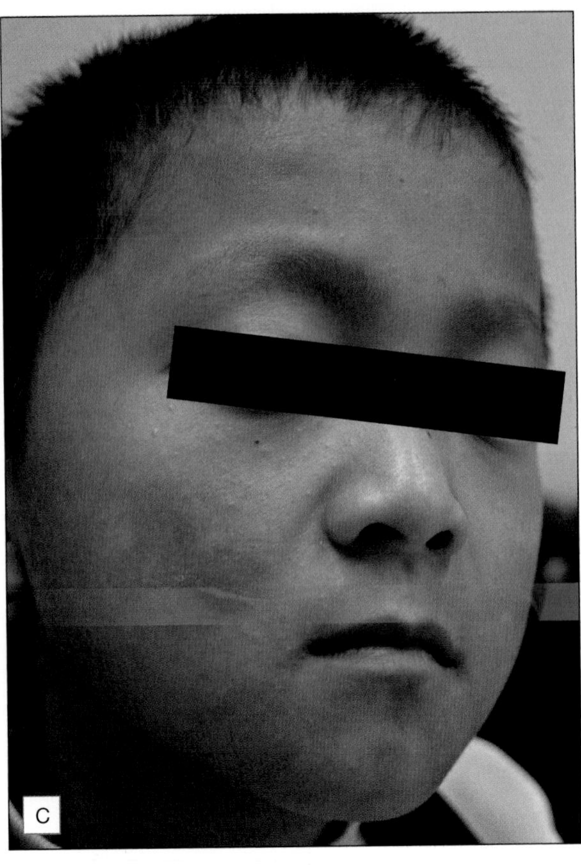

Fig. 14.6 (**A**) A child who received krypton laser PDT at systemic anesthesia. (**B**) Before and (**C**) after views of a boy who received four sessions of krypton laser PDT

but a longer interval is advisable. Each session's result was permanent without recurrence, which is different from the experience with PDL therapy. Physical damage to the vessels showed some repair of endothelial cells and no evidence of lesion recurrence was found in the PDT-treated lesions. Clinical observation also revealed good therapeutic result. There was a 96% effective rate. The clearance degree improved with every session (Fig. 14.7).

Lesion clearance is dependent on the thickness of the blood vessels in the lesion. Even in severe cases, such as Sturge–Weber syndrome, the treated area faded to near normal skin color after 10–12 sessions (Fig. 14.8).

Clinical follow-up revealed good results. Between October 1999 and July 2002, 538 cases of PWS were treated using krypton laser PDT. Treatment ranged from one to 14 sessions, with a mean of 6.32 sessions. Of the patients, clearance of more than 75% was seen in 285 (52.97%); of 50–74% in 231 (42.94%), and of 25–49% in 22 (4.09%). Therefore, 96% of patients had successful treatment. Thirt-two patients had temporary adverse effects of hyperpigmentation (5.95%), which completely

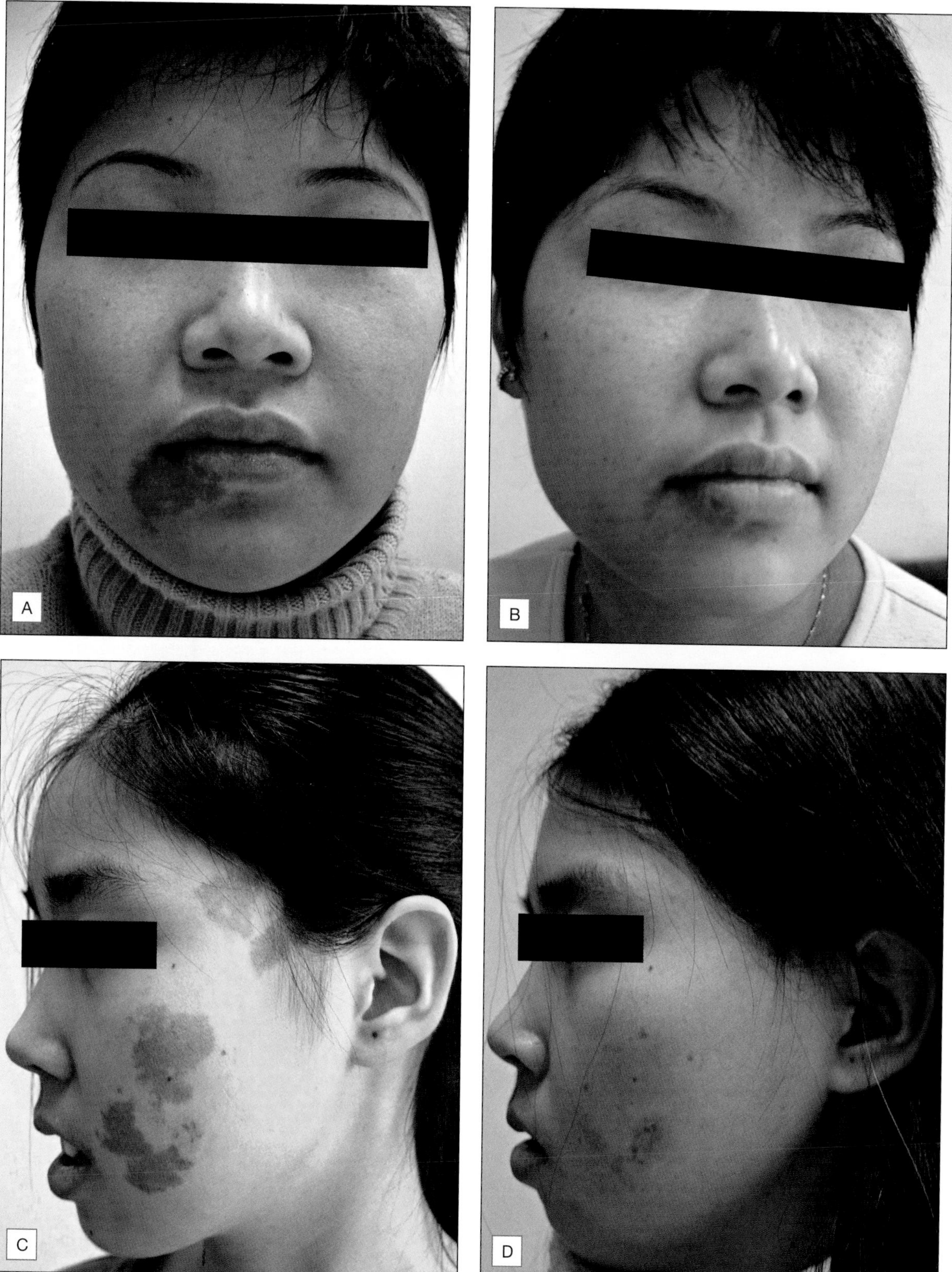

Fig. 14.7 (**A**) Before and (**B**) after views of a woman treated with two sessions of krypton laser PDT, with a good result. (**C**) Before and (**D**) after views of a girl who received three sessions of krypton laser PDT, with a good result

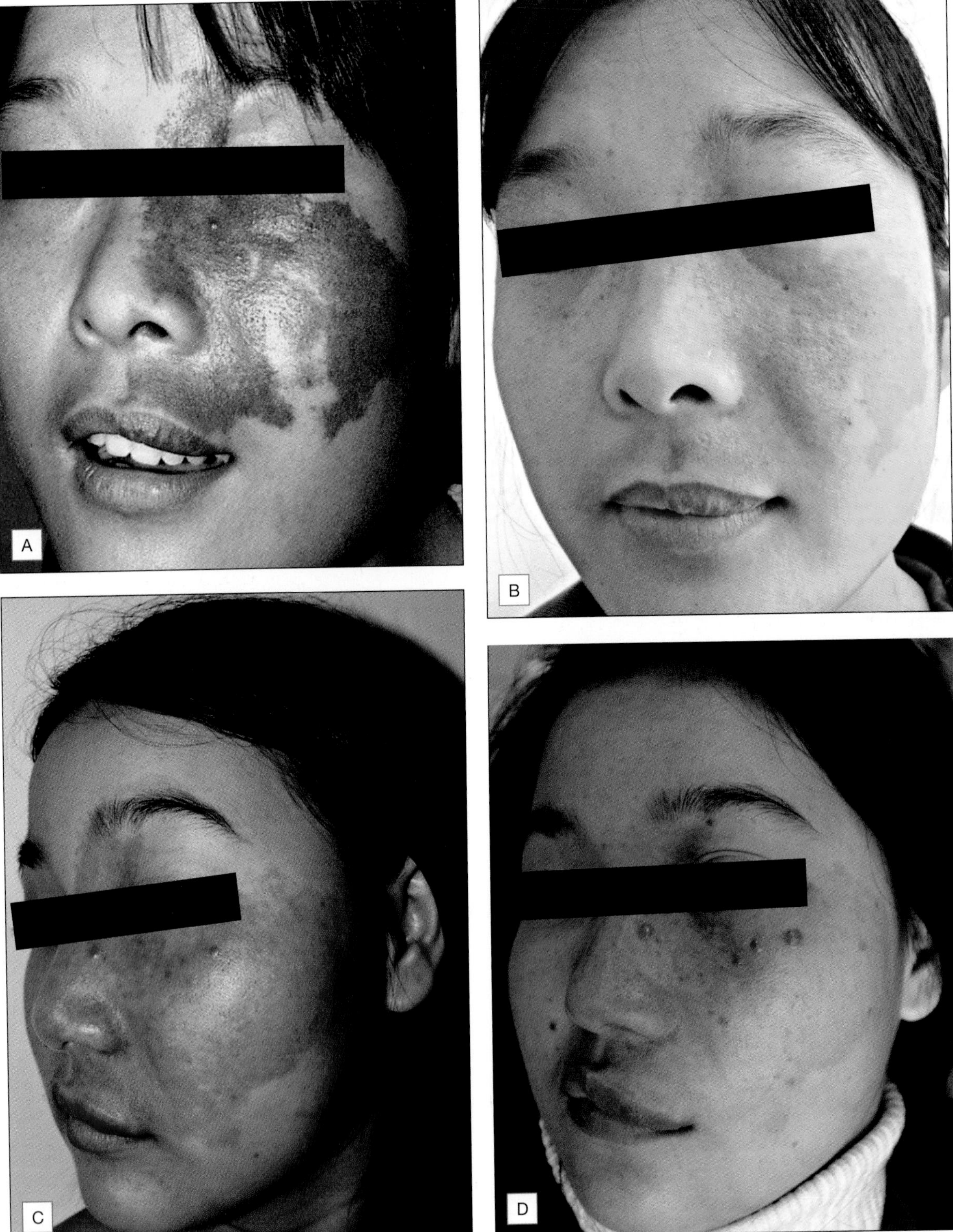

Fig. 14.8 (**A–D**) Two girls with Sturge–Weber syndrome who received multiple krypton laser PDT (7 and 11 sessions, respectively) show marked improvement between the before (**A,C**) and after treatment views (**B,C**)

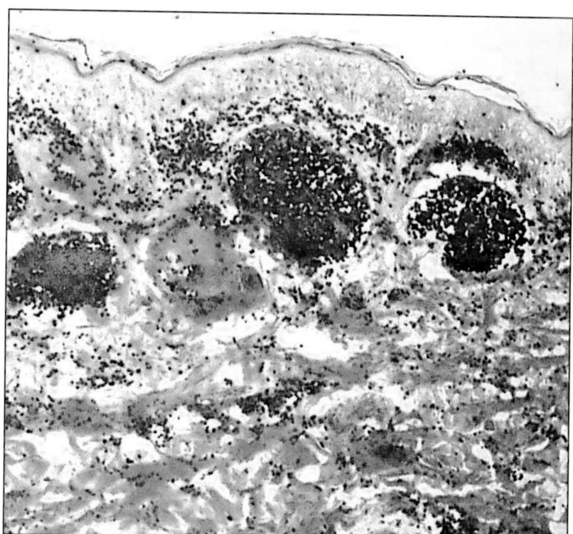

Fig. 14.9 Histopathology of a volunteer's biopsy stained with H&E shows red blood cell extravasation to the surrounding tissue after destroying the endothelial blood vessel wall, 2 weeks after krypton laser PDT, and no dermal damage

and spontaneously regressed 2 years post-PDT. No patient experienced permanent side effect

Pathologic findings revealed endothelial blood vessel cells destroyed with erythrocyte extravasation but no surrounding tissue damage. This was confirmed in a volunteer's skin biopsy 2 weeks post krypton laser PDT, showing selective destruction of the target lesion (Fig. 14.9).

This strongly supports our hypothesis that PWS vessels can be destroyed layer by layer: when the superficial layer becomes normal, the krypton laser photon can penetrate to the deeper layers of the lesion to activate the photodynamic reaction in these layers. Although the 413-nm light can physically penetrate to a depth of 0.2 cm, the clinical result shows deeper penetration, because this kind of laser therapy depends on photon-activated photodynamic reaction, which produces singlet oxygen that destroys endothelial cells. In contrast to selective photothermalysis, the laser energy indirectly impacts on the therapeutic result.

• Advantages and disadvantages of nonthermal effective PDT in the treatment of PWS

The significant advantage is the selective target destruction. There is no risk of pigmentation changes, texture alteration or scar formation. The disadvantages are the complicated procedure compared with PDL; also sun exposure is forbidden and TV and PC screen exposure limited for 1 month post treatment, a regimen more difficult to enforce in Western societies.

FUTURE DEVELOPMENTS

We believe the most important factor in the future development of PDT in the treatment of vascular lesions will be the photosensitizer. There are many kinds of photosensitizers, e.g. porphyrin, porphyne, and second-generation of photosensitizers such as chlorine e_6, benzoporphyrin derivative monoacid (BPD), and 5-aminolevulinic acid (ALA). A safe photosensitizer that is metabolically active only for a short time is needed. Photosensitizers that absorb reddish light will have a greater penetration depth and more efficacy. Among them, BPD has strong absorbance at 576 nm (molar extinction coefficient 15 000 M/cm) and 690 nm (30 000 M/cm). The copper vapor (578 nm) and krypton (676 nm) are the matched wavelength lasers, so the potential applications are predictable. As yellowish and reddish laser light can penetrate deeper than krypton 413-nm light, improved results can be expected.

It has been noted in the literature that, despite full thickness necrosis produced by copper vapor laser PDT, healing proceeds only after PDT. This might explain the excellent cosmetic results produced after PDT in human skin lesions. We disagree with these views. When full thickness skin necrosis happens, the risks of pigmentation change, skin texture alteration, and scar formation exists. This is counter to the principle of selective treatment of target blood vessels.

Another consideration is the photosensitizer administration method. Photosensitizers can be applied topically or systemically. The latter is helpful for selective target distribution but has the disadvantage of systemic accumulation. The advantage of topical application of photosensitizer is the lack of prolonged post-treatment skin photosensitivity. However, with topical application of ALA there is nonselective target distribution from the epidermis to the dermis and vessels between, which invalidates its use in the treatment of PWS.

CONCLUSION

Nonthermal effective krypton laser PDT is a potential alternative to current laser therapies for PWS. Further study is needed to find a simpler and more available photosensitizer, which has a short metabolic rate, allowing the patient to return to normal social activity soon after PDT. Currently, venous malformation cannot be treated by PDT. A logical approach is needed to explore possible new PDT methods to treat venous malformation and compound venous malformations.

FURTHER READING

Anderson RR, Parrish JA 1983 Selective photothermolysis: precise microsurgery by selective absorption of pulsed radiation. Science 220:524–527

Ashinoff R, Geronemus RG 1991 Flash-lamp-pumped pulsed dye laser for port wine stains in infancy: Earlier versus later treatment. Journal of the American Academy of Dermatology 24:467–472

Gu Ying, Li Junheng, Jiang Yiping et al 1992 Clinical study on the photodynamic therapy as a selective treatment of port wine stains. Chinese Journal of Laser Medicine and Surgery 1:6–10

Gu Ying, Li Junheng, Shan Huanyan et al 1994 Therapeutic analysis of 50 cases of port wine stains treated by copper vapor laser photodynamic therapy. Chinese Journal of Laser Medicine and Surgery 3:215–217

Jeffes EW, McCullough JL, Weinstein GD et al 1997 Photodynamic therapy of actinic keratoses with topical 5-aminolevulinic acid (ALA): A pilot dose-ranging study. Archives of Dermatology 1997;133:727–732

Jiang L, Gu Y, Li X et al 1998 Changes of skin perfusion after photodynamic therapy for port wine stain. Chinese Medical Journal 111:136–138

Kimel S, Svaasand LO, Kelly KM et al 2004 Synergistic photodynamic and photothermal treatment of port-wine stain? Lasers in Surgery and Medicine 34:80–82

Lanigan SW 1998 Port-wine stains unresponsive to pulsed dye laser: Explanations and solutions. British Journal of Dermatology 139:173–177

Lin XX, Wang W, Wu SF et al 1997 Treatment of capillary vascular malformation (port-wine stains) with photochemotherapy. Plastic and Reconstructive Surgery 99:1826–1830

Lucassen GW, Verkruvsse W, Keijzer M et al 1996 Light distributions in a port wine stain model containing multiple cylindrical and curved blood vessels. Lasers in Surgery and Medicine 18:345–357

Mulliken J, Glowacki J 1982 Hemangiomas and vascular malformations in infants and children: a classification based on endothelial characteristics. Plastic and Reconstructive Surgery 69:412–420

Nelson JS, McCullough JL, Berns MW 1997 Principles and applications of photodynamic therapy in dermatology. In: Arndt KA, Dover JE, Olbricht SA (eds) Lasers in Cutaneous and Aesthetic Surgery. Philadelphia: Lippincott Raven, 349–382

Nelson JS, Liaw LH, Orenstein A et al 1988 The mechanism of tumor destruction following photodynamic therapy with hematoporphyrin derivative, chlorin and phthalocyanine. Journal of the National Cancer Institutes 80:1599–1605

Star WM, Marijnissen HPA, van den Berg-Blok AE et al 1986 Destruction of rat mammary tumor and normal tissue microcirculation by hematoporphyrin derivative photoradiation as observed in vivo in sandwich observation chambers. Cancer Research 46:2532–2540

Van der Horst CMAM, Koster PHL, deBorgie CAJM at al 1998 Effect of timing of treatment of port wine stains with the flash-lamp-pumped pulsed dye laser. New England Journal of Medicine 338:1028–1033

Waner M, Suen JY 1999 Hemangioma and vascular malformations of the head and neck, New York: Wiley-Liss, Inc

Xu Deyu, Yin Xiangshen, Liu Jun et al 1984 Study on new photosensitizer agent PsD-007. Journal of the Medical College PLA 5:31–34

Zhou Guoyu, Zhang Zhiyuan 2000 Preliminary clinical study on krypton laser photodynamic therapy for PWS. Shanghai Journal of Stomatology 9:168–170

Zhou Guoyu, Zhang Zhiyuan, Zhang Jizhong et al 2000 Comparative research on mixed and 488nm argon laser PDT for port wine stain. Shanghai Journal of Stomatology 9:173–174

Zhou Guoyu, Zhang Zhiyuan, Zhu Huanguang et al 2000 Continuous Wave Nd:YAG laser in the treatment of oral maxillofacial deep region cavernous vascular malformation. Shanghai Journal of Stomatology 9:168–170

Zhou Guoyu, Zhang Zhiyuan, Zhang Chenping et al 2005 Clinical study on laser therapy of the venous malformations and hemangioma in oral and maxillofacial regions. Chinese Journal of Stomatology 40:200–202

Zhou Guoyu, Shen Lingyue, Tian Kebin et al 2006 Treatment of 133 oral and maxillofacial hemangiomas with long pulsed turnable 1064 nm Gentle YAG laser. Shanghai Journal of Stomatology 15:250–253

15 Clinical Application of Fluorescence Diagnosis

Wolfgang Bäumler, Tino Wetzig

INTRODUCTION

Photodynamic therapy (PDT) is a promising treatment modality to cure nonmelanoma skin cancer. The same photosensitizers used in PDT also can be used for in vivo diagnosis of dysplastic or neoplastic tissue, which is called fluorescence diagnosis (FD). Comparable to PDT, a photosensitizer is applied either topically or systemically, and accumulates thereafter rather selectively in the target tissue. In contrast to PDT, the photosensitizer is excited with very low light intensities to induce fluorescence light and to avoid the generation of reactive oxygen species (ROS). Since the fluorescence exclusively appears in the diseased part of skin, it enables the detection of the superficial tumor in the skin as well as in different hollow organs, e.g. bladder, gastrointestinal tract or lung.

Due to its high selectivity for neoplastic tissue, the substance of most interest for FD is 5-aminolevulinic acid (ALA). ALA is a metabolite of heme biosynthesis, which is taken up actively and at higher concentrations by tumor cells. Under physiologic conditions, ALA-synthase regulates the formation of ALA in the cell. Due to the exogenous application of ALA, this bottleneck is bypassed and the exogenous ALA is metabolized to porphyrins, in particular protoporphyrin IX (PpIX). This process is more likely in tumor cells as compared to normal cells, leading to a concentration ratio of PpIX. The ratio can be used for PDT to selectively destroy diseased tissue and can be used at the same time for FD.

In dermatology, FD may provide a useful tool to highlight precancerous lesions and superficial skin tumors. FD can help to delineate tumor margins for surgery or to detect clinically invisible lesions. Moreover, it can guide clinicians to find the most appropriate point to perform a biopsy for histology. FD can serve as a useful tool to improve the efficacy of PDT.

BASICS OF FLUORESCENCE DIAGNOSIS

When exposing PpIX to light, the light energy is absorbed by and stored inside the molecule for a short time. This process describes the excited state of the PpIX molecule. After a few nanoseconds, the molecule leaves the excited state via three different pathways. The first two options are the return to the ground state by either transforming the stored light energy to heat or by emitting the energy as light, the so-called fluorescence. The fluorescence is shifted to longer wavelengths as compared to the excitation light. For PpIX, blue excitation light at 400 nm is applied, yielding red fluorescence light in the spectral range from 600 to 700 nm. The third pathway is the cross-over to the intermediate state of the photosensitizer and the subsequent generation of ROS for PDT (Fig. 15.1).

The respective quantum yield shows the importance of each pathway. The fluorescence quantum yield is the percentage of molecules that convert the absorbed light energy to fluorescence. With regard to the small fluorescence quantum yield of PpIX (15%), the molecules must be excited with light at 400 nm, which coincides with their maximal absorption. This is ideally performed by applying light of special light sources, such as light emitting diodes (LED), which are spectrally centered at 405 nm and show a spectral half width of about 20 nm (Fig. 15.2). The emission of the LED exhibits an optimal overlap with the absorption spectrum of PpIX and the LED-light is effectively transformed to red fluorescence light of PpIX. The use of Wood's lamp is sometimes mentioned for excitation of PpIX. However, Figure 15.2 shows an incomplete overlap with absorption of PpIX, leading to insufficient generation of PpIX fluorescence.

After excitation of PpIX, its fluorescence is detected by means of digital camera technologies. The use of appropriate optical filters in front of the camera blocks the unwanted blue excitation light, imaging the red PpIX fluorescence only. When correcting the blue channel of the camera for the spectral filtering, a normal color image is possible covering the skin area that is under investigation for diagnostic reasons.

The use of a CCD camera has the following advantages:

- Quantitative data of fluorescence using shading correction and fluorescence standards
- Imaging of the weak PpIX fluorescence under ambient light conditions
- Image analysis and false color-coding

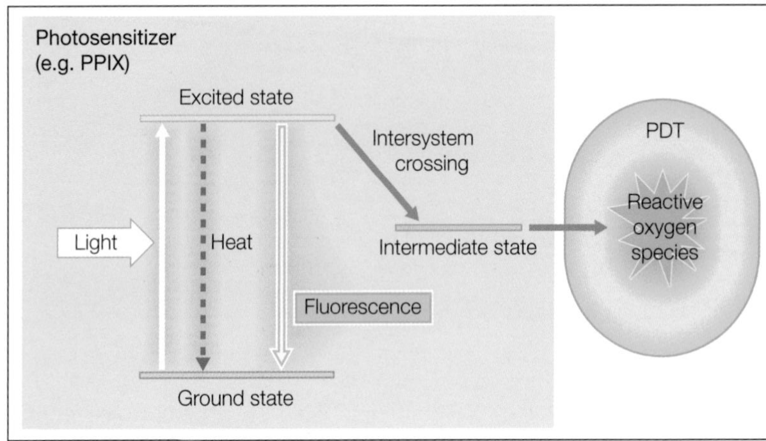

Fig. 15.1 Scheme showing the absorption of light energy by a photosensitizer molecule (e.g. PpIX) and the three main pathways, which lead to the generation of heat, fluorescence or reactive oxygen species

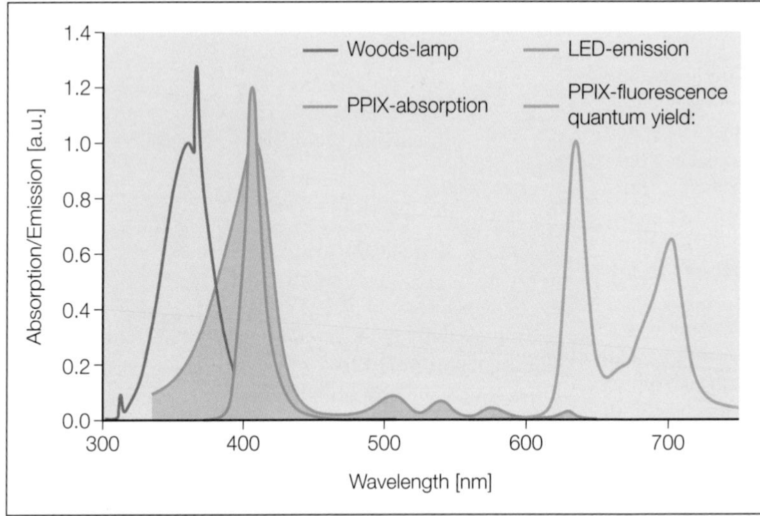

Fig. 15.2 Absorption and emission spectra of PpIX, using different light sources for excitation

- Documentation of the diagnostic findings by storing the images
- Simultaneous documentation of the fluorescence image and the clinical image
- Print out for documentation
- Electronic record of each patient
- Facilitation of patients follow-up

• Equipment

For the use of FD in clinical practice, a complete detection system is recommended that consists of an appropriate light source for exciting fluorescence and a CCD camera for digital imaging. Such a standardized system helps to provide standardized and user-independent decisions when inspecting skin lesions.

The excitation light irradiates the skin area of interest and a CCD camera triggered by the LED monitors the fluorescence of the lesion. Using a short flash excitation, the system enables FD in dermatology in an ambient light situation (Dyaderm, Biocam GmbH, Fig. 15.3). A personal computer or laptop operates the camera, which shows the normal red, green, and blue (RBG) image and the fluorescence images simultaneously in real-time. Moreover, the fluorescence images are processed by image analysis that provides additional information about the lesion. The resulting fluorescent area can be false color-coded and superimposed on the normal RGB-image. This provides the exact position and size of the lesion within the clinical image of the skin.

• Methods

The detection of the fluorescence emitted by the ALA-induced porphyrins (in particular PpIX) may be visible without any additional technical equipment, which has

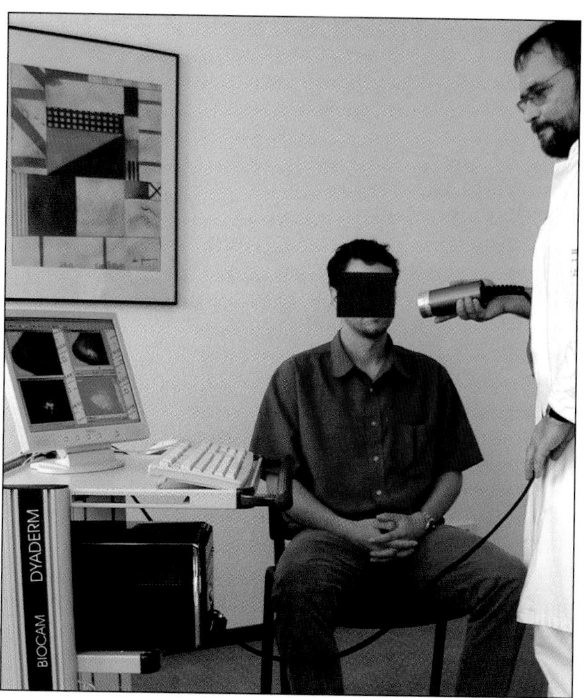

Fig. 15.3 Hand-held system to perform fluorescence diagnosis, which is based on a digital camera connected to a computerized database

some disadvantages. The naked eye can serve as a detector for the red fluorescence using a Wood's light, but this is, if required, also possible with the presented light source. However, inhomogeneity of the irradiation and unspecific background fluorescence lead to a false impression of the distribution of the fluorescence intensity. A quantitative read-out, an objective evaluation, and documentation of the findings is not possible using this method. To enhance the contrast with this simple method of FD, a long-pass filter can be used to avoid interference with the bright excitation light.

For these reasons, camera-assisted systems are usually best in dermatology where large areas of diseased skin are imaged. Moreover, quantification of the measured fluorescence intensities is possible using a reference signal or by calculating the ratio with respect to a reference intensity, e.g. surrounding skin. These calibration methods allow the comparison of the different fluorescent images in different patients, which is a prerequisite for good clinical practice, clinical trials or scientific investigations. On the other hand, calibration to the surrounding tissue enhances the contrast of the specific versus background fluorescence in a single image and the fluorescence intensity is given as a ratio of the reference. Moreover, the FD must be possible in ambient light.

The inhomogeneous irradiation of the investigated skin by the light source (shading) should also be corrected for a quantitative read-out. Additional parameters that influence the measured fluorescence intensity, e.g. age, skin type or inflammation, can thus be considered and corrected by employing respective algorithms. The multiplication of the resulting fluorescence image with certain parameters will make use of the dynamic range of the CCD camera to yield the highest possible contrast. A false-color presentation will make it easier for the investigator to evaluate the distribution of the fluorescence intensity, because the human eye can differentiate colors markedly better as compared to gray shades. In addition, the false color-coded fluorescence images should be superimposed on the clinical image. Thus, a single image contains the complete information of the lesion.

The penetration of the photosensitizer used and the penetration depth of the excitation light limit the detection depth of an FD system. ALA is a small hydrophilic molecule (MW 170) and topically applied ALA penetrates very well into the skin. As described above, blue light was used for irradiation because of the absorption maximum of the induced porphyrins (Soret-band). However, blue light penetrates skin only down to 1–2 mm. Since porphyrins exhibit in addition to the Soret-band other absorption maxima, the Q bands, excitation using deeper penetrating light, e.g. green or red, is theoretically possible, but the Q bands are 10–20-fold smaller as compared to the Soret-band. In light of the low fluorescence quantum yield of PpIX, the blue excitation light is preferred.

BENEFITS IN DIFFERENT MEDICAL FIELDS

FD of dysplastic or neoplastic tissue following the application of ALA either systemically or topically has been used for some time in medical specialties other than dermatology. In urology, a recent study in 104 patients of fluorescence cystoscopy after intravesical instillation of 3% ALA, showed a sensitivity of 96.9% in the detection of bladder tumors as compared to 72.7% for conventional cystoscopy. Better results, i.e. higher sensitivity regarding the positivity of the taken biopsies, using fluorescence endoscopy as compared with conventional endoscopy were obtained in the gastrointestinal tract. In addition, the early detection of tumors in the bronchial tract and longer survival after FD-based resection of malignant gliomas have been reported.

APPLICATIONS AND BENEFITS IN DERMATOLOGY

FD (Box 15.1) and PDT in dermatology are based on the same photosensitizer (PpIX), which accumulates in diseased tissue after application of ALA. The transport of ALA molecules into the tissue and their conversion to PpIX needs usually a few hours, depending on the ALA molecule and its formulation.

Several studies have shown that PpIX fluorescence increases with time and reaches a maximal value 4–6 h after application. However, it is important to consider not only the fluorescence intensity in the diseased tissue but

Box 15.1 Fluorescence diagnosis—dermatologic indications

- Actinic keratoses (including arsenic-induced)
- Bowen's disease
- Initial basal cell carcinoma
- Superficial basal cell carcinoma
- Gorlin–Goltz syndrome
- Psoriasis
- Paget's disease
- Mycosis fungoides
- Lupus erythematosus

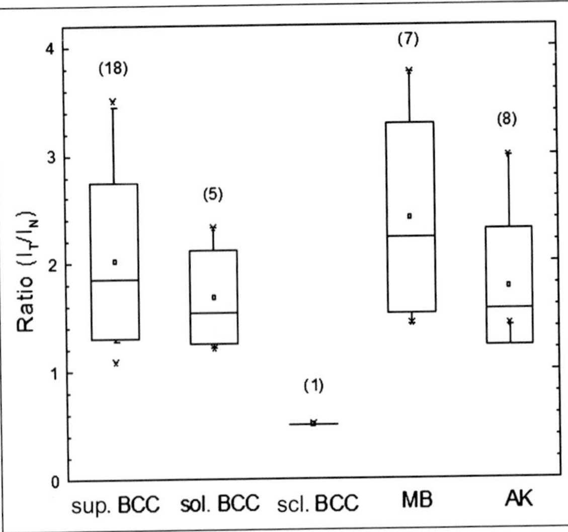

Fig. 15.4 Ratio of the mean fluorescence intensity for tumor versus adjacent normal skin (all incubated with ALA). The small squares represent the respective mean and the large boxes the deviation from the mean. The vertical lines show the 5–95% range and the horizontal lines the median.

also in the adjacent normal tissue. The fluorescence intensity inside the diseased tissue should be maximal, whereas the fluorescence intensity in the normal tissue should be minimal. That is, the ratio of fluorescence intensities should be maximal when comparing diseased and normal tissue. This ratio is determined easily by analyzing digital images of skin lesions.

In a recent study, 24 patients (39 lesions) with histologically confirmed diagnosis (superficial (sup.) solid (sol.) or sclerodermiformic (scl.) basal cell carcinoma [BCC]), Bowen's disease (MB) and actinic keratosis [AK]) were investigated. The entire areas were incubated occlusively with 20% ALA cream (water-in-oil emulsion). The ratio was about 2 for all precancerous and cancerous lesions 3–5 h after ALA application, except for one solid BCC (Fig. 15.4). This ratio is high enough to perform FD using sensitive camera technologies and image processing.

Thus, FD can be performed using more or less the same time course as PDT. In principle, fluorescence images can be taken before, during, and even after PDT. FD can be applied for diagnostic purposes only, e.g. prior to surgery or to check for any tumor recurrence after treatment.

As shown in Figure 15.1, the excitation of PpIX yields fluorescence light (FD) or ROS (PDT). To avoid any PDT effect during FD, the light intensity is kept very low at values usually less than 1 mW/cm^2.

• Evidence for PpIX accumulation prior to PDT

The image processing described above enables the detection of suspicious areas, usually showing a fluorescence ratio greater than 2.0. This indicates the presence of neoplastic transformation of skin as compared to normal tissue. Moreover, the bright fluorescence of the lesions provides evidence for a high amount of PpIX accumulated in the lesions and a good result is expected when performing PDT. Figure 15.5 shows PpIX accumulation in Bowen's disease on a leg.

• Evidence for successful PDT

Under light irradiation, PpIX generates ROS that destroy effectively tumor cells (PDT). At the same time PpIX molecules are cleaved, which is known as bleaching of the photosensitizer. The cleaved PpIX molecules are unable to generate ROS or to emit fluorescence light. While PDT is being performed, the PpIX molecules are destroyed and the fluorescence light decreases accordingly. Usually, directly after PDT, most PpIX molecules are bleached and the fluorescence inside the treated area disappears.

It is noteworthy that complete bleaching of PpIX correlates with a sufficient light dose applied to the entire treatment area. In case of a clear fluorescence signal inside the treatment area directly after PDT, the light irradiation may have been underdosed, in particular at difficult anatomic locations. PDT of disseminated lesions (e.g. AK) is challenging when using a planar light source for a curved surface such as the forehead. Thus, FD is useful to check for photobleaching in the entire treatment area directly after PDT. If there are regions of extensive fluorescence, the PDT light source can be switched on to treat these underdosed regions. FD directly after PDT can help to improve the outcome of PDT.

Figure 15.6 shows a patient with AKs on the forehead. After 4-h incubation with ALA directly prior to PDT, a clear fluorescence signal was seen that correlates with the location of the AKs in the treatment area. One minute after PDT, FD was performed again and hardly any fluorescence signal was seen in the entire area. This image assures a complete and a most likely sufficient PDT of all the AKs.

• Detection of clinically invisible lesions

For several reasons, skin tumors can be clinically overlooked. The clinical inspection of initial lesions or small satellites of visible tumors using the naked eye might not

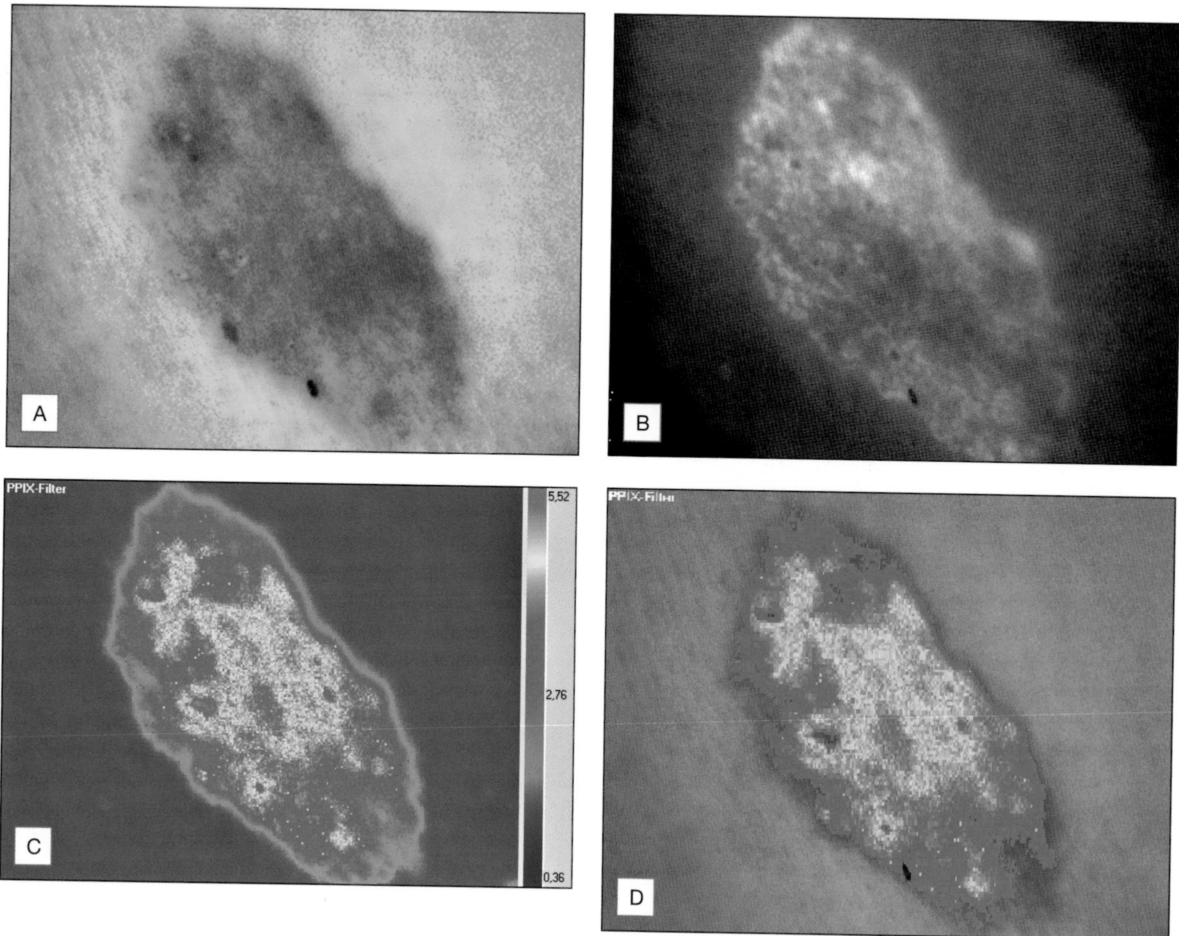

Fig. 15.5 Accumulation of PpIX is exemplary shown by this example of Bowen's disease on the leg of a patient. (**A**) Clinical image, (**B**) B&W image of PpIX fluorescence, and (**C**) false color-coded image equivalent to (**B**). After subtracting the background using a threshold, the relevant fluorescence is superimposed on the clinical image in real-time (**D**)

be sufficient for their detection. Figure 15.7 shows an example of a BCC on the back of a patient. After incubation of the lesion and its surrounding skin with ALA, FD reveals a small fluorescence spot about 1-cm distant to the clinically visible tumor. The fluorescence spot was superimposed on the clinical image and histology revealed a BCC, being either a satellite or an independent lesion. Figure 15.8 is a comparable example showing the excision lines for surgery drawn without prior FD by a surgeon. When performing FD, the fluorescence image shows clearly two suspicious lesions outside these lines. Another example (Fig. 15.9) shows how FD can assist in delineating tumor recurrence after excision of a BCC on the back of a patient.

In pre-treated skin, it is sometimes difficult to detect malignant lesions, which may be new lesions or recurrences. Figure 15.10 shows how FD detects a possible recurrent BCC 2 years after excision.

FD can help to highlight very small skin lesions, showing their extension and location within the normal tissue. FD can help the clinician to find and to treat a new tumor at a very early stage, no matter which therapy is applied. In the follow-up of treated patients, FD can be used to inspect the entire area for any recurrence of malignancies. If the patient has already received FD at an earlier stage, the digital images can be compared to differentiate between recurrences and new lesions.

• Fluorescence-guided biopsy

When looking at an area of diseased skin, the site of highest rate of conversion of ALA to PpIX can be easily detected as it will show the highest fluorescence intensity. This highlighted site will usually concur with the site of highest tumor activity. Figure 15.11 shows FD and histology of the tumor for a case of recurrent BCC after

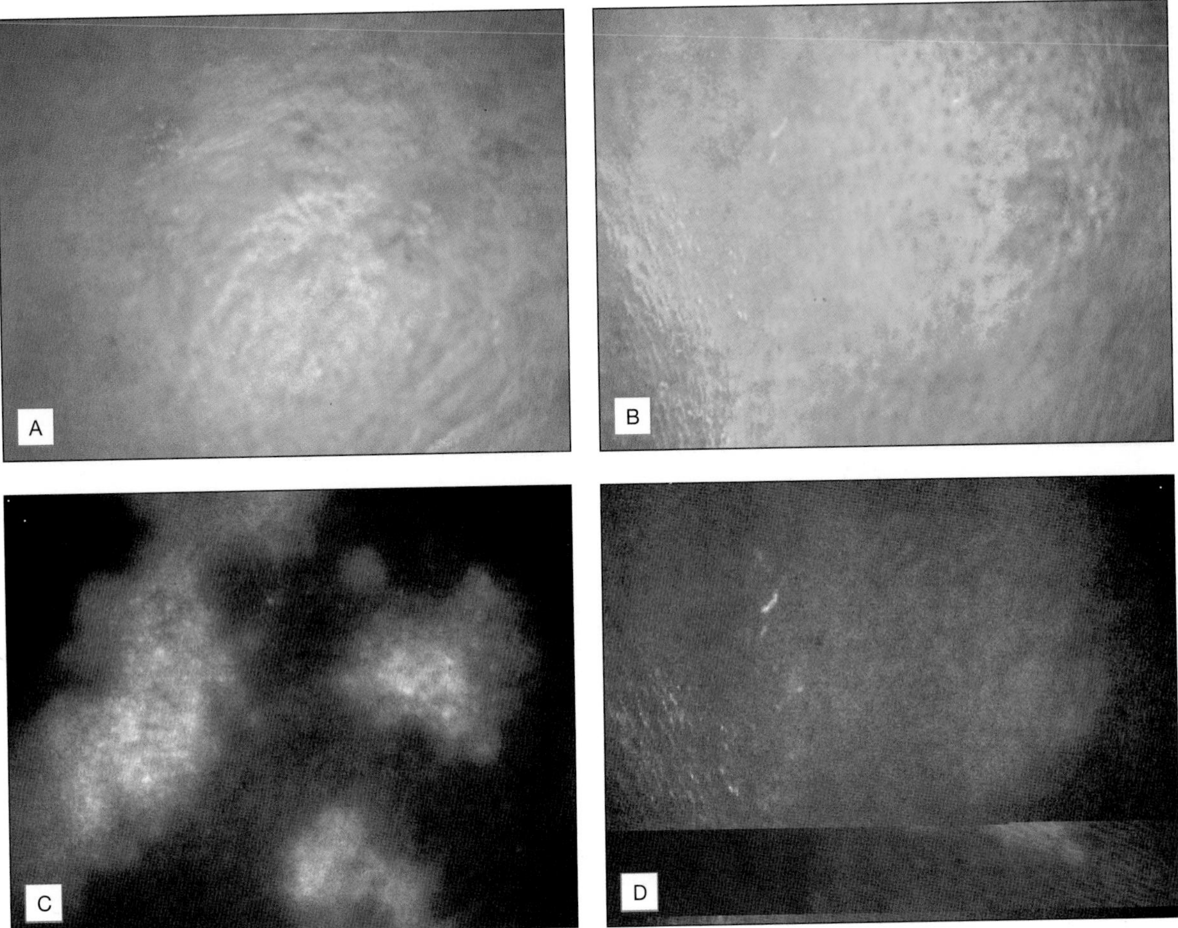

Fig. 15.6 Clinical efficacy of PDT. (**A,B**) Clinical images before and after PDT. (**C,D**) Respective B&W images of PpIX fluorescence. The fluorescence directly after PDT (**D**) has almost disappeared

cryotherapy. Thus, FD can be used as a tool to guide the taking of biopsies in field-cancerized skin or pre-treated areas, when the recurrence of a tumor is uncertain.

• Detection of tumor margins

FD is an attractive diagnostic technique for skin tumor demarcation with potential to move to clinical use. Preliminary studies have shown that fluorescence images and the histopathological tumor boundary of ill-defined basal cell carcinomas can be compared to support Mohs' micrographic surgery. Figure 15.12 shows a clinical example for the use of FD in surgery. The black line represents the clinical tumor boundary, whereas the red line shows tumor boundary with FD. Currently, studies are on the way to prove this concept clinically.

• Improving FD with image analysis

The use of special digital cameras is a prerequisite for image analysis. These can improve the FD images and reveal "hidden" information. When using the FD system, different images are available at the same time: the normal clinical image and the fluorescence image. The clinical image consists of three different color channels detecting the blue, green, and red part of the visible spectrum. With special software, the red channel can be used to simultaneously detect the fluorescence of PpIX, which is located in this spectral region (see Fig. 15.2). The fluorescence is extracted from the red channel and presented as a black and white (B&W) image, which then can be processed by false color-coding. This procedure is usually sufficient to show the clinical and fluorescence images at the same time, as well as their superimposition. The green and blue channels can provide information about the skin and its optical properties that might be used for diagnosis of the lesions.

Beside the PpIX fluorescence, endogenous chromophores such as flavins and collagen also yield fluorescence signals, which can be detected in the blue and green channels. Thus, the fluorescence in the red channel is pro-

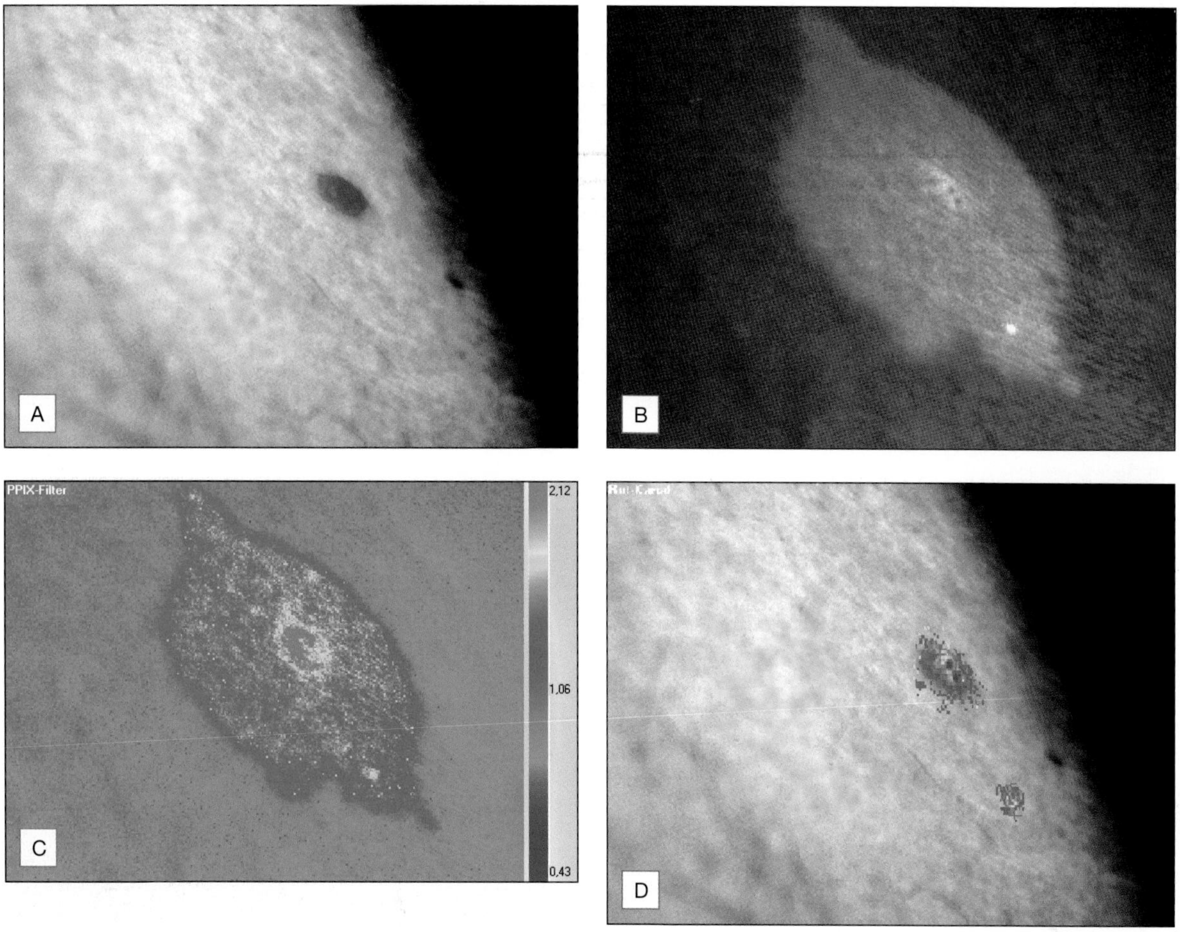

Fig. 15.7 (**A**) BCC on a patient's back. (**B**) B&W image shows PpIX fluorescence in the visible tumor and at a second location. Fluorescence is false color-coded (**C**), digitally processed, and superimposed on the clinical image (**D**), showing a satellite of the BCC

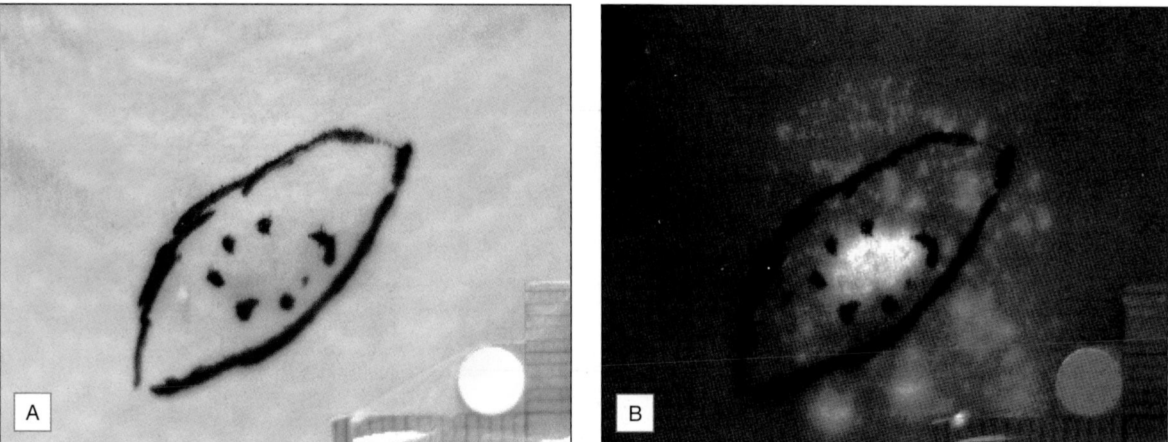

Fig. 15.8 (**A**) BCC with excision lines for surgery. (**B**) Fluorescence images show two suspicious lesions outside these lines

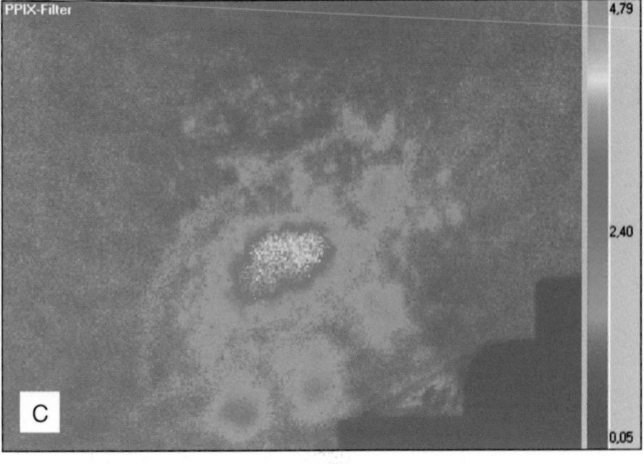

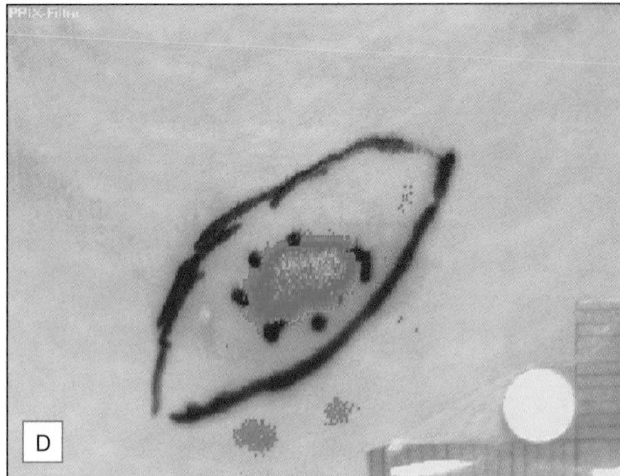

Fig. 15.8 *Continued*

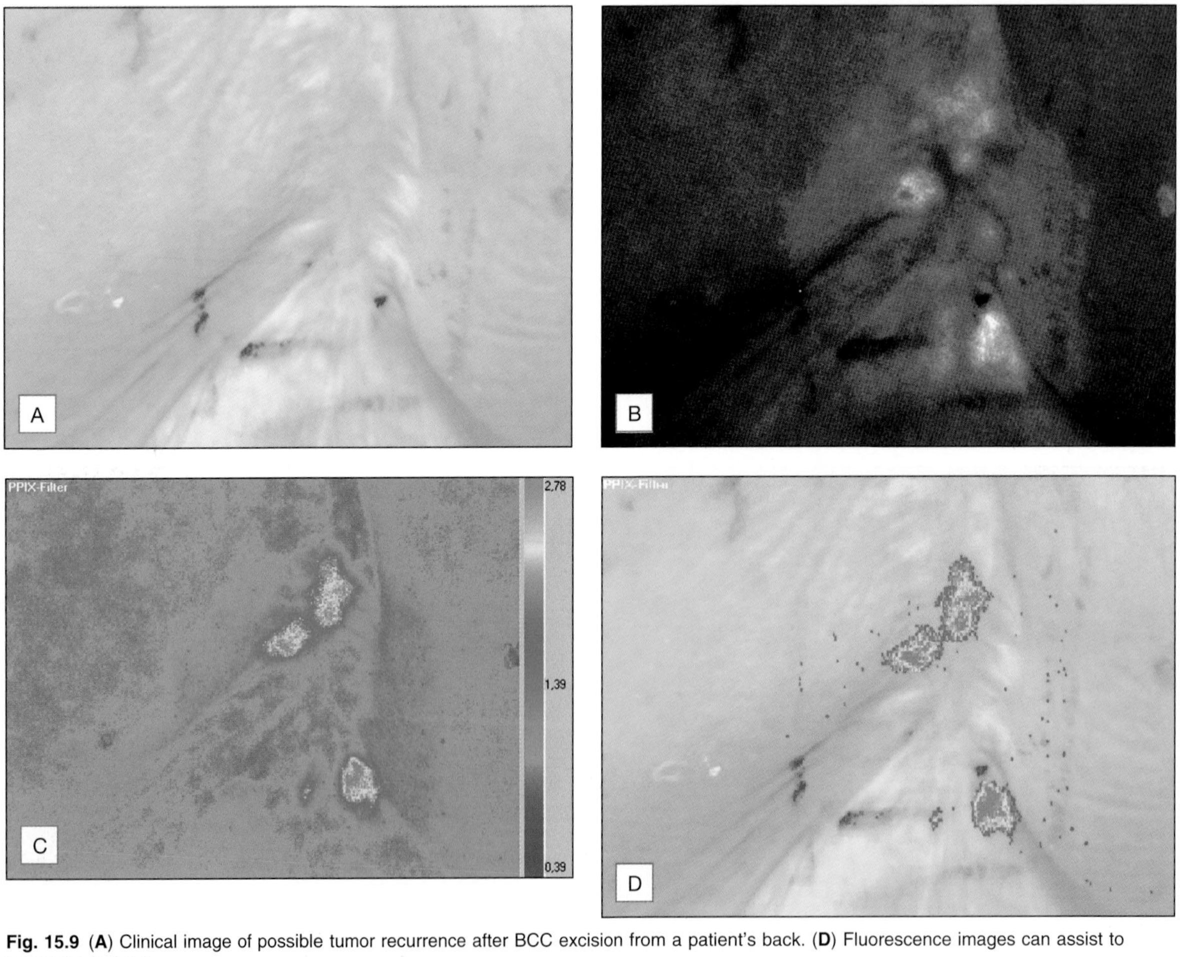

Fig. 15.9 (**A**) Clinical image of possible tumor recurrence after BCC excision from a patient's back. (**D**) Fluorescence images can assist to locate the lesions

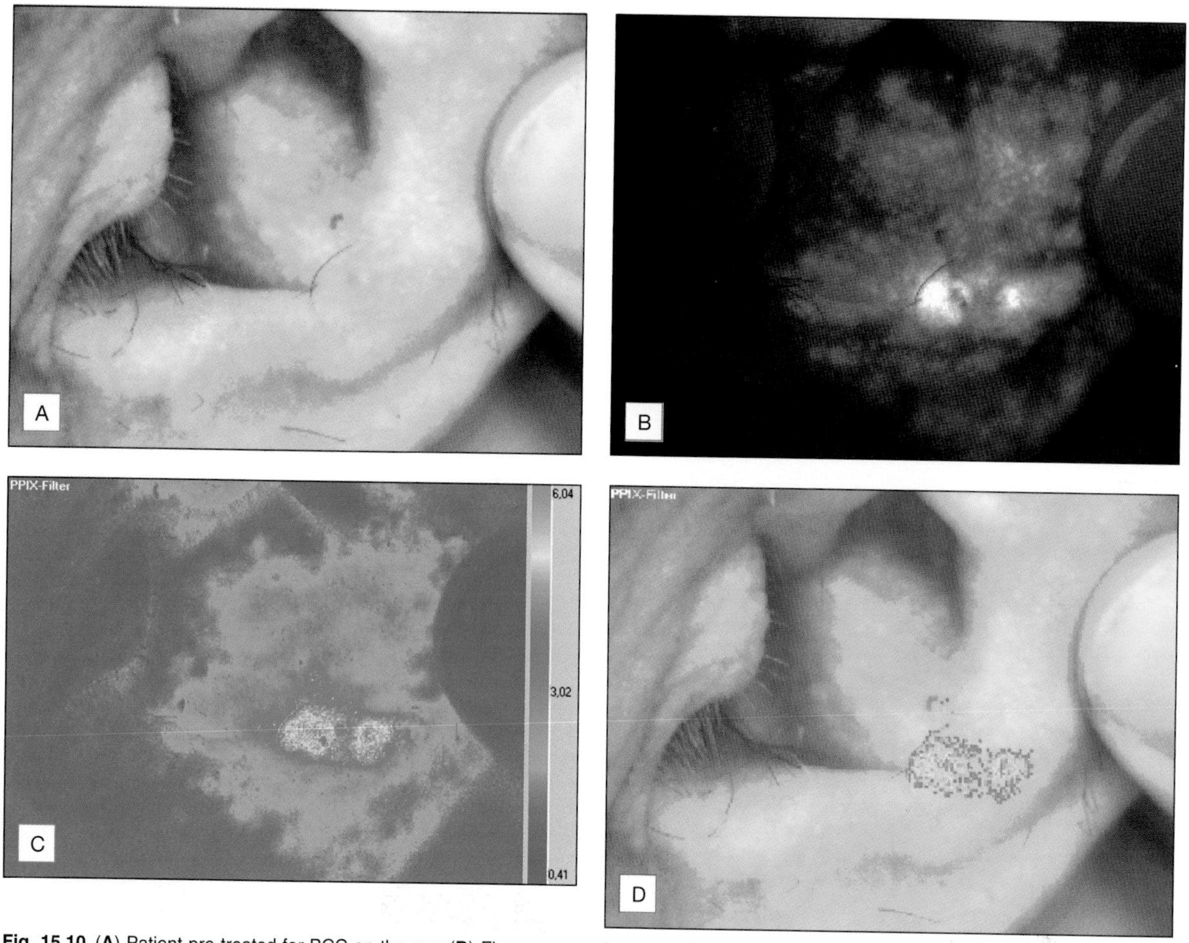

Fig. 15.10 (A) Patient pre-treated for BCC on the ear. (D) Fluorescence shows possible recurrence of the tumor

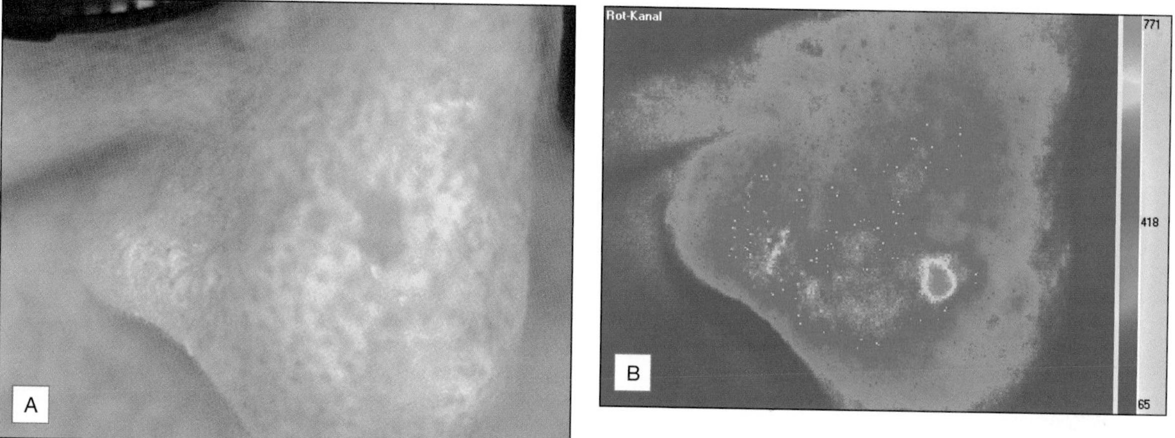

Fig. 15.11 (**A**) Fluorescence-guided biopsy in a patient with BCC recurrence on the nose after cryotherapy. At the location of maximal fluorescence intensity, given by image processing (**B**,**C**), biopsy was taken and histology revealed BCC (**D**)

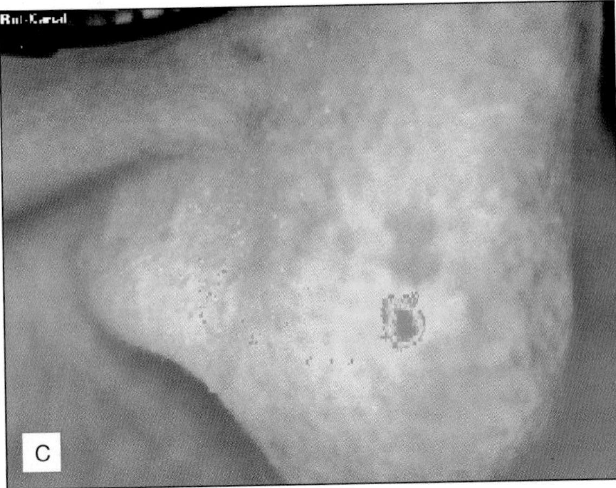

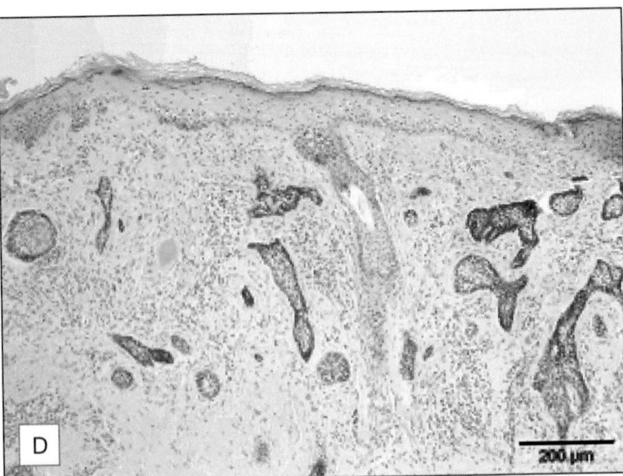

Fig. 15.11 *Continued*

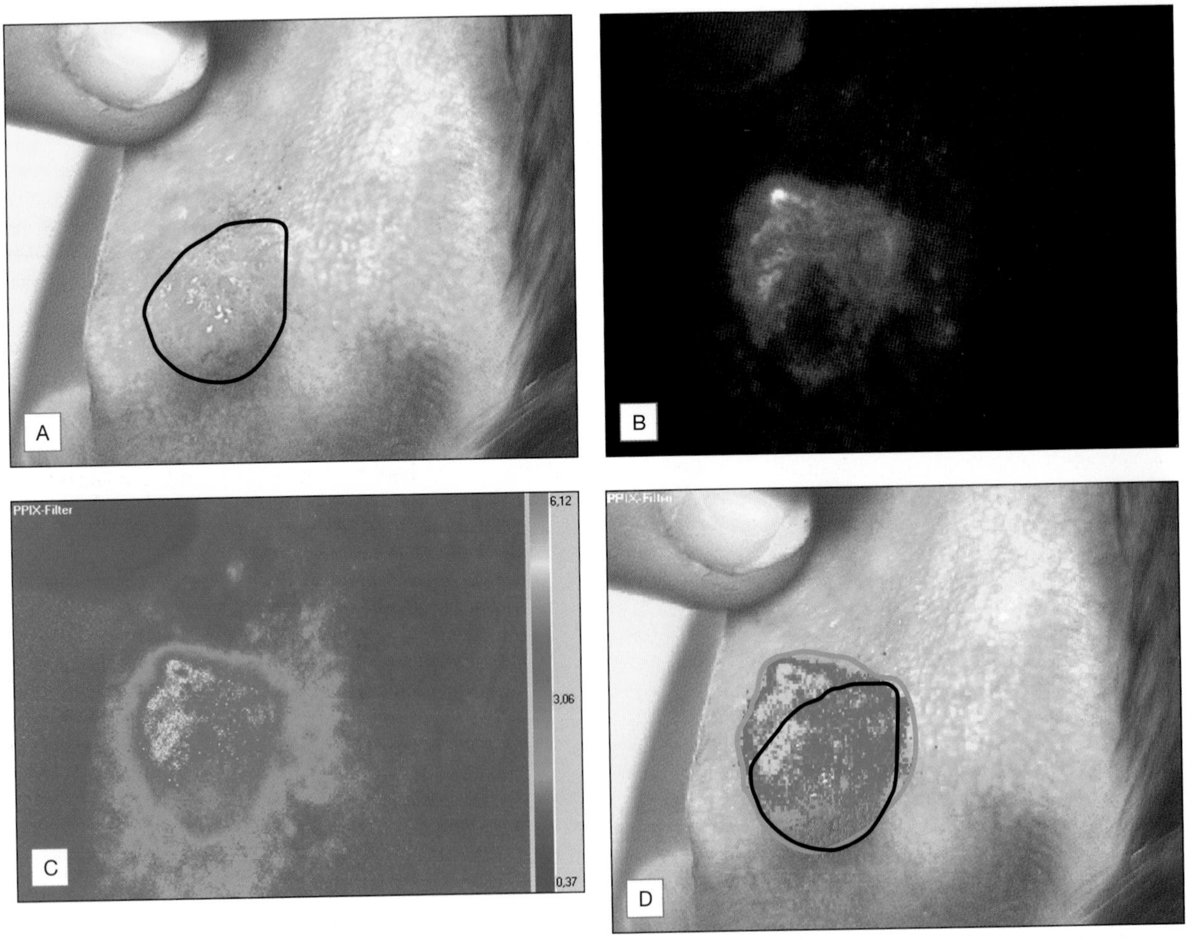

Fig. 15.12 (**A**) Patient with a BCC on the nose who requires Mohs' surgery. The black line represents the tumor boundary drawn by the surgeon without prior FD. (**D**) After FD and image processing, the red line shows a different tumor margin

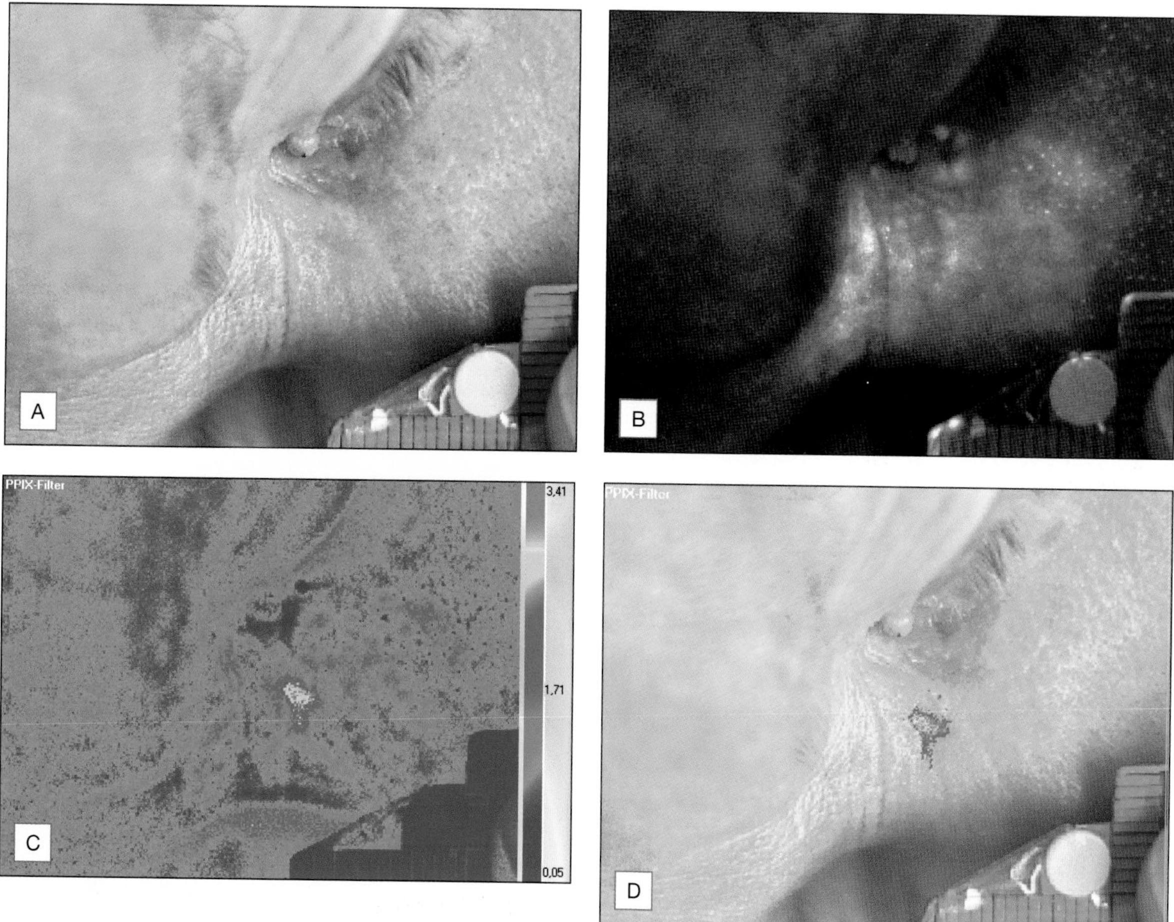

Fig. 15.13 Patient after biopsy for suspected BCC. (**A**) No malignancy was clinically detected. (**B**) FD shows no clear-cut information. (**C**) A suspicious lesion is detected using image processing by calculating the ratio of the camera channels

cessed with data from the congruent blue and green channels. The initial images show improved quality that may have clinical significance, as illustrated in Figure 15.13. After an excision of BCC, clinical inspection revealed no malignancy. Even with normal FD, the B&W image did not clearly show a tumor. When performing image processing by dividing the channels, a tumor residue was detected, which was subsequently excised.

CONCLUSION

FD of skin tumors is not yet a routine procedure, but for clinically difficult cases this method will provide a useful additional device for the detection of malignant melanoma. Digital image processing allows a quantitative and user-independent analysis of the detected fluorescence intensities, and enhances significantly the contrast between tumor and surrounding tissue.

Further investigations will determine a threshold of the fluorescence intensity for different lesions, e.g. BCC or Bowen's disease, which will enable objective discrimination between suspicious and non-suspicious tissue. Having established such an algorithm, FD might provide additional information prior to excision regarding the extension of tumor margins. Moreover, the acquired images (RGB and fluorescent images) will be subjected to different image analysis algorithms, e.g. neuronal networks, for pattern recognition to reveal additional typical characteristics of tumors, which may improve diagnosis.

FURTHER READING

Ackermann G, Abels C, Baumler W et al 1998 Simulations on the selectivity of 5-aminolaevulinic acid-induced fluorescence in vivo. J Photochemistry and Photobiology B 47:121–128

Ackermann G, Abels C, Karrer S, Baumler W, Landthaler M, Szeimies RM 2000 [Fluorescence-assisted biopsy of basal cell carcinomas]. Hautarzt 51:920–924

Akoel KM, Welfel J, Gottwald L, Suzin J 2003 [Photodynamic diagnosis of vulvar precancerous conditions and invasive cancers using 5-aminolevulinic acid]. Ginekol Pol 74:662–665

Ashkenazi H, Malik Z, Harth Y, Nitzan Y 2003 Eradication of propionibacterium acnes by its endogenic porphyrins after illumination with high intensity blue light. FEMS Immunology Medicine Microbiology 35:17–24

Bagdonas S, Kirdaite G, Streckyte G et al 2005 Spectroscopic study of ALA-induced endogenous porphyrins in arthritic knee tissues: Targeting rheumatoid arthritis PDT. Photochemistry and Photobiology Science 4:497–502

Baumgartner R, Huber RM, Schulz H et al 1996 Inhalation of 5-aminolevulinic acid: A new technique for fluorescence detection of early stage lung cancer. Journal of Photochemistry and Photobiology B 36:169–174

Bissonnette R, Sharfaei S, Viau G, Liu Y 2004 Irradiance and light dose influence histological localization of photodamage induced by photodynamic therapy with aminolaevulinic acid. British Journal of Dermatology 151:653–655

Choudry K, Brooke RC, Farrar W, Rhodes LE 2003 The effect of an iron chelating agent on protoporphyrin IX levels and phototoxicity in topical 5-aminolaevulinic acid photodynamic therapy. British Journal of Dermatology 149:124–130

Clark C, Dawe RS, Moseley H, Ferguson J, Ibbotson SH 2004 The characteristics of erythema induced by topical 5-aminolaevulinic acid photodynamic therapy. Photodermatology, Photoimmunology & Photomedicine 20:105–107

Collawn SS, Woods A, Couchman JR 2003 Nondebridement of laser char after two carbon dioxide laser passes results in faster reepithelialization. Plastic and Reconstructive Surgery 111:1742–1750

Ericson MB, Sandberg C, Gudmundson F, Rosen A, Larko O, Wennberg AM 2003 Fluorescence contrast and threshold limit: Implications for photodynamic diagnosis of basal cell carcinoma. Journal of Photochemistry and Photobiology B 69:121–127

Ericson MB, Uhre J, Strandeberg C et al 2005 Bispectral fluorescence imaging combined with texture analysis and linear discrimination for correlation with histopathologic extent of basal cell carcinoma. Journal of Biomedical Optics 10:034009

Fritsch C, Ruzicka T 2006 Fluorescence diagnosis and photodynamic therapy in dermatology from experimental state to clinic standard methods. Journal of Environmental Pathology, Toxicology and Oncology 25:425–440

Gamarra F, Wagner S, Al-Batran S et al 2002 Kinetics of 5-aminolevulinic acid-induced fluorescence in organ cultures of bronchial epithelium and tumor. Respiration 69:445–450

Inoue K, Karashima T, Kamada M, Kurabayashi A, Ohtsuki Y, Shuin T 2006 [Clinical experience with intravesical instillations of 5-aminolevulinic acid (5-ALA) for the photodynamic diagnosis using fluorescence cystoscopy for bladder cancer]. Nippon Hinyokika Gakkai Zasshi 97:719–729

Juzenas P, Juzeniene A, Stakland S, Iani V, Moan J 2002 Photosensitizing effect of protoporphyrin IX in pigmented melanoma of mice. Biochemical and Biophysical Research Communications 297:468–472

Kleinpenning MM, Smits T, Ewalds E, van Erp PE, van de Kerkhof PC, Gerritsen MJ 2006 Heterogeneity of fluorescence in psoriasis after application of 5-aminolaevulinic acid: An immunohistochemical study. British Journal of Dermatology 155:539–545

Kriegmair M, Zaak D, Knuechel R, Baumgartner R, Hofstetter A 1999 5-aminolevulinic acid-induced fluorescence endoscopy for the detection of lower urinary tract tumors. Urology International 63:27–31

Lang K, Lehmann P, Bolsen K, Ruzicka T, Fritsch C 2001 Aminolevulinic acid: Pharmacological profile and clinical indication. Expert Opinion in Investigative Drugs 10:1139–1156

Lippert BM, Gross U, Klein M 2003 Excretion measurement of porphyrins and their precursors after topical administration of 5-aminolaevulinic acid for fluorescence endoscopy in head and neck cancer. Research Communications in Molecular Pathology and Pharmacology 113–114:75–85

Messmann H, Knuchel R, Baumler W, Holstege A, Scholmerich J 1999 Endoscopic fluorescence detection of dysplasia in patients with Barrett's esophagus, ulcerative colitis, or adenomatous polyps after 5-aminolevulinic acid-induced protoporphyrin IX sensitization. Gastrointestinal Endoscopy 49:97–101

Monfrecola G, Procaccini EM, D'Onofrio D et al 2002 Hyperpigmentation induced by topical 5-aminolaevulinic acid plus visible light. Journal of Photochemistry and Photobiology B 68:147–155

Peng Q, Soler AM, Warloe T, Nesland JM, Giercksky KE 2001 Selective distribution of porphyrins in skin thick basal cell carcinoma after topical application of methyl 5-aminolevulinate. Journal of Photochemistry and Photobiology B 62:140–145

Ray R, Hauck S, Kramer R, Benton B 2005 A convenient fluorometric method to study sulfur mustard-induced apoptosis in human epidermal keratinocytes monolayer microplate culture. Drug Chemistry and Toxicology 28:105–116

Robinson DJ, de Bruijn HS, Star WM, Sterenborg HJ 2003 Dose and timing of the first light fraction in two-fold illumination schemes for topical ALA-mediated photodynamic therapy of hairless mouse skin. Photochemistry and Photobiology 77:319–323

Sabban F, Collinet P, Cosson M, Mordon S 2004 [Fluorescence imaging technique: Diagnostic and therapeutic interest in gynecology]. Journal of Gynecology, Obstetrics and Biological Reproduction (Paris) 33:734–738

Smits T, Robles CA, van Erp PE, van de Kerkhof PC, Gerritsen MJ 2005 Correlation between macroscopic fluorescence and protoporphyrin IX content in psoriasis and actinic keratosis following application of aminolevulinic acid. Journal of Investigative Dermatology 125:833–839

Svanberg K, Wang I, Colleen S et al 1998 Clinical multi-colour fluorescence imaging of malignant tumours—initial experience. Acta Radiologica 39:2–9

Szeimies RM, Landthaler M 2002 Photodynamic therapy and fluorescence diagnosis of skin cancers. Recent Results in Cancer Research 160:240–245

Wiegell SR, Stender IM, Na R, Wulf HC 2003 Pain associated with photodynamic therapy using 5-aminolevulinic acid or 5-aminolevulinic acid methylester on tape-stripped normal skin. Archives of Dermatology 139:1173–1177

Zaak D, Karl A, Knuchel R et al 2005 Diagnosis of urothelial carcinoma of the bladder using fluorescence endoscopy. BJU International 96:217–222

Index

Notes

As the subject of this book is photodynamic therapy, all index entries refer to this unless otherwise stated.

Index entries in **bold** refer to information in tables or boxes: index entries in *italics* refer to figures.

To save space in the index, the following abbreviations have been used:

ALA—5-aminolevulinic acid
BCC—basal cell carcinoma
IPL—intense pulsed light
MAL—methyl-aminolevulinic acid
PDT—photodynamic therapy
SCC—squamous cell carcinoma

A

abscess formation, hidradenitis suppurative, 35
acitretin, skin cancer prevention, 105
acne, 11
  alternative treatment, 26
  causative bacteria, 11, **12**
  IPL, 17
acne PDT, 11–27
  active cooling, 25
  adverse effects, **15,** 26–27
    erythema, 14
  ALA
    dose, 20, 25
      stepwise doses, 17
    systemic, 14–15, 20–23, 25, 29
    topical, 15, 29–34, **33**
  algorithm, 20–25, *24*
  antibacterial effect, 31–32
  blue light, 29, 30
  complications, **15,** 26–27
    papulopustular lesions, 17, *23*
    'severe reactive acne,' *20*
  cost-effectiveness, 32
  equipment, 18–20
    light-emitting diode devices, 20, *25*
    metal halide lamps, 20, *24*
  expected benefits, 12–15, *21, 22, 24*
    clinical assessments, **13**
    comedomal lesions, 15
    papulopustular lesion reduction, 13, *19*
  indications, 18
  mechanism of action, 31–32
  patient interviews, 17–18
  patient selection, 12
  post-treatment hyperpigmentation, 11, *12, 13,* 15
  reactive acne, 14
  red wavelengths, 29–30
  time intervals, 17
  tretinoin pretreatment, 18, 20
  ultraviolet examination, **11,** *16,* 17, *20*
  vitamin C iontophoresis, 17, 20, 26–27, *27*
    devices, *23,* 27, *27*
    efficacy, *26*
acne rosacea, treatment indications, 18
actinic cheilitis, 52, *52*
  PDT clinical trials, 59
actinic keratoses, 51–66
  animal models, 106
  clinical presentation, *51,* 51–52
  fluorescence diagnosis, 152, *154*
  histopathology, 52, *52*
  prevalence, 51
  SCC progression, 51, 52
actinic keratoses PDT, 3, 9, 109–110
  active cooling, 111
  adverse effects, 9, 59, 64, 111–112 *see also specific effects*
    exuberant reactions, *60*
    hyperpigmentation, 112
    hypopigmentation, 112
  ALA, *6*
    application, 110–112
    overnight application, 64
  algorithm, *62,* 62–65
    active cooling, 64
    drug application, 63, *63*
    IPL, 64
    skin preparation, 62–63
  benefits, 55–59, *59,* 112, *113*
  BLU-U light source, 53, 61, *61,* 63–64, 110
    clinical trials, 57–59
  clinical trials, 42, 56–59
  comfort/convenience, 59
  complete response rates, 55
  complications, 64
  cost/benefit ratio, 60
  dosimetry, 53, 54–55
    clinical trials, **56,** 57, 59
    incubation time variation, 54, *54,* 59, 64, 111
  drawbacks, 65
  equipment, 61–62
  expected benefits, 125
  future work, 113
  IPL, 10, 59, 61, *62,* 110–111, 115
  Levulan, 4, 56–57, *57, 58,* 59, *59*
  lifestyle preferences, **61**
  light dose, 53, 110
    red light sources, 53

light sources, 110–111
light source, 53
long pulse dye laser/IPL, 61, *62,* 110–111
clinical trials, 59
MAL, 4, 42, 112, 113
medical history, **61**
pain control measures, 64, 111
patient interviews, 61, **61**
patient precautions, 64
patient selection, 55, **55,** 109–110
photorejuvenation, 122
PpIX concentration, 53
rationale, 53–55
session number, 111
skin preparation, 62–63
topical ALA formulation, 53
treatment strategy, 60–64
troubleshooting, 64
active cooling
acne PDT, 25
actinic keratoses PDT, 64, 111
cutaneous T-cell lymphomas PDT, 98
photorejuvenation, 122
warts PDT, 93, *93*
adverse effects (of PDT), 4
see also individual effects; individual treatments
alanine transaminase levels, *21*
alkaline phosphatase levels, *21*
5-aminolevulinic acid (ALA), 3–4
adverse effects, 4
alanine transaminase levels, *21*
alkaline phosphatase levels, *21*
aspartate transaminase levels, *21*
basal cell carcinoma, 80
basal cell nevus syndrome, 81, *81*
intralesional, 81, *82*
bilirubin levels, *22*
cholinesterase levels, *22*
development, 1
dose
acne PDT, 20, 25
psoriasis PDT, 98–99
fluorescence diagnosis, 149
gamma glutamyl phosphorylase levels, *22*
heme biosynthesis, 3
hidradenitis suppurative, 38–39
lactate dehydrogenase levels, *21*
methyl derivative *see* methyl-aminolevulinic acid (MAL)
photorejuvenation, IPL with, 130–131
porphobilinogen formation, 3
properties, **3**
sebaceous hyperplasia, 43–45, **44**
treatment parameters, 46–49
skin cancer prevention mechanisms, 107, *109*
skin penetration, 3–4, 4, *12, 13, 14*
structure, *4*
systemic *vs.* topical, 100
topical, 1–10
treatment experience, 4
animal models
actinic keratoses, 106
BCC, 106–107
port wine stain PDT, 139, *139*
SCC, 106, *106, 107*
anticoagulant therapy, PDT contraindications, 72
antioxidants
avoidance post-PDT, 26
PDT contraindications, 72
skin cancer prevention, 105–106
antitumor necrosis factor medications, hidradenitis suppurative, 36–38
antiviral effects (of PDT), 87
apoptotic cell death, 8–9
argon pumped dye laser PDT, port wine stain, 139, *140*
aspartate transaminase levels, ALA, *21*
aspirin, PDT contraindications, 72

B

basal cell carcinoma (BCC), 67, 105
basal cell nevus syndrome, 79
conventional treatments
cryotherapy, 67
curettage, 67
cytotoxic agents, 67
excision, 67
PDT *vs.,* **72**
radiotherapy, 67
development
p53 gene, 107
PTCH gene, 106
fluorescence diagnosis, 152, *155, 155–157*
incidence, 105
morpheaform, 67, *68,* 80
nodular, 67
pigmented, 67, *68*
prevention, animal models, 106–107
basal cell carcinoma (BCC) PDT, 1, 3, 8, 67, *68*
ALA
adverse effects, **72**
clinical trials, **69,** 69–71
complete clearance rates, 68, 80
cryosurgery *vs.,* 69
alternative therapy *vs.,* **72**
benefits, *70, 71*
cost analyses, 72
MAL, 107
clinical trials, **71**
complete clearance rates, 69, 81, *81*
nodular, cure rate, 67
red light penetration, 67
tumor thickness, 67, 69
basal cell nevus syndrome (BCNS), 79–83, 109
basal cell carcinomas, 79
clinical features, 79, *80*
genetics, 79
management, traditional, 79
basal cell nevus syndrome (BCNS), PDT, 80–81
limitations, 80
photosensitizers, 80
recurrence rates, 80
safety concerns, 81
benzoporphyrin derivative monoacid (BPD), **2,** 3, 147

bilirubin levels, ALA, *22*
bladder tumors, fluorescence diagnosis, 151
blue light PDT, 5
 acne PDT, 29, 30
 erythema, 125, *125–126*
 hidradenitis suppurative, 38, *38*
 nonablative rejuvenation, 116, *117*
 photorejuvenation, 125
 sebaceous hyperplasia, 45–46
 see also individual types
BLU-U PDT, 5
 actinic keratoses PDT, 53, 61, *61,* 63–64, 110
  clinical trials, 57–59
 protoporphyrin IX activating dose, *5,* **6**
Bowen's disease PDT, 67, 74
breast cancer metastases, PDT, 67
breastfeeding, PDT contraindications, 85
Burton scale, acne grading, **11**

C

cavernous hemangioma, 137
cellular necrosis, 9, *9*
cervical intraepithelial neoplasia (VIN), 87
chemiluminescent light patches, 5
chemotherapy, actinic keratoses PDT, 60
cholinesterase levels, ALA, *22*
ClearLight source, 5
 actinic keratoses PDT, 53
clinical trials
 ALA-PDT, BCC, **69,** 69–71
 dosimetry, actinic keratoses PDT, **56,** 57, 59
 Levulan, 56–57, *57, 58,* 59, *59*
 long pulse dye laser/IPL, 59
 photorejuvenation, 125–131
comedomal lesions, acne PDT, 15
complete clearance rates
 actinic keratoses PDT, 55
 BCC ALA-PDT, 68, 80
 BCC MALA-PDT, 69, 80, *81*
condyloma acuminata, 86–87
consent form, photorejuvenation, **133**
contact eczema, MAL-induced, 117
contraindications (to PDT), 72, 85
copper vapor laser, port wine stain PDT, 139–140
corticosteroids
 cutaneous T-cell lymphoma therapy, 95
 psoriasis therapy, 98
cosmesis
 skin cancer PDT, 67, 69, 76
 warts PDT, 85
cost analysis
 acne PDT, 32
 actinic keratoses PDT, 60
 BCC PDT, 72
 photorejuvenation, 122
 warts PDT, 86
cryotherapy
 actinic keratoses, 59
 BCC, 67
  ALA-PDT *vs.,* 69
  PDT *vs.,* **72**
curettage
 actinic keratoses, 64
 BCC, 67
  PDT *vs.,* **72**
cutaneous T-cell lymphomas, 95–98, *96*
cutaneous T-cell lymphomas PDT, **39,** 67, 95–98, **97,** *98*
 active cooling, 98
 application times, 95
 benefits, 95
 light dose/intensity, 95–96
 patient selection, 95
 side effects/complications, 98
 techniques, 95–98
  in vivo fluorescence monitoring, 96, *98*
 treatment tolerance, 96
cytostatic drugs, PDT contraindications, 72
cytotoxic agents, BCC, 67

D

dermatochalasis, 119
Dermatologic Life Quality Index (DLQI), hidradenitis suppurative, 35
desferrioxamine, as penetration enhancer, 75
desquamation, post-PDT, 59, 64, 111–112
dimethylsulfoxide (DMSO), basal cell nevus syndrome, 80
disseminated superficial actinic porokeratosis (DSAP), **39**

E

edema
 actinic keratoses, 57, 64, 111
 skin cancer, 76
EDTA, as penetration enhancer, 75
 basal cell nevus syndrome, 80
emission spectrum
 light-emitting diodes, *25*
 metal halide lamps, *25*
energy density
 light-emitting diodes, *25*
 metal halide lamps, *25*
erythema
 acne PDT, 14, 26
 actinic keratoses PDT, 57, 59, 61, 111–112
 blue light treatment, 125, *125–126*
 skin cancer PDT, 76
ethnicity, ALA skin penetration, 3
evolution (of PDT), 1
excision surgery
 BCC, 67
  PDT *vs.,* **72**
 hidradenitis suppurative, 38
excitation spectrum, protoporphyrin IX (PpIX), 20
expected benefits (of PDT), 5

F

Fitzpatrick skin types, **51**
fluorescence diagnosis (FD), 149–160
 actinic keratoses, 152, *154*
 applications, 151–159
 basal cell nevus syndrome, 81
 BCC, 153, *155, 155–157*
 benefits

dermatology, 151–159
non-dermatologic fields, 151
clinically invisible lesion detection, 152–153
digital cameras, 149–150, 151, 154
equipment, 150, *151*
false color presentation, 151
image analysis, 154, *158,* 159, *159*
indications, **152**
methods, 150–157
naked eye detection, 151
photosensitizer penetration, 151
PpIX accumulation, 152
principles, 149–151, *150*
skin cancer, 152, *152*
successful PDT, evidence for, 152
tumor margin detection, 154, *158*
fluorescence-guided biopsy, 153–154, *157–158*
fluorescence quantum yield, 149
5-fluorouracil (5-FU), 79
actinic keratoses, 57
folliculitis, *17,* 18
fractional resurfacing, 115
fractionation, cutaneous T-cell lymphomas PDT, 96

G

gamma glutamyl phosphorylase levels, ALA, *22*
Gorlin syndrome *see* basal cell nevus syndrome (BCNS)

H

hairless mouse, skin cancer prevention models, 106, *107*
health insurance exclusion, warts PDT, 86
hemangiomas, 137
hematoporphyrin, 1
heme biosynthesis, ALA, 3
hidradenitis suppurative, 35–41
clinical presentation, 35, 36
etiology, 35–36
genetics, 35
histology, 36, *37*
history, 35–36
phases, 36, *36*
prevalence, 35–36
treatment, 36–40
acute flares, 36
medical, 36–38
surgical, 38
hidradenitis suppurative PDT, 38–40
blue light, 38, *38*
clinical studies, 38–40
human papilloma virus (HPV), 85–86
etiology, 85
see also warts
hydrosadenite phlegmoneuse *see* hidradenitis suppurative
hyperpigmentation
acne PDT, 11, *12,* 15
actinic keratoses PDT, 112
port wine stain PDT, 142
psoriasis PDT, 101
hypopigmentation, actinic keratoses PDT, 112

I

immunosuppression, psoriasis therapy, 98
infections, photorejuvenation, 134
inflammatory mediators, 9, *9*
infra-red lasers, nonablative rejuvenation, 115, **116**
intense pulsed light (IPL), 5
acne, 17, 31, *32*
actinic keratoses PDT, 10, 59, 61, *62,* 64, 110–111, 115
photorejuvenation, 115–116, **116,** 122, 125, *128–130,* 128–131
post-acne treatment, 17
protoporphyrin IX activating dose, *5,* **6**
sebaceous hyperplasia PDT, 45, 46, **46**
intraepithelial neoplasia, 86–87
in vivo fluorescence monitoring, cutaneous T-cell lymphomas PDT, 96, *98*
isotretinoin
acne, 32
basal cell nevus syndrome, 79

K

krypton lasers
children, 142, *144*
port wine stain PDT, 141–147, *142*
adverse effects, 141

L

lactate dehydrogenase levels, ALA, *21*
lasers, 5
acne PDT, 18–20
see also individual types
Levulan
actinic keratoses treatment, 4
clinical trials, 56–57, *57, 58,* 59, *59*
costs, 60
development, 4
hidradenitis suppurative, 38
photorejuvenation, 132, **132**
properties, **3**
structure, *3*
lichen planus-like keratosis, 52
lichen planus PDT, **39**
lidocaine, actinic keratoses PDT, 111
light-emitting diodes (LED)
acne PDT, 20, *25*
emission spectrum, *25*
energy density, *25*
fluorescence diagnosis, 149, *150*
skin cancer PDT, 73–74
light sources
acne PDT, 18–20
actinic keratoses PDT, 110–111
photorejuvenation, 125, 128, 134
sebaceous hyperplasia, 45
skin cancer PDT, 73–74
warts PDT, 88
see also specific types
light-tissue interactions, 4–6
alternative light dosing, 5–6
lasers, 5
nonlaser, 5

long pulsed-pulsed dye laser (LP-PDL)
acne, 30–31, *32*
actinic keratoses *see* actinic keratoses PDT
hidradenitis suppurative, 39

M

malignant melanoma metastases, PDT, 67
mechanism of action (PDT), 1, **1,** 95, *96*
metal halide lamps
acne PDT, 20, *24*
emission spectrum, *25*
energy density, *25*
methotrexate, psoriasis therapy, 98
methyl-aminolevulinic acid (MAL), 117
actinic keratoses, 109–110, 112, 113
adverse effects, 117
ALA *vs.*, 117
basal cell nevus syndrome, 80, 81
BCC development in animal models, 107
BCC PDT, 107
clinical trials, 59
development, 4
drug incubation, 40
hidradenitis suppurative, 39, 40
mechanism of action, 117
photorejuvenation, 115–126
nonablative, 115
red light study, 117–118, *118–121*
properties, **3**
regimen, 117
skin penetration, 4
structure, *4*
Metvix, 4
development, 4
properties, **3**
structure, *4*
microdermabrasion
pre-actinic keratoses PDT, 62, *63*
pre-photorejuvenation, 122
mitochondria, targeting of, 8
Mohs' surgery
basal cell nevus syndrome, 79
PDT adjuvant, 68

N

nausea, systemic ALA, 20
nevoid basal cell carcinoma syndrome *see* basal cell nevus syndrome (BCNS)
nonmelanoma skin cancer (NMSC)
incidence, 105
photorejuvenation, 119–120
nonporphyrins, as photosensitizers, 3
non-steroidal anti-inflammatory drugs (NSAIDs)
actinic keratoses PDT, 64
PDT contraindications, 72

P

p53 gene, BCC development, 107
pain
actinic keratoses, 64, 111
psoriasis PDT, 100
skin cancer PDT, 76
warts PDT, 93, *93*
papulopustular lesions, acne PDT, 13, 17, *17, 23*
patient information, **133**
Pc 4, **3**
penetration enhancers, 69, 75
Photochlor, **3**
photocoagulation
hemangiomas, 137
vascular malformations, 137
photodamage, 125
ALA treatment, *6*
Photofrin, 2, 8
basal cell nevus syndrome, 80
cervical intraepithelial neoplasia, 87
photorejuvenation, 125–135
actinic keratoses, effects on, 125
active cooling, 122
applications, 119–122, *122*
blue light, 125
clinical trials, 125–131
consent form, **133**
cost analysis, 122
future directions, 122, 134
home care instructions, **134**
IPL, 10, 115–116, 125, *128–130,* 128–131
light sources, 134
MAL, 115–126
pain management, 122
patient information, **133**
peer-reviewed reports, 130, **131**
post-treatment, 132–134
sunlight avoidance, **134**
pre-treatment preparations, 122
pulsed-dye laser, 131–132
red light sources, 125, 128
MAL, 117–118, *118–121*
side effects/complications, 132–134
infections, 134
phototoxic reactions, 134
sunlight avoidance, 122, 134
techniques, 132, **134**
treatment frequency, 122
treatment strategy, 118–122
photosensitizers, 1–4, **2,** 2–3
basal cell nevus syndrome PDT, 80
bleaching, 152
cytotoxicity mechanism, 2, **2,** 8–9
excitation, 7, *8*
fluorescence diagnosis, 151
ideal properties, 1
incubation times, 8
nonporphyrins, 3
porphyrins, 2–3
vascular lesions PDT, 147
see also individual sensitizers
photothermolysis
hemangiomas, 137
port wine stain, 137, *138*
phototoxic reactions, photorejuvenation, 134
methyl-aminolevulinic acid, 117

phthalocyanine-4, **3**
phthalocyanines, **2**
pigmentation, actinic keratoses, 52
plasma skin rejuvenation, 115
porphobilinogen, formation, 3
porphyria, PDT contraindications, 72
porphyrins, as photosensitizers, 2–3
port wine stain, 101–102, 137–138, *138*
port wine stain PDT
  animal models, 139, *139*
  benefits, *102, 103*
  children, 142, *144*
  clinical results, 142–147, *143*
  development, 138–140
  equipment, 141–142, *142*
  follow-up, 144–147, *147*
  future developments, 147
  krypton laser, 141–147, *143–146*
  lesion clearance, 144, *145*
  nonthermal, 140–141
    advantages/disadvantages, 147
  patient selection, 101–102
  photosensitizers, 140–141
  selective, 140–141
  side effects/complications, **101,** 139, 142
  techniques, **101,** 101–102, 141–147
  time schedules, 141
  treatment intervals, 142–144
pregnancy, PDT contraindications, 85
Propionibacterium acnes, 11, 29
  see also acne
protoporphyrin IX (PpIX), 2
  absorption bands, 53, *53*
  actinic keratoses PDT, 53
  excitation spectrum, 20
  formation, 3
  light-activating dose, 5, **5,** *5*
PsD-007, port wine stain PDT, 140–141
psoralen in combination with ultraviolet radiation (PUVA), cutaneous T-cell lymphoma, 95
psorasis vulgaris, **39**
psoriasis
  alternative treatments, 98
  incidence, 98
psoriasis PDT, 98–101
  application times, 99
  expected benefits, 98, *99*
  patient selection, 98
  side effects/complications, 100–101
  techniques, 98–100, **100**
    ALA concentrations, 98–99
    application times, 99
    multiple treatments, 99
    systemic *vs.* topical ALA, 100
PTCH gene, BCC development, 106
pulsed-dye laser (PDL)
  basal cell nevus syndrome, 81
  hemangiomas, 137
  photorejuvenation, 120–122, 131–132
    nonablative, 115, **116**
  port wine stain therapy, 101–102, 137–138, *138*
  sebaceous hyperplasia PDT, 45
Purlytin, **3**
purpura, post-PDT, 64

R

race, ALA skin penetration, 3
radiotherapy, cutaneous T-cell lymphoma, 95
reaction (to PDT), 6–9
  cellular, 8
  oxidative, 7–8
reactive oxygen species (ROS), 7
  cellular response, 8
red light sources
  acne PDT, 29–30
  actinic keratoses PDT, 53
  basal cell nevus syndrome PDT, 80
  penetration, 67
  photorejuvenation, 125, 128
retinoids
  psoriasis therapy, 98
  skin cancer prevention, 105

S

scarring, post-PDT, 64, 112
scleroderma PDT, **39**
sebaceous glands
  ALA penetration, *12*
  PDT-ALA effects, *15*
sebaceous hyperplasia, 43
sebaceous hyperplasia PDT, 43–49
  adverse effects, 43
  benefits, 43–45
  blue light, 45–46
  light sources, 45
  medical history, 43
  organ transplant recipients, 45
  patient education, pretreatment, 43
  patient selection, 43
  post-treatment care, **49**
  pre-treatment protocol, **46**
  pulsed-dye laser (PDL), 45
  recurrence, 45
  studies, 43–45, **44**
  techniques, 45–46, *47, 48*
  treatment parameters, 46–49
seborrhea, treatment algorithm, *24*
'severe reactive acne,' acne PDT, *20*
singlet oxygen production, 1, **2**
sinus tracts, hidradenitis suppurative, 35
skin cancer
  precursors, 51–66
  prevention, 105–114 *see also* actinic keratoses PDT
skin cancer PDT, 67–78
  advantages, **72,** 75–76
  adverse effects, 76, **76**
  ALA, **76**
    MAL *vs.,* 73–74
  algorithm, *73, 74, 75,* 75–76
    tumor debulking, 73, 75

alternative approaches, 76–77
benefits, **69,** 69–72
cosmesis, 76
complications, 76
fluorescence diagnosis, 152, *152*
light sources, 73–74
MAL, **76**
ALA *vs.*, 73–74
Mohs' surgery adjuvant, 68
pain management, 76
patient interviews, 72
patient selection, 69, **69**
penetration enhancers, 69, 75
photosensitizer application, 74–75
surgery *vs.*, 75–76
see also basal cell carcinoma (BCC) PDT
skin penetration
ALA, 3–4, *12, 14*
race/ethnicity, 3
MAL, 4
skin rejuvenation *see* photorejuvenation
squamous cell carcinoma (SCC), 67, 105
actinic keratoses progression from, 51, 52
animal models, 106, *107, 108*
curettage, *73*
incidence, 105
squamous cell carcinoma (SCC) PDT, 67, 71–72
Sturge–Weber syndrome, 144, *145*
sunlight avoidance/protection
photorejuvenation, 122, 134, **134**
port wine stain PDT, 142
sunlight exposure, skin cancer, 105
sun protection
actinic keratoses PDT, 64
basal cell nevus syndrome, 79
skin cancer prevention, 105
surgery, skin cancer PDT *vs.*, 75–76
systemic 5-aminolevulinic acid (ALA), topical ALA *vs.*, 100

T

T4 endonuclease V, 105
tin etiopurpurin dichloride, 3, **3**
topical vitamin D therapy, psoriasis therapy, 998
tretinoin
acne PDT, 20
basal cell nevus syndrome, 79
tumor debulking, skin cancer PDT, 73, 76

U

ultraviolet A radiation, psoriasis therapy, 98–99
ultraviolet examination, acne PDT, **11,** *16,* 17, *17*
urology, fluorescence diagnosis, 151
uroporphyrinogen I, formation, 3

V

vascular lesions PDT, 101–102, 137–148
future developments, 147
photosensitizers, 147
vascular malformations, 137–138
Verteporfin, **3**
basal cell nevus syndrome, 80
vitamin C iontophoresis, 17, 20, *26,* 26–27, *27*
devices, *23,* 27, *27*
efficacy, *26*
vitamin(s), skin cancer prevention, 105–106
vulva intraepithelial neoplasia (VIN), 86–87

W

warts, 85
histology, 85
see also human papilloma virus (HPV)
warts, PDT
active cooling, 93, *93*
ALA, 87–88
algorithm, 89, *90–92*
benefits, 85–86, **86**
measurement, 85–86, **87**
cost/benefit ratio, 86
equipment, 89, *89*
health insurance exclusion, 86
indications, 88
light sources, 88
patient selection, 85
post-treatment care, 89
recalcitrant, 86
self-administration, 86, 89
side effects/complications, 89, 93
pain, 93, *93*
treatment strategy, 87–89, *88*
wavelength (of light), tissue penetration, 4
Wood's lamp, fluorescence diagnosis, 149

X

xeroderma pigmentosum, 55, 109